CHILLS
and
FEVER

CHILLS
and
FEVER

Health and Disease
in the Early History of
Alaska

Robert Fortuine

University of Alaska Press
Fairbanks, 1992

Library of Congress Cataloging-in-Publication Data

Fortuine, Robert.
    Chills and fever.

    Includes bibliographical references.
1. Public health—Alaska—History. 2. Eskimos—
Health and hygiene—History. 3. Diseases—Alaska—His-
tory. 4. Alaska—History. I. Title.
RA447.A4F67 1989   610'.9798   89-20515
ISBN 0-912006-58-7 (alk. paper)

First printing: 1989, cloth, 1250 copies
Second printing: 1992, paper, 1500 copies
International Standard Book Number: 0-912006-58-7
Library of Congress Catalogue Number: 89-20515

Printed in the United States by Thomson-Shore, Inc.

This publication was printed on acid-free paper which
meets the minimum requirements of American National
Standard for Information Sciences—Permanence of Paper
for Printed Library Material, ANSI Z39.48-1984.

Typeset by Color Art Printing Company Inc.
    in CG Times and Goudy.

Publication coordination and design by Deborah Van Stone
    with assistance from Terrie West.
Copyediting by Sue Keller.
Cartography by Don Haas.
Cover illustrations by Russell Mitchell.

To the Alaska Native people,
who have learned to endure with
courage, strength, and dignity,
this book is respectfully dedicated.

Contents

Illustrations

Figures

Figures

Maps

Foreword

Along with the European trade goods exchanged with American Indians for the products of their environment went a range of infectious diseases. The changes that these diseases brought about in traditional Indian life were probably of far greater importance than all the trade goods together. European diseases such as typhus, yellow fever, diphtheria, influenza, and smallpox killed large numbers of native Americans who lacked a history of exposure and natural immunity, often decimating tribes by as much as fifty to ninety percent.

To damage a native American society severely, disease had to do more than kill individuals. It had to create alterations in the native social fabric that were serious and permanent. Technological skills and leadership were lost and settlement patterns disrupted as survivors reorganized in new locations. Illness of epidemic proportions often destroyed a society's ability to produce and distribute food and to care for the sick. A functioning subsistence system was of vital importance, for without it a culture could not remain intact.

The native peoples of Alaska, although contacted by Europeans much later than natives of other areas of North America, were not spared the devastating effects of disease. Although true epidemics may have occurred fairly infrequently, as the tempo of culture contact increased, patterns of health were permanently altered and the specters of ill health and death were constantly present. Until well into the present century, treatment was far from professional in quality and there were only a few individuals with even rudimentary knowledge of medicine to care for a widely dispersed and, for the most part, apathetic population resigned to the ravages of disease.

Aleuts, Eskimos, and Indians were baffled by the onset of an illness that failed to respond to traditional ministrations of the shaman. The early missionaries, representing several denominations, most of them without formal medical training, would attempt to treat the sick unless they found the shaman in attendance. Sometimes the patients would consult with the shaman and village elders before deciding to accept the missionary's treatment. Once acceptance had been decided upon, there was a tendency to believe that a single dose of any medicine ought to cure any illness immediately. When medicine failed to achieve an instant cure, the patient frequently stopped following instructions for its use or turned back to reliance on traditional medical practitioners. Since native peoples did not understand the nature of contagion, they were unwilling to curtail their normal traveling and visiting, and this was probably as much a factor in the spread of disease as any other.

Sources for the study of health and illness in Alaska are abundant but not necessarily obvious, and they have received little attention from students of human behavior, particularly in the crucial area of the impact of disease on society. Undoubtedly the most convincing evidence is provided by the pathologies evident in excavated skeletal material or, more rarely, in the fortuitously preserved frozen or mummified human remains that have been discovered in the Aleutian Islands and northwest Alaska. Information provided by these sources is particularly helpful in reconstructing the disease and trauma that were present in late prehistoric and protohistoric populations. Most illnesses, however, leave no trace in skeletal remains and broad inferences derived from autopsies performed on a few preserved remains are risky.

Modern ethnographic literature is another important source for the study of health and disease which, thanks to increased research during the past thirty years, now provides detailed studies for virtually every native group in Alaska.

The most comprehensive ethnographies, however, are unlikely to provide detailed information sufficient to satisfy the requirements of the medical historian, and even the best accounts require careful evaluation and interpretation.

The most abundant and intriguing source materials are the first-hand observations made by contemporary observers of native life from earliest contact through the nineteenth century. These include explorers, missionaries, traders, and government officials. Most of these eyewitness accounts contain only incidental references to health problems and are usually based on limited interaction with native peoples. Few observations were made by trained medical personnel and even those that were, such as occur in the reports of ships' physicians, government doctors, nurses, or medical missionaries and teachers, are based on a knowledge of medicine far removed from what it is today. Although many early observers of native Alaskans expressed appreciation of and sympathy with their way of life, few are free of the prejudices and value judgments characteristic of nineteenth century Euro-American culture, and their accounts must be judged accordingly.

The study of health and illness based on these sources requires special prerequisites. The ideal investigator should combine the talents and training of the historian, anthropologist, and physician. Dr. Robert Fortuine more than fulfills these requirements. He is a physician trained in public health who has worked for many years in Alaska and with Alaska's natives. At the same time, he has had a long and abiding interest in the history of Alaska, its native inhabitants, and the Euro-Americans who came later and were the agents for culture change. His thorough familiarity with the historical and anthropological literature and his broad, practical experience has enabled him to combine sympathetic cross-cultural understanding with rigorous scientific methodology.

Dr. Fortuine firmly believes that the history of medicine provides "a unique perspective on history" in that it examines "the role of health and disease in daily life and as factors that shape historical events." An important new dimension has been added to our understanding of Alaska's history. It is a fascinating story, well told in this fine book.

James W. VanStone
Department of Anthropology
Field Museum of Natural History
Chicago, Illinois

Acknowledgments

Most of the research for this book was done at the Alaska Room and the Alaska Health Sciences Library of the Consortium Library of the University of Alaska Anchorage. Other libraries used include the Elmer E. Rasmuson Library at the University of Alaska Fairbanks, the Heritage Library of the National Bank of Alaska, Anchorage, the Z.J. Loussac Library of the Municipality of Anchorage, the Library of the Arctic Institute of North America (when it was still based in Montreal), and the Stefansson Collection of the Dartmouth College Libraries in Hanover, N.H. To the helpful staffs of all of these institutions I owe special thanks.

Many individuals were kind enough to read all or part of the manuscript and to offer their helpful comments, encouragement, and criticism. Most of their suggestions have been incorporated into the final text, but I alone am responsible for any errors. I am especially grateful for assistance to the following (listed alphabetically): Robert Arnold, Richard P. Barden, Ernest S. Burch, Jr., Mary Core, Tanya DeMarsh, J. Kenneth Fleshman, Carla Helfferich, Sue Keller, Theodore A. Mala, Frederick A. Milan, Claus-M. Naske, Naomi B. Pascal, Cynthia D. Schraer, Robert K. Singyke, David W. Templin, and James W. VanStone. I recognize also a special debt to former Alaska State Senator Willie Hensley and his legislative assistant Robert Arnold for their invaluable encouragement and support in the publication of this book.

To Joan Phair Thorp (Quel-Quel-La-Mit) I am personally grateful for her continuing interest in the project and her hard work in bringing the book to the attention of various Alaska Native organizations.

Finally, I would like to offer my cordial thanks to Debbie Van Stone of the University of Alaska Press for her skill, persistence, and enthusiasm in seeing this book through the production process.

In a true sense this book has been a family project. My son Alex Fortuine gave indispensable assistance by designing a computer program that permitted the storage and retrieval of large amounts of information essential for the organization and writing of the book. My daughter Willa Ryan typed several drafts of the holograph manuscript—no mean feat considering the text was written by a physician schooled in the art of illegibility. My son

Andrew, who shares my word-processor for his school work, patiently deferred his turn at the keyboard on occasion to allow me to meet editorial deadlines. But I owe the greatest debt to my wife Sheila, who constantly encouraged me, patiently bore my preoccupations and occasional ill-humor, and listened to long recitations from earlier drafts with attentiveness and good critical judgment. Most of all, however, she has been a constant and supportive companion who also believed in the importance of what this book is trying to say.

-- R.F.
Anchorage, Alaska
August 1989

CHILLS
and
FEVER

Introduction

Henry Sigerist (1951, 1:7), perhaps the greatest modern scholar of medicine, once wrote that medical history studies "health and disease through the ages, the conditions for health and disease, and the history of all human activities that tend to promote health, to prevent illness, and to restore the sick, no matter who the acting individuals were." Far from being a narrow, arcane corner of historical research, therefore, the history of medicine properly encompasses the whole range of human life, society, and endeavor. It has, to be sure, a unique perspective on history, which is all the more important for having been neglected: namely, the role of health and disease in daily life and as factors that shape historical events.

Alaska and its diverse peoples afford an unusual opportunity for studying the interactions of disease and history. Although a vast land, with extremes of topography and climate, Alaska has certain features that render it a giant microcosm, if such a paradoxical expression may be permitted. These factors include geography, culture, time, and history itself.

Geographically, Alaska comprises a huge land mass and large offshore islands, with forbidding mountain ranges, great river systems, and seemingly endless stretches of tundra, taiga, and forest. Both the land and the seas around it are rich in animal and plant life, not to mention mineral wealth and, as we now know, petroleum. The climate varies widely, from the cool, damp regions of the Panhandle and Aleutian Islands, to the moderate climate of the south-central region, the seasonal extremes of the interior, and finally the true arctic climate of the northwest and north coasts. Despite the diversity of topography and climate of the region as a whole, however, the settled parts of Alaska share a cool, largely maritime environment in which the people maintain an especially close relationship with animal life. These factors are basic to an understanding of the disease and death patterns that were manifested not only by the original inhabitants of the land but also by those who came after.

The aboriginal cultures of Alaska developed their distinctive traits over many centuries in response to geography, climate, and resources. Basic needs such as food, clothing, and shelter were satisfied by the efficient and often ingenious use of the materials at hand, including all kinds of animal products, wood, and stone. Although practices differed in detail among the scattered and often isolated populations of Natives, definite affinities and sometimes striking similarities in customs can be discerned, due not only to independent convergence but also to the cultural diffusion resulting from trade. Similar cultural traits usually result in similar patterns of disease and injury.

The third unifying factor in Alaskan medical history is time. The recorded history of Alaska effectively began with the first voyage of Vitus Bering in 1728, little more than two and a half centuries ago. During this brief period medicine has moved, at least for the Native peoples, from the typical characteristics of preliterate societies to space-age health technology in the hospitals of Anchorage and Fairbanks. Western civilization made the same transition over a period of several thousand years, although far more has been accomplished in medicine in the last two centuries—indeed, the last few decades—than in all prior recorded history.

The fourth unifying factor is the nature of Alaskan history itself. For a large region with a small and scattered population, much historical documentation exists, perhaps in part because the land's natural beauty and remarkable people compelled the interest and attention of visitors. The relatively brief span of recorded Alaskan history also simplifies the historian's task, especially considering that only two nations have exerted hegemony over the region. Thus, the record of diseases and their impact, and of the development of health services, is relatively easy to trace.

The focus of the present work is on the role of health and disease in the history of Alaska from the earliest times to 1900. The primary emphasis is on the Alaska Native people, who after all were the sole occupants of the land until the middle of the eighteenth century, and for the rest of the period under consideration far outnumbered the Europeans and Euro-Americans.*

Historians in the past (with a few exceptions) have viewed early Alaska largely in terms of European exploration and settlement, the fur trade, the gold rushes, and the exploitation of fish, timber, and mineral resources. Human interest has focused on explorers, missionaries, miners, and politicians, rather than on those whose lives were most radically changed by this so-called "development."

* Elsewhere in the texts the term "American," although not strictly correct, will refer to Euro-Americans or citizens of the United States. The Alaska Natives did not acquire citizenship until 1924.

Although the Natives rightfully take center stage in this study, health and disease in the lives of the Europeans—and later the Americans—will not be neglected, not least because most of the available information is told from their perspective. Furthermore, the health and habits of the Europeans and Americans, in the last analysis, had a profound and often detrimental effect on the later health of the Natives.

The specific objectives of the present work are

1. To reconstruct as fully as possible the diseases from which the Alaska Natives suffered around the time of first European contact and before Western culture had a strong influence on health;

2. To discuss health aspects of the early recorded history of Alaska, including the beginnings of medical care and the impact of disease and death on historical events; and

3. To trace in chronological fashion the introduction and spread of certain diseases which have had a profound influence on the lives of the peoples of Alaska, both Native and Caucasian.

The year 1900 was chosen as a termination for this analysis for several reasons. That year itself was a momentous one, including as it did the peak of the Nome gold rush and, more important medically, a terrible influenza and measles epidemic that devastated western Alaska. In addition, by the turn of the century the exploration of Alaska was virtually complete and probably all Alaska Natives had encountered Whites for at least a decade or more. With the thousands of prospectors and camp followers who had poured into Alaska during that final decade, it was obvious to Native and White alike that there was no turning back from the rapid cultural changes that were engulfing the territory.

SOURCES

Health and disease, despite their importance, have received scant attention from historians, anthropologists, archeologists, and even physicians writing about Alaska. Few historians have given more than a courteous nod to health matters, limiting their discussion to such subjects as scurvy on shipboard, epidemics (especially the smallpox epidemic of 1835 to 1840), the liquor trade, or to general allusions to the diseased condition of the Natives. Anthropologists, archeologists, and ethnohistorians have written on traditional medicine, shamanism, ethnobotany, and health-related customs, but few have tackled the issue of the impact of disease on society (L. Milan

1974). Nor have physicians rushed in to fill the gap. The modern medical literature on Alaska is extensive indeed, yet very little of it deals with disease or medical care from a historical standpoint. Most physicians cited as sources in this book are contemporaneous with the events and conditions they describe.

Three types of source materials have been used: records of archeological investigations, ethnographic and ethnohistorical accounts, and original narratives of explorers, missionaries, traders, and government officials.

Archeological studies of medical interest have been unfortunately rare in Alaska, but those that exist, mostly by Zimmerman and his colleagues, are invaluable, based as they are on detailed autopsies on fortuitously preserved human remains. Although such studies in most parts of the world are necessarily limited to bones and teeth, in Alaska the practice of mummification among the Aleuts, and the chance preservation in a frozen state of several entire bodies, have led to a detailed knowledge of the health problems of at least a few precontact Natives. (*See* Figure 1.) Broad inferences from such limited material are of course risky, but at least these autopsies can tell with certainty some of the diseases that were present in aboriginal times.

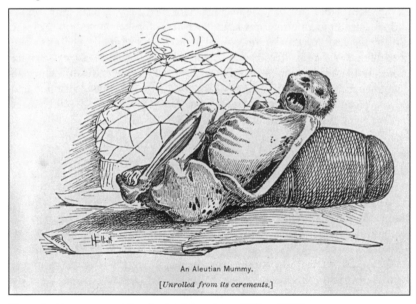

An Aleutian Mummy.
[*Unrolled from its cerements.*]

Figure 1. Aleut mummy, showing burial position. (Elliott 1886.)

Anthropologists have studied in detail nearly all the Native groups in Alaska. They have analyzed the material, social, and intellectual aspects of these cultures, not only from artifacts, but from early historical materials, by participant observation, and by systematic interviews of contemporary carriers of the cultures. These efforts have indirectly produced considerable information of medical value.

Far more valuable for the history of medicine, however, than these more or less contemporary studies are the many early narratives and eyewitness accounts of life in Alaska from 1728 through the end of the nineteenth century. Few writers make more than incidental reference to health, but in the aggregate they give a fairly comprehensive picture of the diseases and health hazards that they themselves and the Natives faced. They also give a fresh, contemporaneous view of the beginnings of medical care in Alaska. Not a few of these narratives are by physicians who were often, curiously, serving in another capacity such as naturalist, explorer, miner, missionary, or teacher.

Eyewitness accounts, despite their fundamental importance as primary source material, also have distinct limitations. Very few writers seem to have made specific inquiries about the diseases that were prevalent in the areas they visited. Contacts with the Native people were likely to be brief and not infrequently hostile, or at least shrouded in mutual suspicion. The Natives, moreover, were appropriately clothed for a cold climate, thus affording little scope for observation beyond the face and general body contour. Only the most obvious diseases and deformities would have been apparent in such encounters; the sick and disabled were in any event likely to have been left behind in the village.

Differing languages and value systems also impeded understanding of health matters. Interpreters, when they could be found at all, were rarely skilled in both languages. Many of the early visitors were bound by the cultural conventions of their own time and country, and some of their writings betray a blatant or only thinly disguised prejudice against the "savages" they encountered. More were prepared to castigate the Natives' habits of personal cleanliness than to praise a clever Native surgical technique. Even those with a positive or sympathetic frame of mind, however, had little opportunity to observe Native life firsthand.

It must further be remembered that few of these writers had any knowledge of medicine beyond that of a well-informed citizen of the time. Even those who were physicians were trained in a wholly different system of medical theory and practice from what we know today. Their ideas on causation, diagnosis, and treatment of diseases seem quaint or even absurd to us today, just as ours may be to some future medical historians.

Finally, it is nearly inevitable that my own perspective—that of a physician trained in public health with a long experience working with the Alaska Natives—will creep into the narrative from time to time. No author, and probably few readers, can remain wholly dispassionate when deeply immersed in the subject matter of this book. The topic has its tragic and even sordid side, from whatever set of mind it is approached. I have tried hard to write an evenhanded account, by largely letting contemporary witnesses speak for themselves. These sources, as noted, are not without bias and nearly all are culture-bound by the Euro-American tradition. If this book seems to emphasize the viewpoint of the Alaska Natives, it is because their story has had few chroniclers.

THE NATIVES OF ALASKA

Throughout this book the Alaska Natives are discussed under six major groupings, a compromise between the oversimplified traditional classification of "Eskimo, Indian, and Aleut," and the ponderous schema that might be adopted in a scientific treatise. The grouping used here, namely Aleuts, Pacific Eskimos, Yupik Eskimos, Inupiat Eskimos, southeastern Alaskan Indians, and Athapaskan* Indians, has the virtue of being simple and of corresponding relatively well to the major geographical and climatic regions of Alaska.

In the available space it would be inappropriate to give more than a brief outline of selected aspects of these cultures, particularly those that have a direct or indirect bearing on health. Most cited references are necessarily secondary sources.

Aleuts

The Aleuts originally inhabited the entire volcanic Aleutian Chain and outer third of the Alaska Peninsula. Their homeland is treeless, with cool summers and relatively moderate winters. The islands are swept by frequent

*The spelling "Athapaskan," used here, is the one preferred in the ethnographic literature from which this book draws. The people themselves generally spell it "Athabascan," whereas the Alaska Native Language Center at the University of Alaska Fairbanks favors "Athabaskan."

storms and high winds, but remain mostly free of permafrost and shore ice. The seas abound in fish, shellfish, sea mammals, and maritime birds. The land is largely devoid of large animals, except for brown bears and caribou on the Alaska Peninsula.

Aleut culture is related to that of the southern Eskimos and their languages show certain affinities. In precontact times the population was probably in the range of 12,000 to 16,000, scattered in dozens of villages, largely on the southern, or Pacific coast (Lantis 1984a, 163; Laughlin 1980, 15). The people lived in large semisubterranean structures, known as *barabaras,* constructed of driftwood logs or whale bones, and covered with skins, grass, and sod. The houses were heated by oil lamps and contained many cubicles, separated by hanging mats, for the members of the extended family (Lantis 1984a, 166-67; Laughlin 1980, 52).

The people wore parkas with standing collars and fashioned with some artistry from fur, birdskin, and sea mammal intestine. Most of the year they went barefoot, although in the eastern parts they sometimes wore boots and trousers in the colder seasons. The hunters wore elaborate wooden hats, shaped like an inverted scoop, which served as a shield against sun and rain (Lantis 1984a, 170-71).

Most food came from the sea and included sea mammals, fish, shellfish, and waterfowl. In some seasons the diet was supplemented by eggs, seaweed, greens, roots, and especially berries. The men hunted sea mammals, including whales, from one- or two-holed skin boats known as *baidarkas.* Their hunting implements included harpoons, sometimes tipped with poison, throwing boards, and retrieving hooks. Gathering of plants and shellfish, the latter especially important in lean times, devolved on the women (Laughlin 1980, 27-49).

During pregnancy a woman was under the close supervision of her mother or grandmother. At the time of birth she was taken to a special hut, where all male influences could be removed. The mother gave birth in a squatting position, assisted by the women, who massaged her abdomen that day and repeatedly over the next few days. The baby was also massaged, then washed, warmed, and induced to vomit before being put to the breast. The child was breast-fed for at least a couple of years, or until the teeth erupted (Merck 1980, 174-75; Veniaminov 1984, 189-90).

The Aleuts practiced extensive body ornamentation, although the details of when and under what circumstances it occurred are often unclear. Labrets, or lip ornaments, were especially conspicuous, and usually consisted of pieces of bone or stone in the shape of teeth placed in slits or perforations in the lower lip. Most men wore long narrow bones, sometimes festooned with

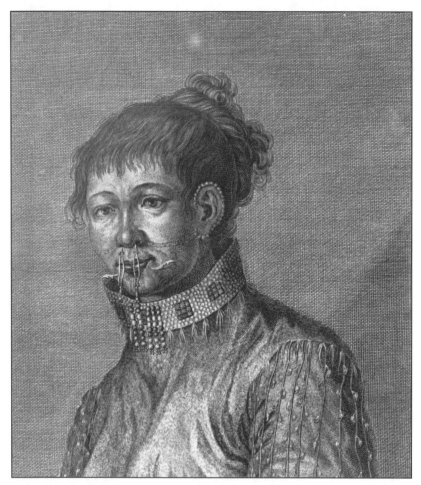

Figure 2. Aleut woman, with labrets, nose and ear ornaments, and tattoos. (Sarychev 1802, Rare Book Collection, Archives, Alaska and Polar Regions., University of Alaska Fairbanks.)

beads, through a perforation in the nasal septum. Both men and women wore feathers or bead-like pieces of shell or bone in perforations in the pinna of the ear. Tattoos of the face, arms, and backs of the hands were also common (e.g., Coxe 1787, 68, 76; Ellis 1782, 1:289; Laughlin 1980, 57). Preparation for all these methods of ornamentation required skillful surgical techniques (Fortuine 1985, 24-28). (*See* Figure 2.)

An Aleut girl at the time of her first menstrual period was immediately taken to a separate hut or a special section of the family dwelling. There she remained for thirty to forty days and was permitted no visitors except her mother or other close female relative. The girl's joints were bound with a special waxed cord said to prevent arthritis and senility, and to protect the village water and food supply. At the end of her seclusion she washed herself for five days and returned to society, although some restrictions continued to apply. Later menses required shorter periods of isolation (Veniaminov 1984, 210; Marsh and Laughlin 1956, 84; Merck 1980, 174, 178).

The Aleuts probably had the most highly developed system of traditional medicine of any of the Alaska Natives. Healing was performed by male or female shamans and other types of practitioners, including surgeons, masseuses, and herbalists. The shamans used largely magical methods but also employed plant remedies or surgical procedures. The surgery of the Aleuts, in fact, was particularly sophisticated, for their knowledge of anatomy was based not only on the dressing-out of animals, as in other cultures, but also on their practice of making human mummies and performing autopsies on dead slaves or enemies (Marsh and Laughlin 1956). They sutured wounds, removed arrows and other missiles, bled their patients, and used a technique known as "piercing" to let out bad humors. Old women were particularly skillful in the use of abdominal massage for various internal disorders. The Aleutian Islands, being green most of the year, provided a variety of medicinal plants, but often the first and indeed only method of treatment for injuries and illness was fasting (Laughlin 1980, 103-4; Bank 1953; Fortuine 1985, 29-36; Lantis 1984a, 176).

The Pacific Eskimos

The term Pacific Eskimos, in this book, refers to the inhabitants of Kodiak Island, or Koniag, and to the people of Prince William Sound known as Chugach. In precontact times these southern Yupik Eskimos extended from the mid-Alaska Peninsula and Kodiak Island, across the southeastern shores of the Kenai Peninsula to as far east as Kayak Island. Little is known of any of these people, however, except the Koniag and Chugach. Both of the latter used a similar language known as Pacific Eskimo, or Alutiiq, and their cultures showed other common traits (D. Clark 1984, 185). The Pacific Eskimos lived in coastal villages and around the time of contact numbered about 8700, most of them living on Kodiak Island. In fact, the population density of the Koniag was probably the highest of any of the Alaska Natives

(Oswalt 1967, 25, 115). Both the Koniag and the Chugach were warlike and often engaged in armed conflict with their neighbors.

The Pacific Eskimos, like the Aleuts, lived in a relatively mild maritime climate, although their coastline is also subject to severe and often unexpected storms. These Eskimos are the only ones who live on the edge of dense forests, which cover large areas of their habitat, especially around Prince William Sound and on the eastern third of Kodiak Island.

Their homes were large, accommodating as many as twenty persons from several families. The dwellings were semisubterranean, fashioned from logs and turf on Kodiak Island, or sometimes from wooden planks in Prince William Sound. Inside, a main room had a central hearth and could be used as a living area, as a workshop, or for ceremonies. Small side rooms were heated with hot rocks and sometimes served as sweatbaths (D. Clark 1984, 191).

Clothing was similar to that of the Aleuts, with long hoodless fur or birdskin parkas, and rain parkas *(kamleika)* fashioned from strips of seal intestine. Gloves and trousers were apparently not worn and most people went barefoot in the warmer months. Hunters wore slanted conical hats made from twisted spruce root (D. Clark 1984, 194-95).

The Pacific Eskimos depended largely on fish and sea mammals, including whales, for their food supply, but they also caught birds and gathered eggs, shellfish, and many kinds of plants in season. Caribou were sometimes taken for food and fur on the Alaska Peninsula. Larger sea creatures were harpooned from a one- or two-holed *baidarka.* Both the Koniag and the Chugach also employed a large skin boat known as a *baidara,* similar to the umiak of northern Alaska (D. Clark 1984, 187-89).

A pregnant Koniag woman at the time of childbirth was taken to a small hut away from the main building, where during labor an old woman stretched or pummeled her abdomen (Davydov 1977, 164). After delivery, during which the Chugach woman remained on her hands and knees, the baby was washed and wrapped. Mother and child were then isolated for several weeks. The child was regularly nursed at least until the age of three and sometimes among the Chugach to the age of eleven or twelve (Birket-Smith 1953, 87).

The Pacific Eskimos were extensively ornamented in a manner similar to the Aleuts. Lip ornaments were particularly elaborate, often placed in a long horizontal slit on the lower lip. The nasal septum was perforated during infancy and later the aperture held ornaments of feather, bone, or shell. The margins of the ears likewise often contained small ornaments. Tattooing was particularly favored among Koniag women (Cook 1967, 3(1):250; Merck 1980, 103; Shelikhov 1981, 53; Fortuine 1985, 24-28).

At the time of her first menstrual period, a Koniag girl was sequestered for six months in a tiny hut away from others, and was not allowed to return to full participation in community life for a year. Among the Chugach menarche was less of an ordeal, and involved only a ten-day stay in one of the sleeping rooms in the main house (Holmberg 1985, 53; Birket-Smith 1953, 154).

The traditional medical practices of the Pacific Eskimos were highly developed, especially among the Koniag. Shamans could be either male or female, and on Kodiak Island, at least, were not infrequently transvestites (Gedeon *in* Pierce 1978, 135). Koniag surgeons were especially skillful and courageous, performing operations for boils, wounds, urinary stones, and cataracts. Bleeding and piercing were also widely employed, often by women, for the treatment of internal illnesses (Fortuine 1985, 31-36). Massage was a modality favored by Chugach women practitioners. Both groups used many types of plants and other substances for healing (Birket-Smith 1953, 117; Davydov 1977, 177; Pierce 1978, 129-30).

The Yupik Eskimos

The Central Yupik Eskimos (hereinafter called simply Yupik) are a large group inhabiting parts of the Alaska Peninsula, the Bristol Bay region, the Yukon-Kuskokwim Delta, Nunivak Island, and the southern and perhaps eastern shores of Norton Sound. A closely related group, known as Siberian Yupik, live on St. Lawrence Island in the Bering Sea.

The climate of this large area is variable, with cold, damp winters and cool summers along the coast, and higher summer temperatures and lower winter temperatures in the river valleys. Most of the coastal areas consist of level, treeless tundra with thousands of small lakes and meandering sloughs. Further inland, especially along the rivers, are stands of stunted spruce, willow, cottonwood, and birch.

According to one estimate, the Central Yupik population numbered approximately 11,000 around the time of contact (Oswalt 1967, 114). They were distributed into two major groups—those who lived in coastal communities in Bristol Bay and along the Bering littoral, and those who inhabited villages along the major river systems such as the Nushagak, Kuskokwim, and Yukon. Although they spoke a common language, called

Central Yupik, they had major differences in their subsistence patterns and their material culture. Most lived in permanent winter villages, but also went to spring camp on the tundra, and to fish camp in the summer.

Village dwellings consisted of a small outer room, connected to the main room by a tunnel either at ground level or below. This passageway was designed to keep cold air from penetrating into the main room, the entrance to which was covered by a skin or grass mat. The walls were constructed of driftwood logs and four posts supported the roof, in the middle of which was a hole to admit light and allow ventilation. On the outside of the log walls were placed sheets of birchbark, or grass, then a layer of sod to provide extra insulation. Inside, a fireplace was in the center of the floor and sleeping or storage benches were distributed along the walls. In the spring camps and fish camps the people lived in smaller sod huts or tents (VanStone 1984, 229-31).

The winter dwelling was occupied by the women and children only, for the men lived and slept communally in the *kashim,* or men's house. This large building, similar in design to the other houses, served as the center of social and ceremonial life in the village. It was also here that the young men learned the skills necessary to hunt, fish, and fashion tools and weapons (VanStone 1984, 233). (*See* Figure 3.)

Winter clothing consisted of a long parka, usually but not always hooded, made from the fur of ground squirrels or marmots and trimmed with strips of fur. Underneath the people wore belted trousers that reached to the knees. Instead of a hood some used a fur or birdskin cap. A woman's parka was slit up the sides and decorated with ground squirrel tails. Footwear included socks of woven grass and fishskin or sealskin boots (Oswalt 1967, 141-42).

The annual subsistence cycle for those who lived along the rivers began in the spring with trapping small fur-bearing animals and taking migrating birds by means of snares, nets, and spears. By mid-June the people were devoting all their energy to the major runs of salmon, which they caught using drift nets, or in some areas basket traps. Most of the fish were dried on racks for later use. In the fall the men turned to caribou hunting and beaver trapping, then retired to their winter villages (VanStone 1984, 228-33).

In coastal villages the subsistence cycle was somewhat different. In the spring the men hunted seals, including the bearded seal, in their kayaks, and occasionally were able also to kill belugas or walruses. In the summer they fished for salmon at the river mouths, often with a pronged fish spear. Bird eggs were a late spring delicacy, as were nesting birds themselves, which

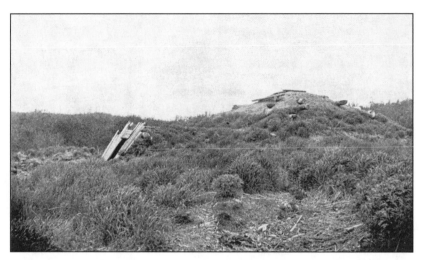

Figure 3. Eskimo semisubterranean *kashim,* on the lower Yukon. (Cantwell 1902.)

were caught by a net on their breeding cliffs. Both the coastal and riverine Eskimos gathered many types of plants, especially berries, some of which they preserved in seal oil for the winter (Lantis 1984b, 213-14).

At the time of childbirth a woman was attended by her mother or an older woman from the village. For delivery she usually lay on her left side, although other positions were also used. After the birth the mother was expected to continue to lie on her side for several more days. The infant was nursed for the first time almost immediately, even before being washed. The mother breast-fed her child for three or four years, although she also offered solid food, beginning with premasticated fish liver, dried fish, and fish soup, at a much earlier time (Lantis 1959, 31-35).

Ornamentation among the Yupik was less elaborate than among their southern neighbors. Simple round labrets of stone, shell, or bone were worn at the corners of the mouth in perforations made in infancy (Khromchenko 1973, 60; Lantis 1959, 32). The nasal septum was also pierced in childhood and often contained a piece of sinew from which beads were suspended. Ear ornaments were sometimes large and complex. Only the St. Lawrence Island Yupik used extensive tattoos (Nelson 1899, 51-52). (*See* Figure 4.)

An adolescent girl was considered unclean for forty days after her first menses. During this time she was secluded, with her face to the wall and a parka over her head. She was expected to work diligently at her daily tasks

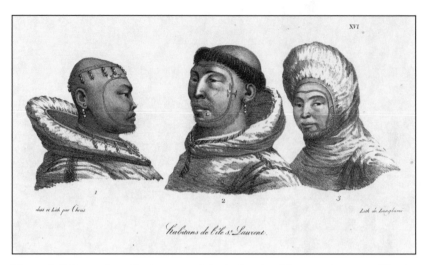

Figure 4. Eskimos from St. Lawrence Island, showing labrets and tattoos. (Choris 1822, Rare Book Collection, Archives, Alaska and Polar Regions Dept., University of Alaska Fairbanks.)

and was permitted to go outside only at night. At the end of this period she bathed, put on new clothing and was considered eligible for marriage (Nelson 1899, 291).

The Yupik ascribed serious illnesses, as did other Natives, to several supernatural causes, including sorcery, soul loss, and object intrusion. Such illnesses required the services of a shaman, who could be male or female and usually held a position of some wealth and prestige in the community. Common minor illnesses and accidents were treated by a family member or by an old woman skilled in the use of plants and other remedies.

Shamanistic healing techniques included dancing, chanting, and the performance of various types of legerdemain, all carried out in an impressive and dramatic setting (Lantis 1946, 200-202). Empirical healers used many types of plants, among which stinkweed *(Artemisia tilesii)* and willow *(Salix* spp.) were preeminent (Ager and Ager 1980; Oswalt 1957; Lantis 1959). Animal products used medicinally included seal oil, human milk, urine, and the anal glands of the beaver (Lantis 1959, 89). Surgery was not highly developed in this region. Bleeding and piercing were employed for internal illnesses, cuts were sutured, and sometimes an amputation was performed for frostbite (Fortuine 1985, 31-36). Heat and cold also found therapeutic uses (Lantis 1959, 10; 1946, 202).

The Inupiat Eskimos

The Inupiat, or north Alaskan Eskimos, are primarily a coastal people, occupying the Seward Peninsula and the offshore islands, the shores of Kotzebue Sound, and the northern coast of Alaska. An important subgroup, however, had their winter homes inland along the Noatak, Kobuk, and Colville rivers, or even further inland reaching to the northern foothills of the Brooks Range. This last group, known as the Nunamiut, was in some ways culturally distinct because of its dependence on the caribou for food and clothing. All speak variations of the same language, Inupiaq, which is closely related to the language of the Canadian and Greenlandic Eskimos. Around the time of contact the Inupiat have been estimated to number 6350, including 1500 Nunamiut (Oswalt 1967, 114).

The climate of northern Alaska is characterized by severe winter temperatures, usually aggravated by a wind-chill, and short, cool, damp summers. In the interior the winter temperatures plunge even lower, although the summers are somewhat milder. Nearly all of the habitat of these Eskimos is low tundra underlain with permafrost, with much standing water in the summer months. Along the river valleys are small stands of stunted trees.

The northern Eskimos in early times did not have closely integrated communities, but rather loosely associated settlements of extended families, with primary loyalty to the kindred group (Spencer 1984, 326-27). Among the Nunamiut, who were often on the move, the social organization was even more loose (Hall 1984, 341).

The winter houses of the coastal people were solid structures built partially underground from turf and driftwood, with a long passageway, at a lower level, leading to the main room. The hearth was located centrally, below a smoke-hole, and sleeping and storage benches were arranged along the walls. Storage rooms often opened into the main passageway (Burch 1984, 307; D. Ray 1984, 290; Spencer 1984, 327). A men's house, here called *karigi*, was of similar construction but larger. A Nunamiut winter dwelling consisted of a ground-level willow frame covered with skins, sometimes insulated by moss or sod (Hall 1984, 342). Summer homes among the northern Eskimos were usually tents made from walrus skin, sealskin, or caribou hides.

The clothing of the Inupiat varied somewhat according to geographic location and hence the availability of materials. Most of the coastal peoples wore long hooded parkas of sealskin and caribou hides trimmed with wolf, although they also used ground squirrel and ermine on occasion. In winter an inner parka was worn with the hair inward. Both men and women wore inner and outer pants, with skin socks and boots (D. Ray 1984, 289; Burch 1984, 309). The Nunamiut fashioned their clothing largely from caribou skins (Hall 1984, 341).

The subsistence pattern of the northern coastal Eskimos was organized around the spring hunt of the great bowhead whale, although other types of food, especially seals and fish, were taken through the year. Further south around Kotzebue Sound and the Seward Peninsula, fish and various types of seals were the staples, as were caribou in the inland area. Walrus were important around the Bering Strait during their annual spring migration. Eggs, birds, and a variety of fresh and salt water fish were available seasonally. Greens, roots, and berries were important additions to the diet in the warmer months. In the interior caribou provided as much as ninety percent of the food supply, which was also supplemented by bear, moose, mountain sheep, ptarmigan, and fish (D. Ray 1984, 287; Burch 1984, 306; Spencer 1984, 328; Hall 1984, 341).

Eskimo women of the north coast gave birth in a small hut, sometimes made of snow, away from the main dwelling. She was assisted by a single female relative and usually delivered in a kneeling position. After childbirth the mother remained in her hut for four or five days, during which she observed various dietary restrictions. The baby was not permitted to nurse for two days, but instead was given small amounts of warm oil and water (Spencer 1959, 231-33). Other groups had slightly different practices, particularly with regard to the length of isolation following delivery (P. Ray 1885, 46; Cantwell 1889, 82). In some areas the mother gave birth unassisted ([Jarvis] 1899, 120-21; Giddings 1961, 153).

The northern Alaskan Eskimos used fairly simple body ornamentation. Labrets were fashioned from bone, ivory, wood, and stone, and usually worn as a round disk in a perforation below the corners of the mouth (J. Simpson 1855, 921-22; Cook 1967, 3(1):438). Most women wore baleen or beads in their perforated nasal septum. Beads or small pieces of bone were also commonly worn in ear perforations (D. Ray 1975, 91; Beechey 1831, 1:393; Ellis 1782, 1:330). Simple tattoo patterns, usually vertical lines on the chin of women, were widespread (Merck 1980, 190; M'Clure 1857, 63).

Most groups, except the Nunamiut (Gubser 1965, 208), required a girl at the time of her first menstrual period to undergo a time of isolation ranging from five to forty days. During this time the girl was expected to wear a special caribou skin hood to shade her eyes, and to observe certain dietary restrictions. She also was expected to learn the skills and responsibilities of womanhood during her seclusion (Spencer 1959, 243-44; Giddings 1961, 20-21, 154).

Traditional medicine in northern Alaska was similar in broad outline to that of the Yupik Eskimos. The shaman was the most important healer and held considerable power and authority among the people. Most (although not all) were men who seemed predestined for the task because of their unusual set of mind and their apparent ability to commune with the spirits around them. Other types of healers were few, most of the empirical healing being performed by relatives or ordinary members of the community. (*See* Figure 5.)

Because of the rigorous climate and short summer, plant remedies on the northern coast were few (Spencer 1959, 328; DeLapp and Ward 1981). Some were employed along the rivers and in the interior further south, however, particularly stinkweed (*Artemisia* spp.), willow (*Salix* spp.), and yarrow *(Achillea borealis)* (Cantwell 1889, 83; Lucier et al. 1971, 254; J. Anderson 1939; Gubser 1965, 239-40). The universal remedies of the region were seal oil and whale blubber, each of which had numerous uses (e.g., Spencer 1959, 328; Stoney 1900, 89; Lucier et al. 1971, 254). Surgical techniques were sometimes employed by shamans, but also by others in the community. Among the practices reported were perforations for labret holes, and bleeding and piercing (often called "poking"), used for a variety of internal and external illnesses (Dixon and Kirchner 1982). A few cases of major amputation for frostbite are known (Fortuine 1985, 24-36).

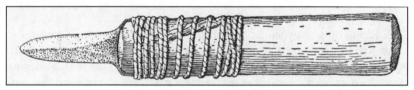

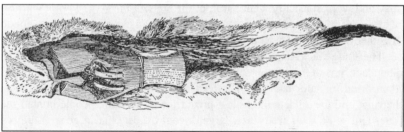

Figure 5. Eskimo lancet, pointed with nephrite; Shaman's doll fetish, used in healing. (Nelson 1899.)

Southeastern Alaskan Indians

The Indians of southeastern Alaska included the dominant Tlingit, the closely related Kaigani Haida on the southern half of Prince of Wales Island, and the Tsimshian, a Canadian tribe that emigrated to Alaska only in the late nineteenth century. Although all groups had their distinctive cultural traits, they shared much in common with each other and with tribes of the British Columbia coast. At the time of contact the Tlingit numbered about 15,000 and the Alaskan Haida another 1800 (Langdon 1987, 61). They lived in relatively permanent villages in the bays and inlets during the winter months and dispersed to fishing villages to spend the spring, summer, and fall.

The southeastern part of Alaska consists of several large islands, with many smaller islands and a narrow mainland strip. The entire area is mountainous, with impressive glaciers in the northern St. Elias Mountains. The climate is moderate, but heavy precipitation occurs in the form of rain, drizzle, and fog, especially in the late summer and fall. The islands are densely forested, largely with Sitka spruce and other tall conifers. The region abounds with wildlife, including sea mammals, land mammals, birds, and a rich resource of salmon that ascend the short rivers to spawn.

Tlingit and Haida permanent homes faced the ocean and were substantial structures built of roughly hewn cedar planks. The interior consisted of a central excavated area with a hearth, and ground-level sleeping platforms along the walls. Twenty to thirty persons from several closely related families often occupied a single house. Summer dwellings were smaller and less solidly built (Langdon 1987, 65).

Clothing was fairly simple and unadorned. The men wore a deerskin loin cloth and the women a skirt or apron of deerskin or woven cedar bark. Outer garments included a fur robe, sometimes made of sea otter skin. A conical hat of woven spruce roots was useful for warding off the heavy rains. Both men and women usually went barefoot throughout the year. Tlingit warriors wore a visored wooden helmet and a cuirass made of wood slats bound together (Drucker 1955, 81-83).

The Tlingit and Haida were above all fishermen, depending chiefly on the abundant runs of salmon, which were caught in traps at the river mouths and then dried for later use. Other important food fish were halibut, haddock, herring, and the eulachon, the last prized for its oil. The people hunted sea otter and some seals from their large dugout canoes, but in general did not tackle large sea mammals such as whales or sea lions. Other important products of the sea were shellfish, seaweed, and fish roe. Occasionally the people of this area hunted larger land mammals such as deer, mountain goat, sheep, and bear. Roots, greens, and especially berries were important seasonal supplements to the diet (Krause 1956, 121-25; Langdon 1987, 61).

A pregnant Tlingit or Haida woman nearing delivery was moved to a small hut of logs and branches, where she was assisted by her mother, another female relative, or a midwife. Following birth of the child she was considered unclean and confined to the hut for up to thirty days, during which time stringent dietary restrictions were imposed (Krause 1956, 151; Khlebnikov 1976, 27). The infant was rubbed with grease, washed in urine, and tightly wrapped in skins (R. White 1880, 36). The midwife induced the baby to vomit by manipulating the abdomen, in order to remove impurities (Holmberg 1985, 20-21). The child was apparently breast-fed for only ten to thirty months, less than for any other Alaska Native group (Veniaminov 1984, 415).

Tlingit and Haida women wore conspicuous facial ornaments. The most notable was a large wooden disc in the lower lip that not only caused considerable facial distortion, but also interfered with talking and eating. The lip was pierced in childhood and the wound kept open by a wire, and later by progressively larger wooden plugs. Other types of ornamentation involved piercing the nasal septum and the ears for insertion of metal rings or feathers (Krause 1956, 94-100). Tattoos were particularly favored among the Haida (Niblack 1888, 370).

The customs associated with a Tlingit girl's first menstruation were harsh indeed. She was secluded in a tiny hut built of evergreen branches for as much as a year, during which time she was required to wear a special cloak and hood that prevented her from looking at the sky. Her mother brought food to her, but she was only permitted to drink water through the hollow wing-bone of an eagle. At the end of this ordeal a celebration was held in her honor (Holmberg 1985, 21-22; Krause 1956, 152-53). A Haida girl at the onset of menstruation was secluded in a corner of the main house for only a month or two (Krause 1956, 210).

Tlingit and Haida traditional medicine was solidly rooted in shamanism. Disease could be due to soul loss or the malevolence of sorcerers, or it could be inflicted on humans because of the anger of the creator. The shamans, who could be either male or female, were held in fear and respect because of their spiritual powers in the community, powers they had gained through a long and difficult apprenticeship. They used amulets, chants, dances, and a trance-like state to commune with the spirits and identify which one could help effect the cure (Holmberg 1985, 32-34). Sometimes such sessions ended

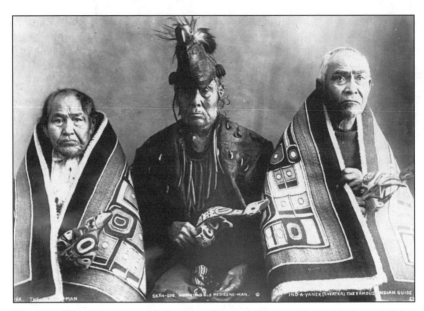

Figure 6. Tlingit shaman with brothers. (Vertical File, Archives, Alaska and Polar Regions Dept., University of Alaska Fairbanks.)

in the dramatic naming of a sorcerer, who was then appropriately punished by the community, usually with torture and death (Krause 1956, 200-201). (*See* Figure 6.)

Empirical medicine was probably less important than shamanistic healing in southeastern Alaska. Certain plants, notably devil's club *(Echinopanax horridum)*, had multiple uses (Justice 1966), some of them magical in nature (De Laguna 1972, 7:655-65). A favorite among animal substances was "hooligan" oil, rendered from the eulachon fish (McGregor 1981, 66). Another was bear gall, which was thought to be especially effective against arthritis (R. White 1880, 37). Little information on surgical techniques is available except for those relating to ornamentation (Fortuine 1985, 24-28, 35). The Tlingit often resorted to the warm mineral springs south of Sitka for the treatment of skin diseases and joint pains (*see* Chapter 7).

The Athapaskans

The Athapaskans are a large and diverse family of Indians who live not only throughout much of central Alaska, but also over a vast region of western Canada. In Alaska, classification by language reveals eleven groups, which may be conveniently divided culturally among those of the major river drainages (Ingalik, Holikachuk, Upper Kuskokwim, Koyukon, and Tanana), those of the cordillera, or uplands (Kutchin, Han, Tanacross, and Upper Tanana), those of the Pacific coast (Tanaina), and those of the Copper River basin (Ahtna). In addition, the related Eyak Indians lived around the mouth of the Copper River east of Prince William Scund (VanStone 1974, 15-20; Krauss 1982). All of these linguistic groups shared many cultural traits, although the details of their daily life differed somewhat, particularly among the four main geographic areas. At the time of contact the total population of Alaskan Athapaskans has been estimated at between 6000 (VanStone 1974, 11) and 10,500 (Langdon 1987, 50).

The home of the Alaskan Athapaskans stretches over a huge area of interior Alaska, bounded by the Brooks Range on the north, the Pacific littoral around Cook Inlet on the south, the lower Kuskokwim and Yukon river valleys on the west, and the Canadian border on the east. The geographic features include mountains, plateaus, and flatlands. Most areas are forested with spruce, birch, cottonwood, alder, and willow. The climate is severe, with extremes of cold in the winter and temperatures ranging as high as 90° Fahrenheit in the summer. Precipitation is fairly light over much of the habitat.

Athapaskan houses took several forms. Most populations were seasonally on the move and hence avoided complex permanent buildings. A common type of summer home was a rectangular structure consisting of sheets of bark laid between upright poles, with a flat or gabled roof. Even more temporary or portable dwellings were in the form of a simple lean-to, or in the eastern areas, a skin-covered conical teepee. For winter use two types of houses predominated. One popular form was a semisubterranean dome-like structure consisting of upright poles bent inward and covered with skins. Another type resembled a log cabin (Hosley 1981, 538-39).

The people wore tailored skin clothing throughout the year, using principally hides from the caribou, moose, and mountain sheep. The garments consisted of a long sleeved hairless shirt and legging moccasins in the summer, and with fur trousers, moccasins, mittens, and a hood or cap added in the colder times of the year. The outfit was often decorated with dentalium shells or porcupine quills (Hosley 1981, 539).

Subsistence patterns depended on the seasonal availability of food in the various geographic regions. In the high country near the Canadian border, big game hunting, particularly for caribou, was predominant, although smaller animals and birds provided supplemental sources of food. In the

Yukon Flats in summer salmon fishing took precedence, followed by moose and caribou hunting in the fall. Further downsteam on the major rivers salmon fishing, particularly by the use of basket-shaped traps, became the principal annual subsistence activity. They fished in both rivers and lakes and dried much of the salmon for the winter. The Tanaina, who lived by the sea, depended to a significant extent on the hunting of sea mammals, including seals, sea otters, beluga, and sea lions. The subsistence economy of the Copper River Indians was based largely on the seasonal salmon runs, but also included the hunting of moose, caribou, and small mammals. Plants, especially berries, were used by all Athapaskans, but did not constitute a large portion of the diet (VanStone 1974, 26-31).

Childbirth customs varied somewhat among the different groups. Most women in labor were taken to a small hut erected for childbirth, apart from men. One or more women assisted with the delivery, with the woman giving birth assuming a squatting or kneeling position. Following birth the mother remained in the hut, with dietary and other restrictions, for up to twenty days. The newborn was wiped clean with moss and wrapped in rabbit skin or moosehide, and thereafter carried in a cradle-chair or by a carrying strap. Weaning occurred about the age of three or even later (Jetté 1911, 705; VanStone 1974, 76-78).

Body ornamentation was not complex. Lateral labrets were worn by Ingalik men (Zagoskin 1967, 244), who probably adopted the practice from their Yupik neighbors. Most Athapaskans had their nasal septum perforated at an early age and as adults wore dentalium shells or sticks in the aperture. Ear ornaments, usually dentalium shells, were also common, the number correlating roughly with the wealth of the individual (McKennan 1959, 86; 1965, 46). Tattoos were worn by some women for decoration and by some men to indicate hunting prowess (McKennan 1959, 87; Osgood 1971, 95).

The customs associated with a girl's first menstruation were austere and complex, although the details differed widely. From early childhood her mother and other relatives prepared her for this important event, which marked her marriageability. At menarche, the girl was isolated, usually for several months, in a small hut at some distance from the community. Among the Ingalik she was secluded for as much as a year in a corner set apart from the main room of the house by grass mats. During this time she was expected to wear a fur hood and mittens, and not to go outside except at night (Nelson 1978, 41). She had to observe many dietary restrictions and spent the greater part of her time learning the arts and responsibilites of womanhood (Osgood 1958, 183-86). There were a number of variations on this basic pattern (Jetté 1911, 700; VanStone 1974, 80-81).

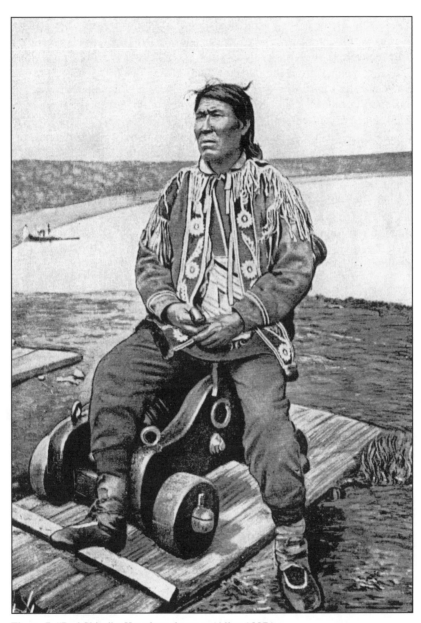

Figure 7. "Red Shirt," a Koyukon shaman. (Allen 1887.)

Healing methods were similar among the various Athapaskan groups. Curing was the principal role of the shaman, who worked, as elsewhere, by frightening away evil spirits (Jetté 1911, 603), or by removing a tangible or intangible object from the patient's body (VanStone 1974, 67). Shamans could be either men or women, and most showed their propensity for this vocation during their adolescence (McKennan 1965, 78), when they first gained their animal helper spirits. (*See* Figure 7.)

Empirical medicine was largely in the hands of family members or elderly women in the community. Some groups, especially the Tanaina (Kari 1987) used many different plant species, but by all odds the favorite Athapaskan plant remedy was the white spruce *(Picea glauca)*, nearly every part of which was employed in healing. The animal products used medicinally included bear gall, wolverine liver, ravens (McKennan 1959, 109), fish eggs, and other fish products (Osgood 1958, 230). Among the surgical techniques were bleeding, scarification, lancing of abscesses, cautery, dental extraction, and the reduction and splinting of fractures (Fortuine 1985, 31-36).

PART I
Health of the Alaska Natives Around the Time of Contact

The four chapters in Part I portray the health status of the Native people of Alaska before, at the time of, or shortly after their first contact with the outside world. Such a reconstruction is necessarily difficult and even hazardous, since it must be made from bits and pieces of information gathered from many disparate sources. Except for the few but very valuable paleopathological studies that bear on the subject, and a few other sources to be mentioned, all the information presented derives from incidental references to health found in the narrative accounts of explorers, traders, scientists, missionaries, and others who described the Natives in the earliest years after contact. Most of the observations are by nonmedical people who had very limited understanding of even common diseases. Although the scarce reports by physicians are especially valuable, they too are not always completely intelligible, since eighteenth- and nineteenth-century concepts of pathology often differ markedly from our own.

Each of the major Native cultural groups were "discovered" at different times by Europeans. The first were the Aleuts (or possibly the Eskimos of St. Lawrence Island or the Diomedes) in the first half of the eighteenth century. They were followed by the peoples of Kodiak, southeastern Alaska, Cook Inlet, and Prince William Sound—all contacted before the end of the eighteenth century. Although initial brief encounters with the Yupik Eskimos had occurred in the eighteenth century, intensive contact did not take place until the Russians opened up trade with the peoples of Bristol Bay, the Yukon-Kuskokwim Delta, and Norton Sound in the first half of the nineteenth century. The northern Eskimos likewise had brief encounters with Europeans in 1778, or even perhaps a half century earlier, but only sporadic contact thereafter until the time of the Franklin search and the beginnings of intensive whaling in the Bering Sea in the 1840s and 1850s. A few isolated bands, such as those on the Kobuk and Noatak rivers, had no significant outside contact until the 1880s. Some Athapaskans encountered Russians as early as the 1780s around Cook Inlet and at the mouth of the Copper River, but the majority had little exposure to Europeans until the 1830s and 1840s, with some having no regular interaction until the 1880s.

In this section the varying experiences with respect to outside contact have been taken into account in an attempt to reconstruct health conditions. It is apparent that a brief isolated encounter with another culture will do nothing to endanger even a fragile health status, unless a highly virulent infectious agent is introduced. Only prolonged contact with another culture, including changes in food, dress, clothing, weaponry, or customs, is likely to alter patterns of health, particularly for the chronic and degenerative diseases. Even most infectious diseases, with a few notable exceptions such as smallpox, measles, and influenza, are not highly contagious and are not spread by a brief or casual encounter.

In light of these considerations, therefore, the assumption has been made in these chapters that the original disease patterns of the Alaska Natives can best be reconstructed from a study of precontact human remains, and from descriptions of diseases as they were observed by the earliest visitors before intensive cultural change had taken place. These assessments can be refined, although with greater risk, by two further sources of information—the evidence of traditional medicine and the judicious use of inference from modern scientific evidence. Multiple traditional remedies for certain conditions suggest that the conditions were common in that society. Moreover, modern knowledge of the ecology or natural history of diseases, such as those carried by wild animals, can lead to reasonable assumptions about the prevalence of such diseases in earlier times.

1

General Health Status

HEALTH, STATURE, NUTRITION

Many of the earliest European visitors to Alaska made general comments on the health of the people they encountered. These writings must be used with caution, since they usually resulted from short meetings with Native leaders or hunting parties, and probably did not reflect conditions as they were in the villages and homes where the sick and disabled would tend to congregate.

One of the first encounters between Europeans and Alaska Natives occurred in the Aleutians in 1741. In September of that year Georg Steller (1988, 103), the naturalist on the returning Bering expedition, described nine Aleuts on the Shumagin Islands as "of average height, strong, and stocky, but rather well proportioned and fleshy on arms and legs." Shortly afterward Alexei Chirikov (1922, 1:305), in command of Bering's other vessel, also met some Aleuts, whom he characterized as being of fair size, seemingly healthy, and resembling the Tartars. A report from 1764 described the Aleuts as either medium in height or quite tall, and "healthier and tougher" than the indigenous peoples of Asia (M. Lazarev and P. Vasiutinsky *in* Andreyev 1952, 29). Captain James Cook (1967, 3(1):459) considered the Aleuts "rather low of stature, but plump and well-shaped." His surgeon William Ellis (1782, 2:45-46) was more precise, estimating the height of the men to be from five to five and a half feet, with the women generally shorter. (It is well to keep in mind that the average European of the time was probably also in the same general range.) Two other accounts from the late eighteenth century described the Aleuts as being of medium stature. Martin Sauer (1802, 154), on the Billings expedition, further noted that their complexion was "dark brown and healthy," and the women were chubby. His colleague Dr. Carl Heinrich Merck (1980, 199-200) described the men as stately, agile, and with a good physical build, and the women as sturdy and well-built.

The earliest observations on the health of the Koniag came from Grigorii Shelikhov (1981, 53-55), who in 1784 founded on Kodiak Island one of the first European settlements in Alaska. He described the people there as "tall, healthy, and well-fleshed" and free of communicable diseases except for venereal disease. Most early visitors, in fact, found the Koniag to be taller than the Aleuts (Sarytschew 1807, 2:18; Merck 1980, 105; Langsdorff 1814, 2:62), but others considered them to be of only medium height. Hieromonk Gedeon (in Pierce 1978, 134) thus described them and noted that many of them were stooped, or round-shouldered. In the early nineteenth century G. I. Davydov (1977, 148) thought that only a few Koniag were tall, but found them in general well built and healthy, even in old age. Both he and Dr. Merck, however, then went on to catalogue the diseases from which they suffered (Davydov 1977, 177-79; Merck 1980, 107).

Very few early reports on the Chugach Eskimos have survived. Cook (1967, 3(1):351) called them "small of stature, but thick set good looking people," while Ellis (1782, 1:236) considered them to be "fat and jolly, as if they lived well." Nathaniel Portlock (1789, 248) thought they were for the most part short in stature and "square-made," whereas Gavriil Sarychev* described them as "of middle-size" (Sarytschew 1807, 2:22).

The first European contact with the Yupik Eskimos of southwestern Alaska came in 1778 during the voyage of Captain Cook. John Ledyard (1963, 85), while the ships were in the vicinity of Kuskokwim Bay, described the Eskimos he saw as "tall, well-made and wild fierce looking people." Nearly a half century later the Russian explorer Vasilii Khromchenko (1973, 53, 60, 63, 71) characterized the Yupik of Bristol Bay as medium in height, stately, and with a proud manly gait. The Nunivak men were well built but spare, while the women were said to be fat and to walk with a heavy step. Further north at Stuart Island, both the men and women were described as spare and having a "weak constitution." A couple of decades later Lt. Lavrentii Zagoskin (1967, 211, 106) noted that the people of the Yukon-Kuskokwim region were of medium height, with the men chubby, but not obese, and the women rather stout. Around Norton Sound the people were also of middle height and well-proportioned. On St. Lawrence Island Otto von Kotzebue (1821, 1:191) found the Eskimos to be

---

* Here and elsewhere in the book the reader will note that the spelling of Russian names in the text sometimes differs from that in the reference citation. The names in the text proper are spelled according to the accepted modern transliteration, while those cited as references correspond to the spellings found in the original books, usually early English translations.

of middle stature, but of "robust make and healthy appearance." Karl Hillsen, sailing with Gleb Shishmarev in 1820, on the other hand, considered them to be short (*in* D. Ray 1983, 31). Both Edward W. Nelson (1899, 27) and Sheldon Jackson (1886, 58) thought of the Kuskokwim Eskimos as the shortest ones whom they knew.

The first description of the northern Eskimos comes again from Ellis (1782, 1:330). In Norton Sound he found the men stout and well made, but in general below middle size, although three of four were nearly six feet tall. At Cape Denbigh the men were said to be "very plump and full of flesh" (Ellis 1782, 2:12-13). Some years later, at Cape Rodney, Lieutenant Sarychev of the Billings expedition found the people to be of middle stature (Sarytschew 1807, 2:45), while another on the same ship considered them to be often tall and healthy-appearing (Merck 1980, 190). The discoverer of Kotzebue Sound noted its inhabitants to be "of a middle size, robust make, and healthy appearance" (Kotzebue 1821, 1:209), while Frederick Beechey (1831, 1:360) found some Eskimos near Cape Thompson to be as tall as five feet, nine inches. William Hooper (1853, 223) considered these people to be strongly built, well formed, and even taller than the average European. Capt. C. L. Hooper (1881, 56) reported that many were over six feet; one he saw at Cape Krusenstern was "fully six feet and six inches in height." Unusually tall Eskimos were also known from Norton Sound (Dall 1870, 136) and the Noatak region (J. W. Kelly *in* Hrdlička 1930, 224; Seemann 1853, 50). Lt. John C. Cantwell (1889, 81) described the people of the upper Kobuk as "quick in their movements, active and strong in youth, but growing aged-looking rapidly." In Barrow Dr. John Simpson (1855, 920) actually measured a number of men and found their heights varied between five feet, one inch, and five feet, nine and a half inches, with their weights ranging from 125 to 195 pounds. In general, he considered them to be robust, muscular, and inclined to spareness rather than corpulence, an opinion shared by John Murdoch (1892, 33) a couple of decades later.

Among the first visitors to southeastern Alaska to comment on the Tlingit was Captain George Dixon (1789, 171), who in 1787 found them "about the middle size, their limbs straight and well shaped." After persuading a young woman to wash her face, he was surprised to find that it had "all the cheerful glow of an English milkmaid." The Spanish explorer Alejandro Malaspina (*in* Cutter 1972, 48) noted their height to be at least equal to that of the Spaniards and their build to be proportionate except for relatively underdeveloped thighs and legs. One of his officers described them as of medium height but robust and strong (Suría 1936, 254), an opinion shared by the Frenchman C. P. Claret Fleurieu, chronicler of Etienne Marchand's voyage (Fleurieu 1801, 1:217). A Russian visitor described them as "fairly tall, virile, and well-proportioned" (N. I. Korobitsyn *in* Andreyev 1952, 174), but the French explorer J. F. G. de La Pérouse (1799, 1:405), in contrast, thought the Tlingit of Lituya Bay were so feeble in body frame that the weakest of his sailors could wrestle the strongest Indian to the ground.

The evidence of the narratives is also conflicting with respect to the stature of the Athapaskans. Much of the information is rather late, although of course features such as height and body structure do not change much in a couple of generations unless there is a marked change in diet and culture. The first Russian explorer among the lower Yukon Indians called them tall in stature (A. Glazunov *in* VanStone 1959, 43), while Zagoskin (1967, 243) a few years later considered the same people to be of middle stature, adding that they had a spare build but were well proportioned. The first American citizen to explore the Yukon described the Indians of the Shageluk River who came to trade as a "fine, healthy, vigorous, energetic race" (Raymond 1870-71, 173). Nelson (1978, 37) found some to be six feet or over, although these stood out over their fellow "almost stunted" tribesmen. The Indians of the upper Kuskokwim and the coastal Indians around Cook Inlet were said to be rather short in stature, especially compared with those of the interior (Mendenhall 1899, 339; Learnard 1900, 666; Spurr 1899, 72). The Indians of the interior were described by C. E. Griffiths (1900, 726, 732) as hardy and healthy-appearing, and taller in stature than other Indians he had encountered. The chief of the Matanuskas, according to J. C. Castner (1900, 703), was six feet, two inches in height and weighed 220 pounds. Several others were said to be at least six feet, four inches tall.

LONGEVITY

Early narratives assert that not a few Natives survived to old age, despite the hazards of their existence. The Aleuts, in particular, were long-lived. According to church records kept by Father Veniaminov, some twenty percent of Aleuts lived past the age of sixty and a few survived to the age of ninety or more (Laughlin 1980, 10-13). A visitor to Unalaska in 1816 met and talked with an Aleut reputed to have been more than one hundred years old (Chamisso 1986, 44). The elderly were treated with respect and kept active as long as possible. The men continued to hunt in protected bays and shallows, while the women carried on such tasks as sewing and berry-picking, as their strength and skills permitted (Laughlin 1980, 15). The

Koniag, likewise, were said to live to an advanced age, sometimes a hundred years or more (Shelikhov 1981, 55). They grew so old, according to one observer, that they could hardly walk under the burden of years (Merck 1980, 107). Another remarked that the elderly often performed the same duties as the young, and that even in old age they did not seem feeble (Davydov 1977, 148).

Other Eskimos were not so fortunate. Aleš Hrdlička (1931, 132) found few skeletal remains of the elderly in his excavations of burial sites along the Kuskokwim. In the later nineteenth century a population study revealed that less that one percent of the population were sixty-five or older (U.S. Department of the Interior 1893, 175), although by this time the effects of introduced diseases can not be discounted. Nelson (1899, 29) attributed the lack of longevity of the Yupik to the constant wetting and exposure to which they were subjected. The hard struggle for existence also took its toll on the appearance of the people. One visitor to southwestern Alaska found it rare that a woman of twenty-five did not appear to be elderly (Zagoskin 1967, 108).

The Inupiat were also said to look older than their years. Beechey (1831, 2:303) thought that the women "lost their comeliness" early in life and that age was accompanied by a haggard and care-worn appearance. At Barrow an early visitor remarked that most of the people died by the age of forty and that by sixty the survivors were very decrepit (P. Ray 1885, 45), a view echoed by an explorer of eastern Kotzebue Sound (Stoney 1900, 85). Others noted that a few individuals reached a great age (Murdoch 1882, 39; J. Simpson 1855, 924; Cantwell 1887, 76). Older persons were treated with great respect and given loving care. They engaged in sedentary pursuits, such as carving and sewing, and rarely complained of their lot (Stoney 1900, 87; Spencer 1959, 252).

La Pérouse (1799, 1:405) thought that the Tlingit were not particularly long-lived and that they rarely reached the age of sixty. On the other hand, Dr. Eduard Blaschke (*in* Krause 1956, 163), who had much greater experience, felt that once a child escaped the hazards of infancy, he or she was usually strong and healthy and often lived to a ripe old age. The elderly were attended with great care and respect by members of the community (Khlebnikov 1976, 27).

The Athapaskans also seemed to show signs of age beyond their years, and few were said to live to a great age, at least in earlier times (Herron 1901, 69; Dall 1870, 196; Brady 1900, 59). Although consideration was shown for the superior wisdom of years (McKennan 1965, 54), by and large the elderly were felt to be a burden, especially among the nomadic bands, and some were even treated with overt disrespect (VanStone 1974, 82-83).

PERSONAL AND COMMUNITY HYGIENE

Native homes, according to the early narratives, were often crowded, dirty, and poorly ventilated, to the extent that some visitors were unable to remain inside for more than a few minutes. And most of these visitors were themselves used to the crowded, smelly accommodations on board ship and thus must have had a rather high tolerance for poor hygienic conditions.

Thomas Edgar (*in* Cook 1967, 3(2):1351-52) one of Cook's officers, spent a night in an Aleut sod house at Samganoodha Harbor, but got very little sleep because of flea bites. He confided to his diary that "their homes stink very much and even swarm with Maggots and the People themselves are very filthy and Dirty." Even the Orthodox missionary Father Ivan Veniaminov (1984, 180), who always tried to reflect sympathetically the conditions of traditional life, called the Aleuts slovenly. "All refuse," he wrote, "is thrown out at the entry of the yurta. . . . Household utensils are almost never washed. Even from places where they fetch water for food and drink there is frequently disgusting foulness. Children are almost always dirty, soiled, their hair tangled." In contrast, Sauer (1802, 155) found the Aleuts to be "very clean in their persons." Other early visitors report that the Aleuts often bathed in the sea or in hot volcanic springs (Merck 1980, 176), or regularly washed with urine (*in* Masterson and Brower 1948, 57).

The Koniag, according to an early nineteenth-century ethnographer, had a strong odor about them, due in part to the animal fat remaining in the skin clothing, in part to the whale blubber they ate, and to the fact that they rarely washed themselves (Davydov 1977, 150). Another wrote, "They will not go a step out of their way for the most necessary purposes of nature" (Lisiansky 1814, 214). Other accounts from this period confirm the unhygienic conditions of their houses and villages (Campbell 1819, 78; Lisiansky 1814, 215).

As for the Chugach, Dixon (1789, 68) remarked that the greatest beau among them was he "whose face is one entire piece of smut and grease, and his hair well daubed with the same composition," a description echoed by other visitors of the time (Portlock 1789, 249; C. L. 1789, 32). A much later writer noted that the constant exposure in their houses to dampness, dirt, and cold made them unusually susceptible to pulmonary disease (Abercrombie 1900b, 399).

About the Eskimos of northern and western Alaska, Dr. Merck (1980, 190) remarked as early as 1791 that the people around Cape Rodney "don't seem to be friends of washing." Likewise, early visitors to St. Lawrence Island and Nunivak Island were struck by their dirty clothing (Kotzebue 1821, 1:191), sooty skin (Khromchenko 1973, 63), and the strong odor of whale oil about them (Choris *in* VanStone 1960, 146). In Barrow Dr. John Simpson (1855, 921) observed that their faces were relatively clean but seemingly little effort was applied to the rest of the body, probably due to a shortage of water during most of the year.

The winter dwellings of the northern and western Alaskan Eskimos were noisome and likely to breed disease. They were smoky and poorly ventilated, to the extent that the air could be suffocatingly hot (Maguire 1857, 376; Beechey 1831, 1:367). The entrance to such dwellings was usually a semi-subterranean passage only high enough for crawling. It was the usual practice for members of the household to urinate and defecate in the hallway (Spencer 1959, 57). Lieutenant Zagoskin (1967, 114) wrote that it was necessary to crawl on all fours "through filth which is unimaginable to an enlightened mind and indescribable in words: there is dog dung, frozen human urine, ashes, bones, hair, etc., etc., etc." According to Captain Hooper of the Revenue Marine Steamer *Corwin* (1884, 103), "the Eskimos' appearance when they first emerge from their houses after a long winter of hibernating in the smoke filth and vermin is disgusting in the extreme, their skin being fairly covered with scales of dirt, their eyes sore, and their hair and clothes alive with vermin." A visitor at Ikogmiut, on the lower Yukon, found the village filthy, with refuse everywhere and six dead dogs prominently in evidence (Dall 1870, 227).

The situation was similar among Alaskan Indians. Early visitors to the Panhandle found the hair, skin, and clothing of the people to be covered with dirt and grease (not to mention paint applied for decoration) (Rollin *in* La Pérouse 1799, 2:364; Fleurieu 1801, 1:217). A missionary some years later (Green 1984, 35) described the Tlingit "with their long hair filled with fish-oil, . . . their faces daubed with dirt and paint and their blanket, which they wear unwashed till covered with filth and vermin." The houses were described in comparable terms in the eighteenth century. La Pérouse (1799, 1:400) wrote of the dreadful sanitation of their summer fish camps, and Tomás Suría (1936, 254), on Malaspina's expedition, likened their homes to pigsties. Captain Dixon (1789, 173), after describing their "wretched hovels," which were so poorly constructed that they did not keep out the snow or rain, wrote: "The inside of these dwellings exhibits a compleat picture of dirt and filth, . . . in one corner are thrown the bones, and remaining fragments of victuals left at their meals; in another are heaps of fish, pieces of stinking flesh, grease, oil, &c."

Nor did the Athapaskans spend much effort on cleanliness in earlier times. Frederick Whymper (1868, 153) likened the passageway to an Ingalik house to a sewer, with an overwhelming odor from fish, meat, and old skin clothes. Nelson (1978, 40) in his travels along the Innoko River found the women to be "excessively filthy." William Healy Dall (1870, 98, 194, 221), who traveled extensively in the interior, repeatedly remarked on the lack of personal hygiene of those he encountered.

It is apparent from these accounts that many early visitors were impressed and often dismayed by the vermin, dirt, and stench they found. Their descriptive comments, unfortunately, usually betray thinly veiled attitudes of superiority, condescension, or even contempt toward those whom many of them considered to be unenlightened savages.

That the standard of hygiene and sanitation was sometimes no better among the Europeans of the time, however, is demonstrated by Sir George Simpson's comment in 1842 (1847, 2: 190) about the capital of Russian America:

> Of all the dirty and wretched places that I have ever seen, Sitka is pre-eminently the most wretched and most dirty. The common houses are nothing but wooden hovels, huddled together without order or design, in nasty alleys, the hotbeds of such odours as are themselves sufficient, independently of any other cause, to breed all sorts of fevers.

Or consider the account of Capt. George Vancouver (1798, 3:140-41) when he visited a Russian trading post in Cook Inlet in 1794. Walking up the path, he noticed a terrible stench "occasioned, I believe, by a deposit made during the winter of an immense collection of all kinds of filth, offal, etc., that had now become a fluid mass of putrid matter."

And, those who might think that such problems were confined to isolated areas of the North American continent should read the recent account by Jack Larkin (1988, 50, 52), which vividly details the dirt, vermin, pungent smells, and appalling sanitation of early nineteenth-century America.

Filth, decaying food, human excreta, contaminated drinking water, close contact with animals, crowding, and poor ventilation can assist the spread of disease wherever they occur, whether in a Native village or in a European urban slum. Thus, there seems little doubt that the unhygienic conditions of traditional life in Alaska Native villages contributed to the prevalence of infectious and parasitic diseases among their inhabitants (*see* Chapter 3).

FAMINE AND MALNUTRITION

Probably the people of all Alaska Native cultures suffered from hunger and malnutrition at some time or other, but a few of them, notably the Aleuts, Athapaskans, and Inupiat, were particularly vulnerable to the vagaries of weather, seasons, and animal migrations.

Long before the arrival of the Russians the Aleuts were subject to periodic starvation, especially during times of warfare. Even in times of peace the nature of the food supply and the damp climate made it difficult to preserve foods for long periods. A missed or unsuccessful hunt or a long siege of stormy weather, therefore, could quickly bring hunger to a community. Food scarcity often came during the winter months; in fact, according to Veniaminov (1984, 257), the Aleut word for the month of March meant "when they gnaw straps." During these lean times the whole family would often go to the shore and collect seaweed, crabs, or mussels to sustain them (M. Lazarov *in* Coxe 1787, 87). Sometimes they were lucky enough to find the remains of a sea lion or even a whale that had been washed ashore (Vasiutinsky *in* Andreyev 1952, 31). But in times of hardship the Aleuts freely shared whatever food was available, with the most generous share going to the children. The adults bore hunger patiently and without complaint (Veniaminov 1984, 172; 1972, 51). Because of a similar climate and similar food resources, the Koniag also suffered periodic food shortages, which forced them to subsist largely on shellfish in the winter and spring (Lisiansky 1814, 173). From archeological evidence it is apparent that the Chugach Eskimos also knew periods of starvation (Lobdell 1980, 83).

Nor were the Eskimos of western and northern Alaska strangers to hunger, especially during the winter months. Those most susceptible to starvation were those who depended largely on one source of food, such as salmon for the people of the Yukon-Kuskokwim Delta, or caribou for the Nunamiut. When the salmon runs were small, or when the caribou migration was missed, Eskimo hunting and fishing technology, no matter how ingenious, was inadequate to assure a food supply sufficient for the lean months. Cantwell (1889, 54), for instance, described a village along the Kobuk River where many of the inhabitants had starved during the previous winter. Occasionally tribal warfare led to the loss of many hunters and a subsequent period of starvation, as happened near Point Hope around 1800 (Jackson 1893a, 1278).

When their regular food was in short supply, the Eskimos changed their eating habits to accommodate the situation. An example is the Nunamiut, who depended more on ptarmigan, rabbits, squirrels, and fish when they could not obtain caribou or other large game. When even these alternative resources were lacking, family groups might spread out over the country in a last desperate search for food (Gubser 1965, 93, 248; Spencer 1959, 138). Dr. Simpson (1855, 935) noted that in 1853 the hunters at Barrow took only seven small whales, causing the inhabitants to use flesh and blubber from a dead whale that had drifted ashore more than two years before. Even this resource was insufficient, however, and many died of starvation that winter. In 1891 the Revenue Cutter *Bear* found that the people of King Island had killed and eaten all their dogs and were subsisting solely on seaweed broth (Jackson 1895, 1709). The Eskimos along the great Alaskan rivers depended almost entirely on the summer salmon runs for their winter sustenance, and when these failed, hardship and even starvation ensued (Oswalt 1967, 143). There were reports of cannibalism in rare times of extreme famine (Weyer 1932, 114-18).

As a rule the Indians of southeastern Alaska had plentiful food supplies from the sea and thus infrequently faced hunger. Life among the Athapaskan Indians of the interior, on the other hand, was frequently balanced precariously on the edge of disaster. Game was often scarce and always unpredictable. As early as 1828 there is a report of a hundred deaths among the Ahtna due to the failure of the caribou herds (Wrangell 1970, 7). Around the same time Kyrill T. Khlebnikov (1976, 29) told of a tribe north of the Anikats (presumably Athapaskans) who had resorted to cannibalism in times of famine. The tribes of the lower Yukon also knew the pangs of hunger nearly every winter (Nelson 1978, 39, 44). Heavy losses from starvation occurred periodically, perhaps every ten to fifteen years. One Ingalik woman was said to have stayed alive by eating the lice from the dead bodies of her fellow villagers (Osgood 1958, 148).

MENTAL HEALTH

The mental health of the Alaska Natives in earlier times must for several reasons remain ill-defined. First, the earliest visitors to Alaska probably did not even see the mentally disturbed, if they indeed existed, since such individuals were unlikely to be conspicuous outside the villages. Second, the barriers of culture and language would have made it most difficult for a European to have discerned mental aberration when it occurred, since many aspects of Native behavior were already quite beyond their previous experience. Third, mental disorders as we know them today only began to be scientifically described by Freud and his circle toward the end of the nineteenth century. Fourth, by the time many early accounts were written, the Natives were already showing signs of reaction to the great cultural stresses they were undergoing in a rapidly changing world. The present discussion will be limited to two general areas, namely suicide and "insanity" in general.

Among the Aleuts suicide sometimes resulted when an old man felt he had become a burden to his people. Such an individual might drown himself or ask his friends to kill him (Merck 1980, 80, 176). Veniaminov (1984, 170) remarked that the Aleuts of Unalaska were formerly very prone to suicide but that he had never heard of a case in his sojourn there from 1824 to 1834. He speculated that some of the apparent suicides of earlier times might have been self-destruction when warriors were trapped in a hopeless position by the enemy. Yet elsewhere (1984, 368-69) he noted that the Atka Aleuts sometimes committed suicide under the influence of strong emotions, such as in sorrow over the death of a near relative, or when consistently unsuccessful in their endeavors. Despair was also a cause of suicide, as demonstrated by the fourteen Aleut girls who drowned themselves when taken to Kamchatka by Gavriil Pushkarev in 1762 (Berkh 1974, 26). Despair suggesting a true depression was observed by Dr. Merck (1980, 132) in 1790 in an Aleut taken on board a Russian vessel. This unfortunate individual tried to cut his throat when he heard some sailors threaten to throw him overboard. When Merck examined him, the man was withdrawn and "melancholic," lowering his eyes when being approached. After his neck wound was repaired, the man made a gradual but not complete recovery.

Suicide was said to be not rare among the Koniag, who sometimes took their own lives for what seemed to the Russians to be insignificant reasons. A Koniag could not bear the humiliation of imprisonment or physical punishment and not infrequently took his own life instead (Davydov 1977, 160-63; Tikhmenev 1979, 68). Sometimes wives killed themselves to avoid reproach after unfaithfulness to their husbands. Others took their own life as a result of grief for the loss of a loved one (Pierce 1978, 16-17, 128). When an individual decided to commit suicide, no one tried to talk him or her out of it or interfere in any way with the act itself (Davydov 1977, 150).

A few informants state that suicide was rare among the western and northern Eskimos (H. Weinland *in* Oswalt 1963, 99; Stoney 1900, 87). When it did occur, it seemed to be more often the result of a broken taboo than a depressive state. For example, a Barrow man hanged himself when he learned that he had married a woman who had been the wife of his brother. Another fell on his own seal spear when tension developed between himself and a cousin, both of whom were married to the same woman (Spencer 1959, 257, 106). Similar grounds for suicide are cited for the Nunamiut (Gubser 1965, 66, 221). An elderly or sick person who felt he could no longer contribute to the community welfare also sometimes took his own life or asked another to assist in performing the deed.

Suicide among the Tlingit was less the result of despair and depression than an act of calculated defiance. If an injured person saw no possibility of revenge or other satisfaction, he might kill himself, perhaps by drifting out to sea without a paddle, so that his antagonist would be publicly held responsible for his death (Krause 1956, 155). The other person must then either follow the suicide's example or pay the full indemnity to the family of the dead man (Beardslee 1882, 177). Sometimes the family exacted the death of the antagonist or that of a blood relative (Oberg 1966, 216).

The Athapaskans did not condone suicide, and a victim's body was given no regular funeral or burial. Most suicides were thought to be the result of insanity, except for the elderly people who died in order not to be a burden to the community. Women who committed suicide usually hanged themselves from a tree, while men strangled themselves with a snare, or drove a knife or arrow into their heart (Osgood 1936, 144; Osgood 1958, 148).

Only a few early narratives make reference to mental aberration or insanity. Dr. Merck (1980, 177) described a sick Aleut woman as pale and with a staring expression on her face. Frequently she would burst out into fits of laughter. This woman, whose symptoms and signs are suggestive of schizophrenia, was surrounded by objects that two old women had put into her hands, presumably to divert her. Other mentally ill individuals were not treated so kindly. Although sometimes they were left alone until they had become quite destructive (Edmonds 1966, 66), more often they were deliberately killed, if ordinary traditional methods of treatment were ineffective (Jackson 1893a, 1290-91; Jackson 1896a, 1459; Stoney 1900, 87). Other insane persons were simply abandoned, with a similarly fatal result (Weyer 1932, 138). In 1888 the Moravian missionary Edith Kilbuck told of an insane woman on the Kuskokwim who was deliberately allowed to freeze to death by her nephew, after he was unable to find another to take her life (E. Kilbuck *in* Fienup-Riordan n.d., 169).

Mental illness was sometimes attributed to possession by an evil spirit (Spurr 1899, 75; Birket-Smith 1953, 116). Veniaminov (1984, 217-18) wrote that insanity could result from breaking a taboo, such as speaking lightly about the stars or desecrating a holy place. Treatment of such cases might be attempted by the shaman, who would either try to drive out the evil spirit, or somehow make amends for the violated taboo. Father Iakov Netsvetov wrote of a man on the lower Yukon who had been insane due to a curse, and whom he subsequently converted to Orthodoxy. A shaman attributed the state of another woman said to be possessed to her having prayed (Netsvetov 1984, 31, 51-52).

A rather strange aberration of the northern Eskimos was the so-called "arctic hysteria," first mentioned around the beginning of the twentieth century in Greenlandic Eskimos. This condition has been described as a state of excitement in which an individual, often a woman, temporarily becomes quite aggressive and destructive, talking incoherently, and perhaps even running naked into the cold (Foulks 1972, 18). Clear descriptions of this syndrome are not available from early Alaskan sources except for a passing mention (Rosse 1883, 23). It is likely that most hysterical behavior observed by the Eskimos themselves was not considered an illness but rather a manifestation of shamanic propensities. Such people were both honored and feared (Spencer 1959, 301).

COMPLICATIONS OF CHILDBIRTH AND PREGNANCY

Although Alaska Native women as a rule enjoyed an uneventful pregnancy and easy childbirth, there were invariably times when an abnormality or complication developed. These each Alaskan culture learned to deal with in its own distinctive way.

The earliest sources seem to be in agreement that the Natives were not prolific. Among the factors that might have influenced fertility (which of course can involve either sex) were nutritional state, methods of natural or artificial contraception, abortion, and the presence of disease in one or both parents. Nutrition, as we have seen, was often marginal and there were periods of actual hunger and starvation, known from cultures around the world to be associated with a temporary fall in fertility rates. Although a few specific artificial contraceptive methods are reported for the Alaska Natives, their effectiveness must have been uncertain at best (Birket-Smith and De Laguna 1938, 160; Edmonds 1966, 31). Examples of Eskimo methods of contraception were the use of certain herbs (Edmonds 1966, 31; Lantis 1959, 34), coitus interruptus, or the use of magical methods, such as wearing the belt of a barren woman (Spencer 1959, 229-30). A natural method that was undoubtedly effective, however, was the practice of breast-feeding children for a long period, sometimes up to five years or more (e.g., Lantis 1959, 31-36; J. Simpson 1855, 927; Dall 1870, 196). Although a mother may certainly conceive during this period, her fertility is significantly reduced. Finally, serious disease in either parent, whether congenital, infectious, or degenerative, can impair fertility, although it would be difficult to measure its actual impact in a society, much less an individual.

One of the earliest references to the control of fertility is that of Merck (1980, 72), who reported that an Aleut woman desiring no further children would not bury the placenta, as otherwise prescribed, but throw it on the ground where animals or birds could devour it. The Aleuts also believed that if a postpartum mother's abdomen was not properly massaged, or "collected," she might not be able to bear children again (Veniaminov 1984, 189). In 1790 Sauer (1802, 176) remarked that among the Koniag the most favored of women were those who had borne the greatest number of children. Their neighbors the Chugach believed that a barren woman was "without seeds; her insides were dark." Every woman desired children, especially boys, and a mother with children was considered a lucky omen (Birket-Smith 1953, 83).

During his journeys for the 1880 census, Ivan Petroff (1882, 127) noted that the Yupik Eskimos of Nelson Island were "not fruitful," two children per family being the usual limit, although occasionally he saw as many as four. Zagoskin (1967, 108) described the Eskimos of Norton Sound as "not prolific," most families having only one or two children and none as many as four. At Barrow a decade later mothers were rarely giving birth before the age of twenty and thereafter only at four or more year intervals (J. Simpson 1855, 929). John Murdoch, in a careful study on the north coast (1892, 39) knew of only five pregnancies in two villages over a two-year period.

Although the weight of evidence of the early accounts was that the Natives were not prolific, there were also a few dissenting votes, although from a later period (e.g., Aldrich 1889, 158; V. Gambell 1898, 143). Observations on both sides of the question must be treated with skepticism, however, since they were usually based on brief impressions, and probably did not take into account the pregnancies ending the miscarriage and stillbirth, or the children who died in early infancy. It is also likely that fertility changed from time to time based on the local availability of food and the prevalence of disease.

Abortion was practiced in a few parts of Alaska, although it was apparently not common. Among the Aleuts it was usually an attempt to hide "the fruit of forbidden love," as Merck (1980, 178) delicately phrased it. If the abortion attempt was successful and was discovered, the members of the community, led by the shaman and the woman's male relatives, staged an elaborate ceremony to shame the woman and symbolize her death, in order to prevent poor luck in the hunt or other calamity. The Chugach apparently did not practice abortion as such, but if a miscarriage occurred in an unmarried woman, and she tried to hide the products of conception, the villagers would go to great lengths to find them in order to avert a storm. A married woman who miscarried simply buried or burned the fetus or other tissues (Birket-Smith 1953, 83-85). The Eyak Indians, like their neighbors the Chugach, believed that an abortion caused bad weather (Birket-Smith and De Laguna 1938, 160).

In the north abortion was sometimes attempted by having someone jump on the mother's abdomen, or knead or slap it violently ([Jarvis] 1899, 121). Other methods involved pushing down continually on the fundus of the uterus or pressing it against sharp rocks (Spencer 1959, 229). Unmarried Ingalik women tried to achieve abortion by engaging in strenuous exercise, such as repeated jumping (Osgood 1958, 171). The Inupiat also attributed some cases of spontaneous abortion, or miscarriage, to exercise, such as participation in the blanket toss ([Jarvis] 1899, 121).

Once pregnant the majority of women delivered their infants without difficulty (Nelson 1899, 289; R. White 1880, 36). A certain percentage, however, inevitably suffered complications such as hemorrhage before or after delivery, obstructed labor, or a complicating disease such as eclampsia, which causes convulsions around the time of birth. Any of these could lead to the death of the infant or even the death of the mother. Merck (1980, 72) reported that an Aleut mother who had had a difficult delivery usually sought to limit further pregnancies.

The Aleuts believed that problems attending childbirth were the result of the mother's unfaithfulness. Moreover, if the child did not resemble the father, much domestic strife might ensue, including divorce or cruel punishment of the mother (Veniaminov 1984, 189). Among the Chugach, on the other hand, complications of delivery were blamed on the husband, whose confession would lead to immediate relief of the suffering mother (Birket-Smith 1953, 84). The northern Eskimos usually attributed a long labor to malicious charms performed by another woman before conception (Spencer 1959, 229-30).

Several early clinical examples are known of complications of labor leading to the death of the mother. Dr. Samuel Call (*in* [Jarvis] 1899, 121) knew of a mother in Barrow who died of a hemorrhage from a retained placenta. Another case from the north involved a woman who died in late pregnancy and on whom the shaman ordered a postmortem caesarian section performed (Brower 1960, 57-58). In Sitka in the 1840s Dr. Alexander Frankenhaeuser (*in* Pierce 1974, 22) attended a pregnant woman (possibly not a Native) who died of a stroke the following day. Others died in remote areas without medical assistance (Netsvetov 1980, 130; Golovin 1979, 68; Knapp 1890, 24).

Although Native midwives were often helpless in the face of serious complications of labor and delivery, they employed various special methods to assist in the childbirth process. The most important of these involved manipulation of the fetus *in utero* to bring it into the proper position for delivery. The Aleuts were said to be particularly skillful in this regard (R. White 1880, 41; Laughlin 1980, 11), but such methods were also practiced by the Eskimos (Lucier et al. 1971, 253; Gubser 1965, 211), and the Athapaskans (Osgood 1971, 46). Magical methods, including preventive strategies, might also be employed to avoid or treat difficult labor. If a pregnant Yupik woman got up at night to urinate, she had to continue all the way to the end of the passage before turning back in order to ensure an easy delivery (Lantis 1959, 31). Likewise, in the north a pregnant woman could not walk backward out of a door for fear of having a breech delivery. During labor itself other women busied themselves with untying knots, to facilitate a quick birth (Spencer 1959, 230-33). A Chugach midwife would push a needle under the mother's tongue during labor to make the baby come quickly. In cases of malposition she would feel the baby's head through the abdominal wall and hit it behind the ear to make it turn to the proper position (Birket-Smith 1953, 84).

Although males were generally not welcome at the place of childbirth, a male shaman might be called in to assist in cases of difficult labor and delivery. The shaman did not "lay on hands," but instead, for example among the Yupik or Koyukon, performed certain dances or chants, or left an amulet with the mother (Lantis 1959, 32, 35; Jetté 1907, 169). In arctic Alaska the shaman would perform at the main dwelling house rather than at the birth hut, since close contact with a pregnant woman might cause him to lose his powers (Spencer 1959, 232).

The victim of a pregnancy mishap was most often the newborn, who was subjected to numerous life-threatening hazards in the first minutes, hours, and days of life. The infant might be born prematurely, be subject to hypoxia (shortage of oxygen), have developmental defects, or simply be delivered after a hard labor. The mother's milk was sometimes insufficient, or in the worst case, the mother might herself perish from complications.

Stillbirth must not have been rare since there were cultural practices to prevent it. For example, an Aleut hunter was not permitted to slay a sea mammal with a club, work with a hatchet, or eat the meat of a stranded whale without subjecting his wife to the danger of stillbirth (Merck 1980, 175). According to Davydov (1977, 164) the Koniag custom of pummeling a pregnant mother's abdomen to hasten delivery was a frequent cause of stillbirth.

Infants born alive but prematurely were at special risk. Dr. John Simpson (1855, 929) observed three cases of prematurity during a winter at Barrow, and P. H. Ray (1885, 46) had a similar experience a generation later. An early account of the Kutchin Indians asserted that the declining population was in part due to premature births (Osgood 1936, 150).

Even a normal infant had special dangers to face in the first few days of life. Dr. Call (*in* [Jarvis] 1899, 121) gave vivid examples drawn from his own experience at Barrow. One case was a twenty-eight-year-old unmarried woman with bilateral leg amputations who had to walk about on her knees. When her labor began she was forced out into a snowstorm where she built for herself a tiny shelter. Her baby was born there without outside assistance, and soon froze to death. A second case was that of a woman who went into labor as she and her family group were journeying to the coast from the interior. The expectant mother was left behind alone and delivered her baby on the trail. The placenta failed to be expelled and the mother died of a hemorrhage, following which the infant of course also perished. A third example involved a woman who went into labor unexpectedly while traveling alone. She successfully delivered the infant and placenta and continued on her way. The baby's frozen body was later discovered.

2

Disorders Relating to the Environment

INJURIES

Injuries were a major cause of pain, disability, and death in precontact times. The Natives of Alaska lived out their span in an environment that was fraught with hazards. Theirs was a harsh and unforgiving land intolerant of mistakes, for even minor ones could lead to bodily harm. Injuries are still today the leading cause of death among Alaska Natives.

Injury is defined here to include any bodily harm resulting from physical or chemical agents, asphyxiation, or the effects of heat or cold. An injury can be accidental, inflicted intentionally by another, or self-inflicted. To a larger degree than with most problems, the occurrence of injuries in Native cultures must be reconstructed from indirect evidence. Most injuries were trivial and neither required special treatment nor left permanent effects. More serious mishaps often led to a sudden or lingering death far from help or even far from someone to record the event in memory.

Accidental injuries were commonly associated with the activities of everyday life in the village, camp, on the water, or on the trail. The more serious injuries usually involved subsistence activities such as hunting and fishing. They resulted from sudden storms, aggressive animals, and other unexpected factors that caused a routine event to become dangerous, or even deadly. A momentary lapse of judgment, or simply bad luck, could prove fatal under such circumstances.

Probably the most common fatal accident, then as now, was drowning (e.g., Dixon 1789, 237; Tikhmenev 1979, 2:70; Gedeon *in* Pierce 1978, 143). All Native cultures used boats of some kind and depended at least to some extent on hunting or fishing on the water. The men of some cultures, such as the Aleuts, Koniag, and Tlingit, in fact spent much of their working lives at sea in search of sea mammals or fish. Although their boats were remarkably seaworthy for their size, and the men were skilled sailors, the dangers of Alaskan waters were always close at hand in the form of sudden squalls (Khlebnikov 1973, 57), hidden rocks, treacherous currents, and of course the quarry itself, which might range in size from a hundred-pound fish to a hundred-ton whale. Most Alaska Natives could not swim (Sarytschew 1807, 2:74), nor could they keep afloat very long in their cumbersome clothing. The icy water, in any event, soon overcame even the strongest of them. Sometimes a broken ice floe carried a Native to his death (Adams 1982, 113).

Other types of accidents from subsistence activities might include falls on slippery surfaces, falls from cliffs while gathering eggs (Davydov 1977, 195), falls from moving sleds, the collapse of thin ice, and accidental wounds from knives, lances, and arrows.

Many traumatic mishaps, most of them minor, occurred around the home or village. Falls from walking or running on slippery ice or snow were probably the most common, and led to contusions, sprains, and fractures, especially of the wrist and ankle. Food preparation was another ready source of accidents, for example cleaning fish, dressing out animal carcasses, or cooking over the fire. These led to cuts, scratches, puncture wounds, scalds, and burns, all of which could be complicated by infection. Sometimes the house itself might catch fire and lead to death by burning or by smoke inhalation. A low wood fire, especially in a poorly ventilated tent or sod house, probably led on occasion to carbon monoxide poisoning from incomplete combustion.

Rare but documented cases of injury included volcanic eruption (Davydov 1977, 206) earthquake (Netsvetov 1980, 145), and the collapse of a house due to shifting shore ice (Zimmerman and Aufderheide 1984). Occasionally men fell to their death through volcanic vents (Davydov 1977, 207).

Inflicted injuries, although they could lead to the same types of trauma as accidental ones, are discussed separately in order to stress certain cultural factors in their causation. Such injuries could be due to collective violence, violence against an individual, self-inflicted violence, and the violent attack of animals.

Collective violence often took the form of surprise attacks and brief skirmishes rather than pitched battles. It was prevalent between different ethnic groups, including the Aleuts and Koniag (Laughlin 1980, 54), the Tlingit and Chugach (Oswalt 1967, 18), and the Eskimos and Athapaskans (Weyer 1932, 154; Hall 1975). Clashes also often occurred within a single cultural group, such as the Aleuts (Masterson and Brower 1948, 59), Koniag

(Sauer 1802, 175), Tlingit (Dixon 1789, 237), and northern Eskimos (Burch 1974). The types of injuries sustained in such hostilities were principally knife, spear, and arrow wounds, and burns due to house fires (Weyer 1932, 155).

The most common type of violence perpetrated by individuals on other individuals probably resulted from the tensions that inevitably develop between members of a family or of a small community. Altercations of this type, often about women, were usually brief expressions of anger serving merely to vent hostile feelings, frustration, or to assert dominance, but on occasion they might lead to serious injury or murder (Oswalt 1967, 182; Osgood 1958, 149). This unfortunate outcome in turn nearly always spawned a blood feud between families, with the nearest blood relative of the victim being expected to exact blood in return (Merck 1980, 109; Litke 1987, 86-88; Wrangell 1970, 18; Stoney 1900, 88). Murders might take several forms, but a frequent method, at least among the Eskimos, was by clubbing the victim in his sleep (Weyer 1932, 221-22).

A further form of violence was the abuse of the weaker by the stronger. An example was rape (Holmberg 1985, 20; Spencer 1959, 79), which not infrequently became the basis of a blood feud. A further example was the mistreatment of slaves and other prisoners taken in war. Slavery in some form was practiced among several Alaskan groups, including the Tlingit (Litke 1987, 86), Koniag (Sauer 1802, 175), Chugach (Oswalt 1967, 206), and Aleuts (Merck 1980, 109). Slaves were generally members of a traditional enemy group and were sometimes beaten or otherwise physically abused (Kotzebue 1830, 2:54; Veniaminov 1984, 243; Lisiansky 1814, 238-39). Among the Tlingit it was sometimes the practice to kill a slave when his master died; others might be killed on ceremonial occasions (Litke 1987, 85). Similar practices are known for the Koniag (Shelikhov 1981, 54) and the Aleuts (Merck 1980, 80).

Punishment was another form of trauma intentionally inflicted on another person. Among the Aleuts the principal form of punishment was public ridicule or the payment of an indemnity; sometimes children had food temporarily withheld (Veniaminov 1984, 369). On Kodiak Island children were usually merely lectured for misdemeanors (Gedeon *in* Pierce 1978, 127) although another witness (Davydov 1977, 158) stated that the Koniag sometimes "punish their children till they bleed," apparently to teach them to endure pain. Adult Koniag had a great dread of physical punishment and not uncommonly committed suicide rather than endure the shame (Khlebnikov 1973, 115). In the North Eskimo children were never subjected to corporal punishment, and social deviance among adults was usually dealt with by discussion in the men's house or perhaps by studied ridicule (Oswalt 1967, 178, 182-83). Occasionally, however, a serious crime in parts of Alaska led to a sentence of death by the community (Veniaminov 1984, 242-43; Oswalt 1967, 187). Among the Tlingit a shaman might accuse an individual of sorcery and decree that that person, for example, be tied up on the beach to be drowned by the incoming tide (R. White 1880, 43; Beardslee 1882, 58).

Self-inflicted injury resulting in suicide has been mentioned in the previous chapter. Methods varied, including hanging (Jackson 1897b, 23), drowning (Berkh 1974, 26), jumping from a cliff (Davydov 1977, 160-62), stabbing in the heart with a knife or spear (Stoney 1900, 88), or more passive behavior such as allowing oneself to freeze to death, this last situation sometimes occurring when food was insufficient for the survival of the community (Merck 1980, 80).

Injuries inflicted by animals were often serious and not infrequently led to permanent disability or death. Dogs have been closely associated with some Alaska Native cultures for as long as two thousand years. In earlier times they were probably used for food or for their fur and only later as draught animals (Lantis 1980). Given the characteristics of humans and dogs, however, it is likely that some Alaskan dogs, at least, also served simply as companions. Northern breeds are usually moderately large, strong, tough, and with a recent strain of wolf intermixed. As a consequence they often fight for dominance and also may attack a human when excited, hungry, or sick. Probably the heavy clothing of the Natives, together with their healthy respect for what a dog can do, protected them from more frequent bites.

Injuries from wild animals were the inevitable consequence of the hunt. The North Slope Eskimos harpooned the great bowhead whale, which often reached a length of sixty feet, from a frail skin boat. A flick of the leviathan's tail flukes could destroy a boat and its entire crew (Davydov 1977, 224). Whaling was also practiced by the Koniag, Aleuts, and Chugach. The St. Lawrence Islanders and others hunted walrus, which not infrequently slashed holes in their skin boats with their tusks. Sea lions and northern fur seals were also large enough to destroy a boat under the right circumstances. Although the usual outcome for humans was drowning, such encounters could also lead to bites, fractures, and internal injuries. Dorothy Ray (1983, 27) mentions an Aleut chief whose hand was bitten off by a sea lion. At Unalaska Kotzebue (1821, 2:184) heard of a giant octopus, or squid, that had attacked a Native boat.

Among the land animals, large ungulates such as moose, caribou, or musk-oxen could kill by trampling, but a greater danger was from bears. The polar bear ranged over much of the Arctic and northern Bering coastal areas and was usually hunted with a harpoon. The great white carnivore sometimes gained the advantage and early examples of mauling are known (C. Hooper 1881, 17). The Alaska brown bear was also responsible for occasional deaths and crippling injuries (Jacobsen 1977, 106), although it was not regularly hunted. Hrdlička (1940, 2) mentioned a few Koniag skeletons that showed multiple fractures before death and speculated that they may have been caused by bears.

COLD INJURY

Alaska Natives have developed the means over several thousand years to permit them to live and even thrive in the extreme weather conditions of the Arctic and Subarctic. It is possible (although controversial) that some of the Native peoples, particularly the Eskimos, have also evolved biologically to enable them to adapt more successfully to the cold climate (e.g., F. Milan 1962). Wherever the truth of the matter lies, it is apparent that many features of Native life and culture, including housing, clothing, and footgear, were developed to help them withstand cold temperatures and thus avoid cold injury. Europeans have borrowed such cultural trappings freely from the Natives for nearly two hundred years, thereby enhancing their own ability to survive in northern latitudes. Several Native groups, notably the Aleuts, Koniag, and Tlingit, had the custom of deliberately exposing their children at an early age to icy water and cold temperatures. This seemingly cruel practice was meant to toughen the youngsters and help them to cope more successfully with the hardships and rigors of real life (Veniaminov 1984, 191; Davydov 1977, 164; Khlebnikov 1976, 27).

The earlier narratives seem to be in agreement that the Natives only rarely suffered from serious cold injury. One physician (Rosse 1883, 26) even denied that Eskimos were susceptible to frostbite at all. The Eskimos as well as other Native groups were indeed subject to cold injury, but it was unusual because of the care and respect they exhibited toward the weather and its hazards. They were also better prepared to face these hazards because of the fur clothing and waterproof footwear they had created over the course of time.

Frostbite, in which ice crystals actually form in the tissues, was of course most common in the arctic regions and in the interior, where the lowest temperatures occur. In the far north, moreover, the low temperatures are aggravated by the nearly constant wind sweeping across the unobstructed tundra, causing an added wind chill factor. Frostbite usually resulted when individuals were caught by a sudden storm with no adequate shelter, such as during a journey or while on the trapline. The fierce wind might have blown away a mitten, or lighting a fire to dry wet garments might not have been possible. Spots of frostbite on the tip of the nose, an ear, or a cheek were usually promptly recognized by a companion and treated with the direct touch of warm flesh (Adams 1982, 55). More severe forms were treated by placing the frozen hand or foot in another person's armpit or on the abdomen. A variant of this use of "animal" heat was the application of fresh raw liver, perhaps from a newly killed seal, on the frozen extremity (Zagoskin 1967, 110). Another technique was to rub snow on the frozen part (Osgood 1958, 229), presumably to stimulate the circulation, although this method of treatment is now known to be harmful.

If an area of frostbite was not promptly rewarmed, permanent harm could result. Murdoch (1892, 39-40) saw sores on the faces of Barrow Eskimos from neglected frostbite. Harrison Thornton, a teacher at Wales in the 1890s (1931, 36-37), reported that fully half the men and larger boys in the village at times had skin sloughing from their faces due to frostbite. A more serious sequel was dry gangrene of an extremity from irreversible circulatory injury. After several weeks the devitalized area became clearly demarcated from the intact flesh, at which time it could be cut away with a knife, a task usually performed by a member of the family or a shaman. Examples of such amputations are known from the North Slope Eskimos (Murdoch 1892, 40; [Jarvis] 1899, 121-22), Norton Sound ([Jarvis] 1899, 115), eastern Kotzebue Sound (Stoney 1900, 89), and elsewhere.

Of course many individuals must have died over the years from generalized hypothermia, or the gradual lowering of the "core" body temperature. Infanticide and senilicide deaths, when they occurred, were usually the result of hypothermia (Oswalt 1967, 194; Nelson 1899, 290; Aldrich 1889, 170; Gubser 1965, 122). By far the majority of such deaths, however, were unintentional, as when a person or a party was lost in a storm, or when an infant was born on the trail. Joseph Grinnell (1901, 39) tells of an infant that died from exposure in winter after her sick father had moved into a tent from his house, because of his fear of dying there. Examples of newborn deaths from hypothermia were mentioned in the previous chapter.

EYE INFLAMMATION

Many early narratives blamed the red and watery eyes of the Natives on their constant exposure to smoke in their small, poorly ventilated homes. Certainly the smoke from seal, whale, or eulachon oil lamps, or from driftwood cooking fires, was capable of causing a chronic irritative conjunctivitis. Among the earlier records from southeastern Alaska are those of Frédéric Litke (1987, 95), K. T. Khlebnikov (1976, 29), and P. N. Golovin (1979, 65), all of whom remarked on the red eyes of the Tlingit or the Aleut hunters in relation to smoke exposure. Of the many late nineteenth-century witnesses, a U.S. Army physician (J. Tonner *in* Colyer 1869, 1024) thought that the smoke probably caused both conjunctivitis and "corneitis," or what we would call keratitis today. In the northern region Kotzebue (1821, 1:253) noted the prevalence of eye disease among the Eskimos, attributing it to smoke or glare. Beechey (1831, 1:383) met a "blear-eyed old hag" near Icy Cape, and later Cantwell (1889, 83) blamed the weak and inflamed eyes of the Kobuk Eskimos on the poor ventilation of their winter homes. Dr. John Richardson attributed the excoriated and ulcerated eyelids found among the Eskimos of the North Slope to the smoky seal oil lamps in their dwellings, while Murdoch wrote of the "watery eyes" of old people (*in* Hrdlička 1930, 216, 223).

Several traditional remedies were known for watery, inflamed eyes, including the use of "Alaska cotton" (*Eriophorum* spp.), or willow catkins (*Salix* spp.) to absorb the discharge (Lantis 1959, 17, 22, 60; Ager and Ager 1980, 34).

Another frequent cause of red, watery eyes in the Alaska Natives was snowblindness, an exquisitely painful condition usually caused in the North by the reflection of ultraviolet light from snow or water. This disorder was particularly prevalent in the springtime, when the days were long but snow remained on the ground. The pain and inflammation came on about twelve hours after exposure, and although it could be temporarily disabling, it rarely caused permanent damage to the eye.

The problem is attested from every part of Alaska, but especially from the more northerly regions. The earliest record is from Davydov (1977, 200), who noted it in 1807 among the Kenai (Tanaina) Indians. Kotzebue (1821, 1:253) speculated that the frequent eye disease he saw near the Bering Strait was "occasioned by the long winter, as the snow dazzles their eyes in the open air." Many other accounts are available (e.g., Beechey 1831, 1:345; Murdoch 1892, 39-40; Dall 1870, 195; Scidmore 1885, 89). Dr. Call (*in*

[Jarvis] 1899, 123) considered snowblindness the most troublesome and frequent acute affliction of the long arctic day. At Barrow he saw the first cases around the first of May, and noted they occurred as often on moist, hazy days as they did on bright, clear days. The onset was sudden and intensely painful. According to a miner who suffered from it (Fraser 1923, 77): "You don't know while you are in the sun that anything is the matter, but when darkness comes, your eyes feel exactly as if they were filled with sand. You cannot open them and you suffer terrible agony. You are stone blind for a while."

Some inkling of the prevalence of snowblindness in precontact times can be gained from the many traditional methods to prevent or treat it. The simplest method of prevention was to rub charcoal onto the upper face, much as some football players do today. Such a technique was used by the Athapaskans (McKennan 1959, 109), Tlingit (Krause 1956, 104), Pacific Eskimos (Birket-Smith 1953, 71), and northern Eskimos (Beechey 1831, 1:345). Moreover, it is likely that the long-visored wooden headgear of the Aleuts or the broad-brimmed hats of the Koniag hunters were designed to reduce the glare (Laughlin 1963, 640). A very successful method to prevent the problem was the ingenious snowgoggles developed by the Eskimos in early times (Giddings 1967, 90). This example of simple yet effective technology consisted of a piece of wood, antler, or ivory (Giddings 1964, 44; 1967, 140), made to fit comfortably over the upper face, and provided with narrow slits, or sometimes round or oval openings, for the eyes (Geist and Rainey 1936, 162). Snowgoggles were in use all over the coastal regions north of Bristol Bay (Nelson 1899, 169-170), but apparently not among the Chugach of Prince William Sound (Birket-Smith 1953, 71). William Healy Dall (1870, 195) found them among the Ingalik, who probably borrowed the idea from their Eskimo neighbors on the lower Yukon.

Traditional medical treatment of snowblindness took several forms. Some Athapaskan groups applied animal grease on the eyes, topped by a layer of spruce gum, or held the head over a pot of cooking fish eggs (Osgood 1936, 93; Osgood 1958, 230). The Yupik used cranberry juice, urine, or human milk to soothe the painful eyes (Lantis 1959, 21). Surgical methods were also much in vogue, for example some Athapaskans incised a small blood vessel on the inner side of the upper lids (Osgood 1936, 93; Giddings 1961, 18), or at the outer corner of the eyes (McKennan 1959, 108). Along the lower Kuskokwim the operator might pierce the skin over the bridge of the nose and thence into the underside of the lid near the nose. A second method involved scratching the upper lid along the row of eyelashes (Lantis 1959, 21).

An interesting account of yet another surgical method comes from a miner (who was himself a doctor) treated by an Indian woman around the turn of the century (Grinnell 1901, 71):

> Indian Charley's wife called and looked at the patient's eye, swollen and inflamed and painful to a degree. She pointed to some toothpicks . . . and, being told to "proceed," she whittled three of them to a sharp point. Handing one to the suffering doctor, she bade him thrust it into his nostril. He did so and found to his astonishment that the mucous membrane was without sensation. . . . He continued to thrust in the point of the prick and likewise the two others, when a hemorrhage of considerable severity occurred. . . . In an hour the nose was inflamed and very painful, but the eyes were relieved.

TOXIC SUBSTANCES

The Natives of Alaska were exposed to several types of poisonous substances in their natural environment. Although general experience and cultural taboos protected them from frequent encounters with these hazards, illness and death could result from accidental (or sometimes intentional) exposure.

Paralytic shellfish poisoning, or PSP, is caused by the ingestion of a powerful toxin that is produced by several species of plankton called dinoflagellates. These plankton sometimes "bloom" and are ingested by certain bivalve mollusks, such as mussels and razor clams. When the latter in turn are eaten by humans, a severe illness may result. The disease is characterized by numbness and tingling around the mouth, vomiting, diarrhea, and double vision, followed in severe cases by respiratory paralysis that may lead to death. This problem was first identified in the north Pacific nearly two hundred years ago and still claims periodic victims (Fortuine 1975b).

What was undoubtedly an episode of severe PSP occurred in southeastern Alaska in July 1799, although early accounts differ on the date. Aleksandr Baranov himself, the chief manager of the newly formed Russian-American Company, has left a description of this tragic event, even though he was not personally a witness. A large party of Aleut hunters under his command had left the new fort on Sitka Island and were on their way back to Kodiak in their skin boats, when they stopped for the night at a place called Khutznov

Strait, later called Peril Strait to commemorate the event. Although well supplied with provisions, the Natives could not resist eating some of the small, black mussels that were abundant in the area. Two minutes later about half the party experienced nausea and felt a dryness in the throat. By the end of two hours, says the account, about a hundred hunters had died. Some were saved, according to Baranov, by taking a mixture of gunpowder, tobacco, and spirits to induce vomiting. So far so good, but the chief manager goes on to describe how the illness then became infectious and others died without having eaten the mussels at all (Baranov *in* Tikhmenev 1979, 110-11; Khlebnikov 1973, 26-27).

The unique account of a Native witness—a Koniag named Arsenti—was preserved by Heinrich Johan Holmberg many years later (1985, 43):

> When we found ourselves in Pogibshii proliv (Peril Strait), we turned to eating mussels (Mytilis) because of a shortage of fresh fish. They must have been poisonous at this time of year for a few hours later more than half of our men died. Even I was near death, but remembering my father's advice, to eat smelt (korushki) at such times, I vomited and recovered my health.

Arsenti's version is interesting because it shows that he knew mussels were poisonous in certain seasons of the year, and also knew of a traditional remedy, both of which point to previous experience with the disease.

The account of the same episode by Davydov (1977, 177) a few years later sheds some further light. According to him the Koniag were well acquainted with shellfish poisoning and knew that the mollusks could be harmless at some times and poisonous at others. In describing the events at Peril Strait (which he incorrectly dates in 1797), he recalled that the party camped at the mouth of a stream where there were many shellfish on both banks. Only those from the bank where there was no seaweed covering them caused illness. Within a half hour of eating the mussels a Chugach Eskimo had died, followed shortly by the death of five Koniag. According to Davydov, some eighty persons died that day. All who immediately ate sulfur, rotting fish, tobacco, or gunpowder survived, although some still had tingling sensations in the skin several years later. Davydov heard that pepper boiled in water was also an effective remedy, although no one seems to have tried it at the time. He also asserted that those who were affected felt some relief with the ebb tide.

The disaster at Peril Strait was an unforgettable one but certainly not unique. Veniaminov (1984, 364) mentioned that the Aleuts knew that clams and mussels were sometimes poisonous from May to September, while Holmberg (1985, 42-43) indicated that shellfish poisoning was well known in Kodiak in earlier times.

Botulism is a severe intoxication characterized clinically by drooping eyelids, blurred vision, difficulty swallowing, and, in severe cases, respiratory paralysis leading to death. The offending toxin is produced by a species of bacteria known as *Clostridium botulinum*. Human disease is usually due to the ingestion of improperly preserved foods. Several types of toxin are known, of which type E, associated with fish and sea mammals in northern regions, is the most common in Alaska, although types A and B have also been described. Studies on the environmental source of type E botulinum toxin in Alaska have demonstrated the presence of the organism in the majority of soil samples taken from several northern Alaskan coastal sites. It is significant that Eskimos were butchering marine mammal carcasses on these same beaches (Miller et al. 1972). At least in modern times it appears that contamination of seal, walrus, or whale meat sets the stage for the production of the toxin, which occurs when the food is stored in an airtight container (Eisenberg and Bender 1976).

Although no unequivocal accounts of botulism are known from earlier times, there are a couple of records of people dying after eating partially putrified meat from sea mammal carcasses washed up by the sea. For example, Davydov (1977, 176) knew of several Koniag who died after eating the flesh of a beached whale. Holmberg (1985, 42) states that the Koniag knew a beached whale was unfit for consumption if the gulls avoided the carcass. In 1875 in the village of Kustaten, a beluga whale that had washed up on the beach caused the death of fifty-seven persons who had eaten from it (Aronson 1940). In another episode three families perished in 1901 in the Golovin-Koyuk area as a result of eating flippers from dead seals cast up by the sea (D. Ray 1975, 119-20). Although these reports are suggestive of botulism, they may also represent a more conventional kind of food poisoning, such as that caused by salmonella bacteria (Bender et al. 1972). P. N. Golovin (1979, 65) reported that although the Aleuts often ate tainted meat from whale carcasses, they seemed to suffer only from carbuncles as a result.

Although Dr. Merck (1980, 109) stated categorically that poisons or poisonous plants were unknown to the Koniag in 1790, Davydov (1977, 176) described a species of sweet grass that not infrequently led to the death of whole families who ate it. He speculated that there must be one toxic species among several similar grasses, since many persons seemed to be able to eat them without coming to harm. They did, however, take care not to let the grass touch their lips because the acridity of the juice caused soreness.

Several other poisonous plants are known to occur in Alaska but they are uncommon. The most toxic among them is the water hemlock, *Cicuta mackenziana,* which has been known to cause death in modern times, especially in children (Lantis 1959, 16). Although no deaths have been ascribed to them, two other common plants are moderately toxic, namely the false hellebore (*Veratrum* spp.), which was also used medicinally (e.g., De Laguna 1972, 659), and the death camus *(Zygadenus elegans)* (Heller 1981, 77-85). Other mildly toxic plants are noted by Christine Heller (1963). Certain poisonous mushrooms also occur in Alaska (Kempton and Wells 1968; Wells and Kempton 1961).

Poisoned weapons were not widely used in Alaska, perhaps in part because of the scarcity of known poisonous substances. The Alaska Natives were primarily hunters of large animals and it is understandable that they would seek to enhance the effectiveness of their puny weapons by poison. Whether such weapons were used in warfare is not clear. An early record from the Diomede Islands indicates that the Natives of this region fought with quartz-tipped arrows treated with a toxic vegetable substance. A wound from such an arrow had to be sucked clean immediately or else the victim would die within 24 hours. The eighteenth-century doctor who edited this account speculated that the poison in question was derived from the wolf plant, or *Napellus,* now known as *Aconitum* (P. Pallas *in* Masterson and Brower 1948, 67).

Sauer (1802, 178) noted that the Koniag used aconite, from plants of the genus *Aconitum,* or monkshood, to poison their arrows. "Selecting the roots of such plants as grow alone," he wrote, "these roots are dried and pounded, or grated; water is then poured upon them and they are kept in a warm place till fermented." Such poisoned weapons were used primarily for hunting whales by the Koniag and Chugach (Oswalt 1979, 240; 1967, 130), and perhaps other groups as well (Giddings 1967, 242). Veniaminov (1984, 209-10) wrote that the poisons used by the Aleuts were known only to a few and does not identify them further. A later account indicates that harpoon poisons were made from a mixture of decayed human fat and the crushed bodies of small poisonous worms found in freshwater lakes. Aconite itself may have been added to the mixture, although some studies have shown that it has little or no toxic effect, and may be eaten freely without apparent harm (Bank 1953, 428-29).

BITING INSECTS

No one who has passed a summer in Alaska has failed to notice—sometimes in unprintable language—the myriads of biting insects that swarm around any warm-blooded creature, including humans. These plagues have evoked much comment, and even eloquence, from everyone who has suffered their bites, but it is only the visitors, unfortunately perhaps, whose reactions in the earlier period were recorded for posterity.

Mosquitoes, although present throughout Alaska, were a particular curse in the coastal areas. Petroff (1882, 14), known to exaggerate in some things, was almost at a loss for words in trying to describe mosquitoes: "They hold their carnival of human torment from the first growing of spring vegetation in May until it is withered by frost late in September. . . Language is simply unable to portray the misery and annoyance accompanying their presence." Johan Jacobsen (1977, 91), who traveled to the lower Yukon region around the same time, was moved to write: "One can overcome dangers, and against ambushes one can protect oneself with vigilance, . . . one can overcome all kinds of situations, but against the relentless pursuit during waking and sleeping carried on by mosquitoes, which are constantly replaced by millions of new ones, there is no defense. . . . No philosophy protects against mosquitoes!" On Chamisso Island Dr. Irving Rosse (1883, 24) was prevented by a cloud of fierce mosquitoes from recovering an important message relating to the Franklin search.

Some in their frustration resorted to humor. Dall wrote from the Yukon River that the mosquitoes were like smoke in the air and were distinguished from civilized species by the reckless daring of their attacks (*in* Sherwood 1965b, 29). Dr. Frederick Schwatka (1885, 263), describing how they managed to squeeze through the mesh of their netting, had this to say: "The doctor [Doctor Wilson, surgeon on the expedition], in a fit of exasperation, said that he believed that two of them would hold the legs and wings of another flat against its body while a third shoved it through; but I doubt the existence of cooperation among them. I think they are too mean to help one another."

Beyond the annoyance factor, the bites of mosquitoes could have medical implications. Continuous scratching of bites usually led to skin infections such as impetigo, which could then be spread to other parts of the body or to other persons. Dr. Irving Rosse (1883, 24) mentioned a crew member of the *Corwin* who was so swollen around the face from mosquito bites that he could not see. Another observer (Jacobsen 1977, 91) likened the multiple mosquito bites on the face of a man to the skin of a man recovering from smallpox. Petroff (1882, 14) commented that a man exposed to repeated mosquito bites "loses his natural appearance; his eyelids swell up and close, and his face becomes one mass of lumps and fiery pimples." In modern times it has been demonstrated that the California encephalitis virus can be carried by Alaskan mosquitoes (Feltz et al. 1972).

The ubiquitous mosquito was often accompanied by several other varieties of biting insects, especially in the more wooded areas. These included black flies, chiggers, "no-see-ums" and others, most of which breed in moving water, unlike mosquitoes, which prefer stagnant ponds. Witnesses to their ravages are many, among which a couple of examples may be cited. Capt. Yurii Lisianskii mentioned that his party near Sitka was plagued with gnats and "a small species of flies, with which the woods swarmed. . . . They alight imperceptibly, and occasion a swelling where they bite." A smaller type of fly always seemed to attack below the eyes (Lisiansky 1814, 231). From the Kenai Peninsula a sufferer (probably Ivan Petroff, *in* Sherwood 1974, 88) wrote: "As we approached the big lake . . . the evil [of mosquitoes] was even increased tenfold by the enrollment under the mosquito banner of myriads of small black flies, which left a mark after every bite, red as blood and of the size of a pea." Petroff (1882, 14) also remarked on the unholy alliance of mosquitoes with a small black fly "under the stress of whose persecution the strongest man with the firmest will must either feel depressed or succumb to low fever." Cantwell (1889, 64) was plagued on the Kobuk River with a kind of sand fly "which attacked us with a persistence and violence utterly beyond description."

That the Natives also suffered from these insects is reflected by their methods of protecting themselves from them. The Eskimos often covered their bodies with seal oil to discourage biting (Petroff, 1882, 14). Both Eskimos and Indians used smudge fires to keep the insects at bay (Zagoskin 1967, 162; McKennan 1959, 109), or placed a dish of wet moss and hot coals in the bow of their boat (Dall 1870, 92). One old Indian shaman was observed to be engaged in the endless task of catching and eating the mosquitoes in his vicinity (Castner 1900, 705). When all preventatives failed, back scratchers offered considerable relief (Nelson 1899, 310).

3

Infections

That the Alaska Native peoples before contact were plagued with diseases caused by microorganisms is apparent not only from paleopathological studies, but also from many references to infectious disease in early narratives of the contact period. There is, of course, no inherent reason why the inhabitants of Alaska would not have had their own share of endemic diseases of this kind, just as all other isolated human populations have had. Perhaps the impression has been left not only by historians but by many Native people themselves that all infection was introduced by Europeans on a "virgin" population. Such a belief seems indeed plausible, in light of the terrible devastation seen in later times by the introduction of new diseases such as smallpox, measles, influenza, and syphilis in a population with no previous exposure and hence no immunity.

In this chapter evidence will be presented for the existence of diseases caused by viruses, bacteria, and parasites in Alaska Natives before or at the time of contact. Although individual sources might be reasonably challenged, in the aggregate they demonstrate that such diseases were not only prevalent but often the cause of serious illness and death.

ANIMAL-ASSOCIATED DISEASES

The Native peoples of Alaska had frequent and close contact with many forms of wildlife, including mammals, birds, and fish, and of course insects. Animals and their products were used for food, clothing, transportation, trade, and simply companionship. Animals were shot with arrows, harpooned, caught with traps, and snagged with hooks. Their carcasses were skinned, cleaned, gutted, dressed, and usually eaten, sometimes raw or frozen, and sometimes after preservation and storage for long periods. Some animals, such as dogs, were handled frequently while alive. Natives also inevitably came in frequent contact with the waste products of animals, either by handling their bodies or simply from contact with the contaminated natural environment.

Although evidence for zoonotic (or animal-borne) diseases in Alaska in early times is scarce, proof for a few diseases comes from paleopathology. Adding to this is the extensive evidence for zoonotic illness in Natives compiled in the twentieth century. The organisms causing these diseases usually display a complex life cycle that includes humans, one or more animals, and possibly even an arthropod vector. When these diseases have been found in Alaska in modern times they have been nearly exclusively in Natives or in Caucasians living in the "Native way." There is no reasonable basis for supposing that such diseases were introduced into the wildlife reservoir by Europeans, who rarely suffered from them in the first place. We shall never know the true situation, however, since few if any of these diseases were recognized as entities by medical science more than a century ago, and even if they had been recognized, their relationship to animals was usually unclear.

Taken as a whole, animal-associated diseases were probably never of great importance to the health of the Alaska Natives. Human cases were usually sporadic and only infrequently the cause of death or disability. With a few exceptions the diseases were not transmissible from person to person and hence did not spread in a community or household. Traditional methods of cooking or preserving food probably provided further safeguards against acquiring such diseases.

Human cases of trichinosis have been known in the Arctic since the 1940s (Thorborg et al. 1948). The parasite has been shown to be widely disseminated in nearly every carnivorous animal in Alaska, including some sea mammals, such as walrus (Rausch et al. 1956). In modern times proven cases in Eskimos have been associated with the ingestion of undercooked bear meat or walrus meat (Maynard and Pauls 1962; Margolis et al. 1979). Not long ago evidence of the disease in earlier times was provided by the probable identification of larvae of the causative worm, *Trichinella spiralis*, in the diaphragmatic muscles of the remains of a woman frozen in the ice near Barrow. This individual, definitely from the precontact period, had died of accidental causes (Zimmerman and Aufderheide 1984).

Certain larval roundworms (or nematodes), of the family *Anisakidae*, have been known to cause disease in Alaskan Eskimos in modern times (Lichtenfels and Brancato 1976). These worms normally parasitize sea mammals, fish, and birds, but may be acquired by humans by the ingestion of the larvae found in the flesh of certain saltwater fish, including salmon. The larvae burrow into the lining of the intestinal wall and may in rare instances cause serious illness. This problem may have been what Dr.

Friedrich Eschscholtz was describing during the visit of the Kotzebue expedition at Unalaska in 1816. Noting that the cod caught there abounded in worms, he speculated that the Aleuts escaped infection by cutting the fish in very thin slices. Eschscholtz and another distinguished ship's surgeon of the time, Dr. Karl Espenberg, felt that such worms could lead to human disease (Eschscholtz 1821, 2:334-35; *see also* Sarytschew 1807, 2:72).

More complex parasitic worms called trematodes are also definitely known from early autopsy evidence in Alaska. The eggs of *Cryptocotyle lingua,* normally a parasite of dogs, were recently identified in the frozen remains of an Eskimo woman from St. Lawrence Island (Zimmerman and Smith 1975). Eggs of similar species have been found in the stools of living Eskimos (Hitchcock 1951).

Two species of the *Echinococcus* tapeworm are found in Alaska. Both *E. granulosus* and *E. multilocularis* use several mammals other than humans as their intermediate hosts. Humans break into the cycle by the ingestion of the eggs, usually brought to the immediate environment by the domestic dog, which in turn becomes infected by eating the natural intermediate host harboring the larvae (Lantis 1980). The human, as with many other northern zoonoses, is a "dead-end" host who does not contribute directly to disease transmission.

Echinococcus granulosus is a natural parasite of wolves in Alaska. The adult worm passes hardy eggs that are ultimately ingested by large ungulates, such as moose or caribou, which develop in their viscera cysts containing infective larvae. These in turn are eaten after a kill by wolves and the larvae once more develop into mature worms. The human intrudes into the natural cycle by feeding the raw liver and lungs of moose and caribou to dogs, then ingesting the eggs resulting from inadvertent contamination of hands and household articles with dog feces. In humans the eggs hatch and slowly grow as larvae in the liver or lungs, rarely causing serious disease unless the cysts become large enough to press on a vital structure. Such infections were formerly common among Eskimos and Athapaskan Indians in Alaska. Dall (1870, 195) was probably describing this condition when he wrote of the Athapaskans of the lower Yukon: "Curiously enough, a taenia, developed from hydroids found in the reindeer, is occasionally found among these Indians." The "reindeer" he speaks of were of course caribou, since reindeer were not introduced into Alaska for several more decades.

A second *Echinococcus* species also causes human disease in Alaska, although in the fairly limited geographical area of St. Lawrence Island and the northwestern coastal area of the mainland. In its adult form, *E.*

multilocularis lives in the intestine of foxes. The worm produces eggs which contaminate tundra plants, water, and inanimate objects. Small tundra rodents, such as voles, shrews, and mice, ingest eggs and develop multiple tiny larval cysts in their viscera. These small mammals are a major food item for foxes and, significantly, dogs. Once again humans become accidental intermediate hosts when they ingest the eggs, which develop into cysts in the liver, lungs, brain, and other vital organs. Here, however, the human disease is far more serious, since the masses of tiny cysts invade surrounding tissues like a cancer, not infrequently leading to death (Wilson and Rausch 1980).

A third tapeworm of interest in Alaska is the fish tapeworm of the genus *Diphyllobothrium. Diphyllobothrium latum* and several closely related forms cause human infection in many parts of Alaska, having first been identified in Eskimos in Bethel in 1950 (Hitchcock 1950). Although *D. latum* itself may be exclusively a human parasite in its adult form, other species have been found to infect gulls, dogs, seals, bears, and foxes, in addition to humans. The worm is acquired by the ingestion of the larval forms found in trout, whitefish, blackfish and even spawning red salmon (Rausch and Hilliard 1970). In the 1860s a Koyukon woman unexpectedly passed a large tapeworm following a dose of castor oil administered for a stomach-ache (Adams 1982, 70-71). Further evidence for its endemic nature is its occurrence in many species of animals, its wide geographical distribution in the Arctic, and the infrequency with which Caucasians have been infected.

A few bacterial diseases associated with animals are known from modern times in Alaska, including brucellosis, tularemia, and salmonellosis. None of these could be accurately diagnosed in earlier times, of course, even if they did exist. Again, the association of these bacteria with wildlife suggests that human disease may have occurred in the past.

Brucellosis is a chronic disease in humans, causing fever, weakness, and general debility. It was first reported in an Alaska Native in 1959 (Edwards 1959) and since then several further cases have been published, all from the northern part of the state. The animal reservoir is probably caribou, although some evidence indicates infection in moose and Dall sheep as well. Robert L. Rausch (1972) believes that this was not an endemic disease of Alaskan animals, however, but was instead introduced from Siberia with the domestic reindeer in the 1890s.

Tularemia is another chronic bacterial disease in humans, manifested by fever, swollen lymph glands, and frequently skin lesions. The first cases clinically diagnosed in Alaska Natives did not occur until 1988 (State of

Alaska 1988), although a case was reported in a non-Native as early as 1945 (Williams 1946). In 1960 a serological survey, mostly in Eskimos, showed that five percent had an elevated antibody titer, with the largest concentration of individuals in the lower Yukon area. The investigators felt the animal reservoir was probably muskrats, which were extensively trapped in that region (Philip et al. 1962). A laboratory worker later developed tularemia while working with indigenous Alaskan strains of *Francisella tularensis* from Bethel and Tok (Miller 1974).

In 1969 over one hundred persons in the Eskimo village of Tununak became violently ill after eating uncooked muktuk from the flippers and tail of a beached whale. An intestinal bacterium, *Salmonella enteritidis,* was identified as the causative agent, either from the carcass itself or from external contamination from bird droppings (Bender et al. 1972). In an earlier study from the state laboratories three species of *Salmonella* were isolated from both humans and gulls, and one species, *S. typhimurium,* from humans, gulls, and dogs (Williams and Dodson 1960). These findings suggest that *Salmonella* species are widely distributed in nature in Alaska and could thus easily have been the causative agent of outbreaks of food poisoning in earlier times.

Of viral diseases associated with animals in the Arctic, rabies is by all odds the most important. Again, no early data are available, but the disease has been known to be endemic in arctic foxes and wolves for a long time. The only reasonably well-documented human case occurred in 1942 as a result of severe and multiple bites by a wolf (Pauls 1957). One reason the disease seems rare in humans may be that the heavy fur clothing, boots, and mittens that are worn protect reasonably well from deep bites.

Finally, in recent times the California encephalitis virus, which causes an inflammation of the brain in humans, has been isolated from snowshoe hares in the Tok area near the Canadian border. Though no human cases have been recognized, up to seventy-two percent of residents of certain Athapaskan villages have a detectable antibody titer (Feltz et al. 1972) against the virus, indicating previous exposure and infection.

INFECTIONS OF THE SKIN

Skin infections were mentioned repeatedly in the earliest narratives, suggesting their prevalence. To a certain extent, however, the excellent documentation of these infections may also be explained by their being evident to the casual observer, even in the normally clothed individual.

Zimmerman and his colleagues (1981) found both adult lice and their eggs on the scalp of an Aleut mummy dating from the early eighteenth century. In addition, early narratives from many parts of Alaska described in lurid detail the heavy infestations of head and body lice that the Natives patiently bore. The parasites for their part enjoyed almost perfect living conditions, what with the crowded living and sleeping conditions, the heavy fur clothing the people wore, and the shortage of water for personal hygiene at certain seasons. Two early Russian visitors, Petr Krenitsyn and Mikhail Levashev, described the Aleuts in 1768-1769 as being covered with lice (*in* Coxe 1787, 213). A decade or so later several diarists of the third Cook expedition confirmed the prevalence of the parasites, one attributing infestation to their "wearing Birds and Sealskins, an excellent Harbour for Vermin" (Edgar *in* Cook 1967, 3(2): 1351).

Writing of the Tlingit Indians in southeastern Alaska, Captain Portlock (1789, 286) described in 1787 their practical approach to the problem:

> These poor wretches, by living in so filthy a manner, were entirely covered with vermin; but this they seemed to consider as no kind of inconvenience; for at any time when the lice grew troublesome they picked and ate them with the greatest relish and composure, sometimes indeed, when they were greatly pestered, . . . they would turn their jackets, and wear them inside outwards, by way of giving them a few hours' respite.

Another eighteenth-century observer in southeastern Alaska affirmed that the furs the Tlingit sold were so infested with lice that to take on a cargo of furs was to take on a cargo of lice (Fleurieu 1801, 1:221).

The first Moravian missionaries on the Kuskokwim River found the Eskimos there to be heavily infested not only with body lice but with head lice, one boy having nits so thick he looked as if he had come in out of the snow (Oswalt 1963, 19, 27). Further north the situation was the same among both the northern Eskimos (C. Hooper 1884, 103; Cantwell 1887, 49) and the Indians of the interior (Dall 1870, 221; Adams 1982, 80).

Thus lice were a constant plague to the people of Alaska from the earliest recorded contacts. The practice of picking them off the body or scalp and eating them was widespread in the Arctic and excited much curiosity among those who observed it. Perhaps the basis was simply the need to dispose of the creature in a definitive manner once having taken the trouble to search it out. Another control method observed among the northern Eskimos was to leave their clothing in the outer room of the house each night so that the lice would freeze. The following morning the dead lice could then be shaken out from the doorway (West 1965, 98-99).

Skin ulcers and sores were another problem mentioned repeatedly in the early narratives. Such lesions may have several causes, but it is reasonable to suppose that many were due to chronic infections of the skin. Some of these infections were probably the result of scratching of insect bites, including those by lice. Other infections could have been secondary to such lesions as frostbite, lacerations, or ulcers due to poor circulation.

Davydov (1977, 179) described sores in the Natives of Kodiak in the first years of the nineteenth century: "I have seen," he wrote, "several savages suffering from sores, mostly on the legs and feet. One had had them for seven years; all of the right leg was covered in sores and in between them the flesh was raw. All those infected with this disease give off an unbearable and noxious odor." Around the same time Captain Lisianskii listed "itch" and "ulcers" among the commonest diseases of the Koniag, with hardly anyone on the island to be found without them (Lisiansky 1814, 201).

One of the earliest visitors to Norton Sound described the Eskimos there as having their faces and bodies covered with deep sores, which he took, probably mistakenly, for syphilis (Khromchenko 1973, 71). Another early account described two Eskimo women with deep ulcers of the lower face (J. Wolfe *in* Bockstoce 1977, 122). The fact that two such individuals were observed at one time suggests an infectious etiology, since other possible causes, such as cancer, or injury, would be unlikely to be seen in two individuals simultaneously.

Other such observations are easy to find in the literature but most are of a somewhat later date. One particularly vivid description, though written as late as 1886, originated when the local Native people had just begun regular contact with the outside world. Edith Kilbuck, a Moravian missionary, wrote of the Kuskokwim Eskimos in a letter home (*in* Jackson 1896a, 1460): "We see some of the most loathsome sights that you can imagine—sores that look like some of the extreme illustrations given in surgical books, and then so crusted with dirt that no part of the skin is visible, the sore being angry-looking and full of moving insect life."

Corroborating evidence for the prevalence of skin sores and ulcers comes from traditional medicine. In southeastern Alaska the Tlingit used plant remedies such as "seal's tongue" for sores and boils (Swanton [1908], 70). The Yupik Eskimos had several methods, suggesting that the problem was widespread (or that none of the remedies worked). On Nelson Island they applied a poultice of alder leaves (*Alnus* spp.), which stuck to the sore and helped debride the scabs when they were pulled off (Ager and Ager 1980). Others used yarrow leaves (*Achillea* spp.) as a poultice, or applied spruce pitch (Kari 1987: 33, 142-43 Wennekens 1985, 53). Rancid seal oil or fox grease were other remedies used for sores (Lantis 1959, 8, 18). They were sometimes also washed with urine or sprinkled with the yellow powder from a "puff-ball" fungus (Lantis 1959, 6).

Boils and carbuncles were another common form of skin infection in early times. Davydov (1977, 177) stated categorically that boils were the most prevalent illness among the Kodiak Islanders in the first years of the nineteenth century, sometimes spreading widely over the body and requiring surgical drainage. Father Ioasaf (*in* Black 1977, 82) around the same time wrote that many died of these abscesses, some of which were very large. Both Davydov and Ioasaf described surgical incision and drainage as the usual treatment used by the Koniag themselves. The Aleuts and Chugach Eskimos also suffered from boils but usually treated them with plant remedies instead of surgery (Veniaminov 1984, 291; Bank 1953, 427; Birket-Smith 1953, 117). As early as 1839 boils were described among the "usual diseases" of the lower Kuskokwim Eskimos (Wrangell 1970). Further north an Orthodox missionary mentioned boils as one of the commonest diseases of the lower Yukon Natives only a decade later (Netsvetov *in* University of Alaska 1936-1938, 1:369). Zagoskin in fact ranked abscesses as one of the most prevalent diseases of the people after his journey on foot through the region in 1842-1844 (1967, 110). That Athapaskan Indians also suffered from boils is evidenced by the traditional methods they used to treat them. For example, the Ingalik applied a small piece of rabbit skin to the abscess, and when it ruptured, applied a new piece to absorb the pus. Sometimes they incised the boil with a bone needle (Osgood 1958, 229).

INFECTIONS OF THE EYES, EARS, AND THROAT

Evidence for eye infections is unsatisfactory. In the late nineteenth century there are several references to "granular ophthalmia" sometimes leading to blindness (R. White 1880, 34; Rosse 1883, 23; Petroff 1882, 43); a few observers, in fact, went so far as to call the disease trachoma, normally a disease of the Tropics, but one that can occur wherever sanitation is poor (Young 1927, 159; Thomas 1900, 735).

Other inflammatory conditions of the lids and conjunctivae were also described. Dr. John Richardson (*in* Hrdlička 1930, 216) reported that some Eskimos suffered from ulcerated and excoriated eyelids, and Dr. Rosse (1883, 23) frequently found "ophthalmia tarsi" among the same group. In

Sitka Dr. Frankenhaeuser (*in* Pierce 1974, 28) observed an epidemic of blepharoblenorrhea (inflammation of the lids and conjunctivae) in children in 1848, while at the turn of the century George Thomas (1900, 735) reported ophthalmia neonatorum (usually caused by gonorrhea and thus perhaps introduced) in the Indians of the Susitna valley.

Infectious diseases of the ears and throat also pose difficult questions for the historian. Suppurative middle ear disease and its complications are known to be a curse of modern times among Alaska Natives, especially the Eskimos. Yet for some reason draining ears, or even deafness, were rarely mentioned in the early narratives, although both conditions may be easily recognized by the nonmedical observer with anything more than casual contact. Even traditional medicine is relatively impoverished on the treatment of earaches and draining ears (Osgood 1958, 230; Lantis 1959, 23; Birket-Smith 1953, 117).

That serious middle ear infections did indeed occur in early times, however, is demonstrated by several postmortem studies of precontact human remains. T. Dale Stewart (1979, 268) found no less than fifteen examples of cholesteatoma in his study of Eskimo and Aleut skulls, whereas Michael Zimmerman and his colleagues (1981) found definite evidence of chronic otitis media and mastoiditis in their autopsy of an Aleut mummy. In Kachemak Bay John Lobdell demonstrated evidence of probable mastoiditis in at least two archeological specimens, thus confirming early studies in the same area by Bruno Oetteking (Lobdell 1980, 65).

Infections of the throat are mentioned from time to time in the early narratives, the first account being probably that of Dr. Merck (1980, 107), who in 1790 described a Koniag seriously ill with an abscess of the throat. About a decade later Gedeon observed a Koniag with a dangerous throat infection accompanied by a lip abscess and a sore on his neck (*in* Pierce 1978, 55).

Traditional remedies for sore throat are known for the Aleuts (Bank 1953), Chugach Eskimos (Birket-Smith 1953, 117), Kuskokwim Eskimos (Ager and Ager 1980; Lantis 1959, 23), and Ingalik Athapaskans (Osgood 1958, 230). They involved a variety of extracts of plant and animal substances applied externally, taken internally, or simply chewed.

DISEASES OF THE LOWER RESPIRATORY TRACT

The evidence for respiratory disease in the early contact period is particularly difficult to interpret. First of all, the early narratives speak largely in terms of symptoms, such as cough, spitting up blood, chest pain, and the like, rather than in terms of diseases. The second difficulty is that probably the first diseases to be introduced into the Native populations from outside were those of the respiratory tract, such as colds, influenza, and perhaps tuberculosis, and it is therefore not always possible to distinguish what was new from what was endemic.

Although few autopsies of precontact human remains are available from Alaska, those that are have cast some welcome light on the questions at hand. Studies of an Aleut mummy (Zimmerman et al. 1981), for example, suggest that the individual died of lobar pneumonia with septicemia and multiple visceral abscesses. The recent postmortem examination of the remains of a woman killed hundreds of years ago by the shifting ice near Barrow showed signs of pneumonia and pleural effusions (Zimmerman and Aufderheide 1984).

Chronologically, the first reference to respiratory infections in the narratives comes from Dr. Merck (1980, 177). After a winter of strong winds, he wrote, "many of these [Aleutian] islanders, both men and women, died of chest diseases, pain in the side, coughing and spitting up blood, because they suffer more want at this time and are forced to expose themselves to the weather without adequate clothing."

In the first decade of the nineteenth century Lisianskii observed, after a winter on Kodiak Island, that colds were among the commonest diseases suffered by the Natives there (Lisiansky 1814, 201). Zagoskin (1967, 255), one of the first Europeans to penetrate the Kuskokwim River valley, found that the Natives there, like the Aleuts and Creoles (usually of mixed Russian and Native blood), had weak lungs. "It is the exceptional one," he wrote, "who does not cough blood by the time he is 20." A few years later, in 1847, Father Iakov Netsvetov (*in* University of Alaska 1936-1938, 1:369), listed cough, pectoral pain, bronchial and tracheal pain, and hemoptysis among the commonest symptoms of the people of the lower Yukon. In 1886 Mrs. John Kilbuck, an early Moravian missionary, noted that, "Pneumonia is a dreadful disease here. The people who take it nearly all die. . . ." (*in* Jackson 1896a, 1460). All of these observers had had the opportunity to see the Eskimos of this region in their own villages over a period of time. A Russian doctor in Sitka during the 1850s observed that the Tlingit often had "chronic catarrh" and coughed up blood, but rarely seemed to suffer from tuberculosis (Govorlivyi n.d., 7-8)

Further north, Murdoch found diseases of the lungs very prevalent at Barrow in 1881-1883, especially toward the end of summer, which, of course, was the time when the ice receded from the coast enough to allow the whaling ships to arrive. Murdoch's own opinion (1892, 39) was that the pulmonary infections were due "to the natives sleeping on the damp ground and to their extreme carelessness in exposing themselves to the drafts of wind when overheated." "Nearly everyone," he went on, "suffers from coughs and colds in the latter part of August, and many deaths occur at this season from a disease that appears to be pneumonia." More convincing is the report of Cantwell (1889, 83), who in 1884 was one of the first Caucasians to ascend the Kobuk River. There he found "pulmonary complaints and rheumatism" to be the principal causes of sickness in these Eskimos, who had had virtually no prior contact with the outside world.

Further inland, Dall (1870, 195) traveled extensively in the 1860s among the Indians of the Yukon and its tributaries. Pleurisy, pneumonia, bronchitis, and asthma were some of the diseases he observed among the Ingalik. A decade and a half later Schwatka (1885, 99, 117), a physician by training, said of the same people that pulmonary diseases of various kinds were "very prevalent" and that many died each winter of pneumonia. In another place he made the same observation about the Aleuts, attributing the disease to exposure and adding that other lung diseases were especially prevalent among the children.

The evidence of traditional medicine must not be overlooked in assessing the extent of respiratory disease in earlier times. The first mention may be that of Davydov (1977, 178) who said that the Koniag bled a patient from below the chin for shortness of breath or asthma. In the late nineteenth century several plants were used by the Tlingit for chest inflammation, cough, and pleurisy (Krause 1956, 283), while among the lower Kuskokwim Eskimos seal oil and boiled green spruce needles were used for the treatment of cough (Lantis 1959, 15). Many other plant remedies are known (Fortuine 1988b).

One is left with the uncomfortable feeling that the only early evidence on lower respiratory disease that can be accepted with any confidence is that from paleopathology, since clues from early narratives and traditional medicine may be interpreted in differing ways, and may reflect the early introduction of respiratory pathogens, including *Mycobacterium tuberculosis,* from outside.

INFECTIONS OF THE GASTROINTESTINAL TRACT

Infectious diseases of the gastrointestinal tract do not appear to have been common among Alaska Natives in the early contact period, according to the few narratives that mention them. This paucity of information is particularly surprising in light of the poor sanitation in Native homes and villages repeatedly described by early visitors to Alaska. Food was often left to become putrid before it was eaten, and food wastes were scattered around inside and outside the dwelling. Water for drinking was of doubtful quality and in some areas insufficient for proper personal hygiene.

That diarrheal diseases did exist in early times, however, is suggested by the treatments available in a few accounts of traditional medicine. An early Aleut remedy for diarrhea was the use of an extract of certain astringent roots, which cannot now be identified (Veniaminov 1984, 293). From the lower Yukon area several such remedies have survived, including the use of salmonberries *(Rubus spectabilis),* sphagnum moss *(Sphagnum* spp.), cranberry extract *(Vaccinium vitis-idaea),* and what is probably marsh marigold *(Caltha palustris).* For severe cases the leaves and stems of sourdock *(Rumex arcticus)* were boiled in water and administered twice a day (Lantis 1959, 15). Lt. Henry Allen (1887, 143) described in some detail a shamanistic performance he witnessed in an Athapaskan village to treat a child with diarrhea.

When diarrheal disease was mentioned at all in early narratives, it was usually by someone who had lived among the people for a considerable length of time. Perhaps herein lies the explanation for the seeming low incidence of the disease. The record of a brief or casual encounter with Alaska Natives would not be expected to include observations on the frequency or character of their stools.

Father Veniaminov (1984, 291) wrote that diarrhea was one of the common diseases of the Aleuts in former times. Another Orthodox missionary (Netsvetov *in* University of Alaska 1936-1938, 1:369) agreed that it also had a high incidence among the Eskimos of the lower Yukon, when they still had infrequent outside contact. A generation later a similar observation was made in Barrow, though by that time whaling ships were visiting the north coast in great numbers (Murdoch 1892, 39).

The first scientific studies of enteric microorganisms in Alaska were made in the early 1950s, when most Native families in remote areas were still living in a largely traditional manner. In 1958 Harold Fournelle and his colleagues published findings from a survey carried out in 1955-1956 in ten villages and fish camps of the lower Kuskokwim. Over seventy percent of the people of these communities were interviewed, one-third of whom reported diarrhea in the previous year, usually during the summer months. More than two-thirds of the cases were in children under ten. Five different pathogenic bacteria were found, including two strains of *Shigella* (which causes a form of dysentery), two strains of pathogenic *Escherichia coli,* and *Salmonella typhi,* the latter the causative organism of typhoid fever. Among the many intestinal protozoa identified were cysts of the parasites *Entamoeba histolytica* and *Giardia lamblia,* both of which can cause a severe and prolonged diarrhea. Pinworms and two other kinds of nematode eggs were also found. In 1966 the same investigators did a similar survey in ten Athapaskan villages of the upper Yukon and later added three more villages on the lower Yukon. Although the prevalence of diarrhea was a little less in these villages, many of the same pathogens were found.

Although we can never be certain, it is plausible to assume that these findings are at least representative of the situation as it was two hundred years ago, if not in the specific organisms identified, then at least in the predominant pattern of summer disease in children.

4

Chronic and
Degenerative Diseases

This chapter describes a number of health disorders that do not fit well in the three previous chapters. These conditions have no clear unifying cause, such as cold temperature or microorganisms. Most of them are chronic and most are not directly related to infectious agents, at least so far as is known, although a few exceptions even to these rules will be apparent. To provide at least a modicum of order and consistency, the diseases and disorders have been classified by the portion of the body they primarily affect.

EYE DISEASE

The evidence for chronic eye disease in early times is abundant but vague enough to make any conclusions uncertain. Even the briefest contact with Native people often evoked a comment on the eyes since they were readily visible even in a fully dressed individual. Descriptions of "red," "inflamed," or "sore" eyes probably covered simple blepharitis (infection of the lids), snowblindness, smoke irritation, inflammation from turned-in eyelashes, and the simple changes of aging. Since most observers were not medically trained, however, it is rarely possible to make an exact diagnosis. Infectious diseases of the eye and conditions related to the environment already have been discussed in Chapters 2 and 3.

Cataracts and corneal opacities may be considered together, since medically untrained observers often seemed to confuse a white spot on the cornea with an opacified lens. For example, in Barrow Murdoch (1892, 40) observed several cases of unilateral blindness caused by an opacity of the eye that he thought was either a cataract or a "leucoma," a word which means a dense white scar on the cornea. Others who noted eye opacities in the Natives included Dall (1870, 195) and Dr. H. M. W. Edmonds (1966, 30). Dr. Rosse (1883, 23) described cases of both lens and corneal opacity; in fact, he devoted a large section of his medical report of the *Corwin* cruise to eye disease of various kinds. Several traditional treatments for opacities are known, including an ingenious surgical procedure of the Koniag (Davydov 1977, 178; Black 1977, 84), and the Inupiat (DeLapp and Ward 1981, 14), supposedly using a louse attached to a hair to grasp the whitened area. The Yupik Eskimos sometimes laid a human hair horizontally across the cornea under the upper lid in order to cause chronic irritation and thus rub off the spot. Margaret Lantis's informant for this procedure admitted that it sometimes made matters worse (Lantis 1959, 21-22). The Tlingit tried to draw out the spot by holding the heated broken ends of a certain vine close to the eye (Swanton [1908], 447).

Strabismus, or crossed eyes, was another prevalent condition among the Natives, as attested by several witnesses (Murdoch 1892, 40; Dall 1870, 195).

The most disabling result of eye disease is of course blindness. An individual who was blind could not hunt, fish, sew, or cook, and thus was wholly dependent on the care and support of the family, which itself could be in marginal economic circumstances. From the available early records it would appear that the blind were usually provided loving care and attention by those responsible for them. Captain Cook in 1778 met an Eskimo who was nearly blind near Cape Denbigh in Norton Sound. This man was traveling in a family group that included a crippled boy who himself had one eye destroyed by disease. Later Lt. James King described the same blind man, whose eyes were covered with a whitish film (Cook 1967, 3(1):438; 3(2):1439). In Kotzebue Sound Beechey (1831, 1:394) saw a blind man whose wife showed him a mirror in the vain hope that the reflection could help his sight. Dr. Simpson (1855, 927) at Barrow was impressed with the tender care afforded a blind man by the people of a summer fish camp, and Murdoch (1892, 40) observed the same solicitude for the blind at Cape Smythe. This latter individual was living comfortably with relatives but was said to do his share of the work, for example, as a paddler on a whaling boat. Among the Kobuk Eskimos (Stoney 1900, 87) and at Point Hope (Jenkins 1943, 149), the blind were also observed to be well cared for.

The Natives had various theories on the causation of blindness. For example, Ingalik mothers were careful not to splatter human milk in the eye for fear it would cause blindness (Osgood 1958, 176). The Koniag, on the other hand, believed that blindness could be caused by excessive use of the sweatbath (Black 1977, 99). In fact, blindness was probably caused in earlier times principally by eye injury, cataract, chronic infection, and glaucoma. In 1845 Father Netsvetov (1984, 4) numbered a blind woman among his first converts on the lower Yukon. Elsewhere (1984, 236, 270) he mentions other blind Eskimos, usually elderly. In 1861 Netsvetov (1984, 22, 437) himself, who was half Native, developed a severe chronic eye affliction suggestive of iritis. In the latter part of the nineteenth century the many reports of blindness among Alaska Natives (e.g., University of Alaska 1936-1938, 1:358; 2:63; R. White 1880, 34; Krause 1956, 104; Collis 1890, 108; Rosse 1883, 23) may well have been in part due to introduced infections such as gonorrhea, syphilis, smallpox, and perhaps even trachoma.

One common inflammatory eye disease of later times was phlyctenular keratoconjunctivitis, or PKC, which caused redness, pain, tearing, and, in its later stages, corneal scarring and blindness. PKC is thought to be caused, among other things, by an immunologic reaction to the tuberculosis organism. Whether it occurred in pre-contact times is unknown (Fritz and Thygeson 1951). It has, at any rate, diminished in incidence now that tuberculosis has been brought under control.

EAR, NOSE, AND THROAT DISORDERS

Deafness is only occasionally mentioned in the earlier narratives. According to Murdoch (1892, 39), the chief of the North Slope village of Nuwuk was a feeble old man who was "very deaf and almost blind," but with his mind still intact—probably a case of simple presbycusis, or the deafness of old age. At St. Michael Dr. Edmonds (1966, 31) met a deafmute who was very intelligent, jovial, and communicative. He was said to be a good hunter and fully able to care for himself. Dall (1870, 195) encountered a single deafmute among the Koyukon Indians but some years later Lt. Henry T. Allen (1887, 140) visited a Koyukon village in which four of eleven men were deafmutes, in addition to a woman and a child. It is likely that close intermarriage there had led to the emergence of a hereditary form of deafness. In southeastern Alaska a missionary at Haines knew of three deaf individuals, only one of whom was mute (Willard 1884, 212-23). Quite likely some of these individuals had partial hearing loss secondary to chronic ear infections or possibly meningitis.

Epistaxis, or nosebleed, in the peoples of the Arctic was observed frequently from the earliest European contacts (Fortuine 1971, 100-103). Among the possible causes are trauma, infection, or simply the cracking of the mucous membranes in the cold, dry arctic air. Another possible factor may lie in recent research on the diet of the Greenlandic Eskimos. These studies have revealed that their fish and sea mammal diet is rich in omega-3 fatty acids, which have been associated with a prolonged bleeding time and with a reduced platelet function (Dyerberg and Bang 1979, 433-35).

The earliest report of nosebleed comes from the Aleutians in 1741, when the naturalist of the Chirikov voyage noted that the people wore stones in their noses, which caused them to bleed (Del'Isle de la Croyère 1914, 321). Chirikov's (1922, 305) own explanation of the nosebleeds was that the Aleuts often stuffed roots into their noses, a sample of which roots they brought to him for identification. Coincidentally, Lt. Sven Waxell (1962, 90) of Bering's own ship, visiting another part of the Aleutians that summer, recorded that the people plugged their nostrils with a tough grass of unknown type, which when removed caused a quantity of fluid to flow from their noses and which they licked off with their tongues. Whatever they used to stuff their nostrils, it is evident that the practice caused irritation of the mucous membrane that could have led to bleeding or infection.

Most of the subsequent references to nosebleed come from the northern parts of Alaska (e.g., Rosse 1883, 27; Murdoch 1892, 40). A few mention epistaxis in connection with bleeding from the lungs (Doty 1900, 194; V. Gambell 1898, 144). This may be due to the fact that blood from the nose may drip back into the throat and later be coughed up, or it could mean that hemorrhage from the lung, or hemoptysis, was a separate problem. A particularly graphic description of nosebleeds comes from a teacher-missionary who was at Wales in the 1890s (Thornton 1931, 37):

> A physiological peculiarity of the people (especially the children) is that in winter they exhibit an inordinate tendency to bleed at the nose. Hardly an hour passes . . . without our seeing one or more of them troubled in this way. The slightest blow will induce it, and it frequently begins without any visible cause whatever. Crimson spots may be seen on the snow, resulting from nose-bleeding, that almost look as if they had been occasioned by the butchering of some animal.

The many traditional remedies for nosebleed are a measure of the condition's prevalence. Among the methods used by the Eskimos were to lie prone with the nose in the snow (Thornton 1931, 37), to pack snow, deer hair, or blubber in the nostrils (Spencer 1959, 328), put snow in the mouth (Lantis 1946, 202), or be bled from a scalp vein (Weyer 1932, 324). Other treatments were magical, such as when a Yupik shaman sucked at the back of the neck (Lantis 1946, 202), or when an Ingalik tied up a small bunch of the patient's hair, or streaked the blood from the nose to the hair with a finger (Osgood 1958, 229).

Although the practice of rubbing noses was not a health problem as such, it must have had hygienic implications. Kotzebue (1821, 1:192) was the first to describe this unusual greeting method of the St. Lawrence Islanders: "Each of them embraced me, rubbed his nose against mine, and ended his caresses by spitting in his hands and wiping them several times over my face. Though these signs of friendship were not very agreeable to me, I bore all patiently. To suppress their further tenderness, I distributed some tobacco leaves." Louis Choris (*in* VanStone 1960, 146), an artist with the voyage, confirmed this account and added that the Eskimos wished the visitors to wipe spittle on their faces as a reciprocal gesture. Subsequently, other expeditions (Beechey 1831, 1:323; T. Simpson 1843, 155; W. Hooper 1853, 225; M'Clure 1857, 61, 74, etc.) encountered this practice in one form or another. By 1881, however, the custom had largely died out, presumably under pressure from the Europeans (Murdoch 1892, 422).

A curious bit of cultural evidence suggests that facial palsy, due to loss of function of the seventh cranial nerve, may have been prevalent in earlier times. A number of illustrations of Indian and Eskimo masks collected by Richard Van Wagoner and Tong Chun (1974) seem to show this typical deformity clearly. Such cases may have no known cause, as in the so-called Bell's palsy, or they may be secondary to cold exposure, injury, or an underlying middle ear infection.

DENTAL STATUS

Archeological evidence is particularly helpful in reconstructing the dental health of the Alaska Natives in early times, since teeth and jaws are able to survive many of the vicissitudes of nature. Perhaps the most striking and consistent finding was the constant wear of the teeth, often beginning at an early age and progressing until the crowns were level with the gum margins. This wear, due to the severe occlusal stresses from chewing meat and skins, not infrequently led to exposure of the pulp cavity, periapical abscesses, and ultimate loss of the tooth (Hrdlička 1940, 2). Periodontal disease with receding of the alveolar bone and heavy calculus formation around the teeth also frequently led to tooth loss (Zimmerman et al. 1971, 82; 1981, 638). An Eskimo woman in her forties who was frozen in the ice at Barrow had lost nearly all her teeth, except for a few incisors, and her mandible was atrophic (Zimmerman and Aufderheide 1984, 54). All authorities seem to agree that caries were absent or rare in Alaska Natives (Stewart 1979, 269-70).

Many early accounts describe the appearance of the teeth of the Natives. In the Aleutians one of Cook's surgeons found the peoples' teeth "indifferent, being uneven, and frequently discoloured" (Ellis 1782, 2:45). Veniaminov some years later (1984, 162) noted that the Aleuts had white, clean, and "invariably sound" teeth, although often worn down. Older people, on the other hand, developed yellowish or even black staining of their front teeth, a condition he attributed to their fish-eating. In contrast, the Koniag were said to have white, or "beautiful white" teeth (Gedeon *in* Pierce 1978, 134; Holmberg 1985, 12).

Further north, Lieutenant King, of the Cook expedition (Cook 1967, 3(2):1440) remarked that the people of Sledge Island had black teeth that were "filed down close to the gum," a condition he at first thought was the result of purposeful effort. Ellis (1782, 1:330) also noted that these people had bad teeth that were "worn down to the stumps." Nearly fifty years later Captain Beechey (1831, 2:303) recognized the true state of affairs when he wrote that the Eskimos of Kotzebue Sound had their teeth "worn to the gums by frequent mastication of hard substances." Likewise, W. H. Hooper (1853, 223-24) observed that the young people of Kotzebue Sound had white and regular teeth but that the sand they ate mixed with their food wore their teeth down at an early age. Similar observations were made by others (J. Simpson 1855, 94; Dall 1870, 140; Murdoch 1892, 34; etc.). Dr. Rollin, the surgeon on the voyage of La Pérouse (1799, 2:358), was so impressed with the perfect evenness of the teeth of the Tlingit that he first thought that it was "the effect of art." Upon closer examination, however, he could find no changes in the enamel and concluded that "they are indebted to nature for this regularity." La Pérouse himself (1799, 1:401), however, thought that the Tlingit filed their teeth to the gums by means of a rounded piece of sandstone in the shape of a tongue. In the nineteenth century Holmberg (1985, 37) found their teeth to be beautiful and white. Ens. Albert Niblack (1888, 237) agreed with this assessment for young people, but noted that in old age their teeth were much discolored and worn due to eating the sand and grit found in dried salmon.

Lieutenant Zagoskin (1967, 243) described the teeth of the Athapaskans of the middle Yukon as "white and as even as beads." Just as in the other Native groups, however, Lieutenant Allen (1887, 127) found the Ahtna to have prominently worn teeth, even in middle age. A later ethnographer has described local traditional remedies for toothache, suggesting that dental disease was not uncommon (Osgood 1958, 230; Osgood 1937, 160).

ARTHRITIS AND RELATED DISORDERS

The scientific study of human remains from numerous sites around Alaska has demonstrated that many Alaska Natives suffered from arthritis, particularly of the degenerative type. Such changes have been found in all races, both sexes, and at nearly every stage of life. No doubt they reflect the hard physical life of the people, probably aggravated by the cold, damp weather, and possibly a genetic susceptibility.

Working in several sites on the Aleutians, William Laughlin (1980, 11) found that nearly every skeleton of individuals over forty years of age had arthritic changes in the spinal column, usually "lipping" of the vertebral bodies. The elbows were also frequently affected but with an interesting sex difference: the males showed arthritic changes on the capitellar (lateral) surfaces, whereas the females were affected primarily on the trochlear (medial) surfaces (Laughlin 1963, 641). These differences he attributed to differing daily activities and hence differing bony stresses on the joint. In one Aleut mummy, arthritis of the cervico-thoracic spine was found to be more severe on the left than the right (Laughlin and Aigner 1974, 50, 52), but this finding was not confirmed in another mummy examined in detail (Zimmerman et al. 1971, 82).

In a study of early human remains from Kodiak Island, Hrdlička (1940, 2, 14) described a variety of arthritic changes of the spine and joints, particularly in the elderly. Elsewhere he (1931, 132) found all grades of "arthritis deformans" in the spines of older individuals from the Kuskokwim valley, such changes ranging from simple exostoses (bony excrescences) to a fusion of the entire spine suggestive of ankylosing spondylitis. In a few skeletons just the cervical vertebrae were fused. Only occasionally did he find arthritic changes in the joints of the extremities.

In the Prince William Sound region, archeological work has demonstrated that degenerative arthritis was widespread among the early inhabitants (De Laguna 1956, 86). In more recent years John Lobdell (1980, 63-65) has described osteoarthritic changes, such as lipping and eburnation (dense abnormal hardening) of the bone, not only in the spine but also in the shoulder, ankle, thumb, and knee of human remains from Kachemak Bay in Cook Inlet.

The picture is much the same in the arctic regions of Alaska, where Stewart (1979, 261) found Eskimo remains demonstrating lipping, eburnation, and erosion of joint surfaces in the spine, knee, hip, shoulder, and elbow. Males generally showed more advanced changes than females, probably reflecting their greater physical stresses.

The earliest narrative to mention bone or joint pain in Alaska Natives seems to be that of Dr. Merck (1980, 107), who noted this to be a common finding among the people at Kodiak in 1790. Other early descriptions are distinctly scarce, perhaps because of the intermittent and often mild nature of the disease process in those affected. The best documentation for arthritis comes from southeastern Alaska. In the early days of the Russian-American Company "lumbago" was listed as a common complaint among the Aleut hunters working there (Golovin 1979, 64). Likewise, the medical reports of Drs. Romanovskii and Frankenhaeuser in the 1840s repeatedly mention the problem of rheumatic complaints among the Russians, Creoles, Aleuts, and probably the Tlingit who lived around the capital (in Pierce 1974, 2, 20, 22, 23, 28). In the latter years of the nineteenth century there were numerous reports of arthritis among the Tlingit, often attributed to the damp, cold weather (Teichmann 1963, 184, 196; Colyer 1869, 1024; Wythe 1871, 341; R. White 1880, 35, 37).

Arthritis and "rheumatism" were also said to be widespread on Kodiak Island (H. Elliott 1886, 111), and in the Aleutians (Shepard 1889, 84). In the Yukon-Kuskokwim basin one of Zagoskin's (1967, 232) Native hunters was "seized with rheumatic pains and cramps" and had to be relieved from work. Somewhat later Capt. Charles Raymond (1900, 33) found rheumatism "by no means uncommon" in this region. In the north it was repeatedly described as one of the most prevalent diseases of the Eskimos (e.g., Nelson 1899, 29; Rosse 1883, 23; Murdoch 1892, 39; Cantwell 1889, 83). Dr. Call, however, disagreed. After nearly six months at Barrow in 1897-1898, he concluded that rheumatism was rare, since he had seen only four cases during that period. He did describe, however, a classic case of deforming rheumatoid arthritis in an old Eskimo named McGurty (in [Jarvis] 1899, 123, 127): "He had been confined to his bed with the chronic articular variety for two and a half years. Little remained of him save a skeleton of large and distorted joints covered with skin, reminding one of an Aleutian mummy." Nor were the Athapaskans spared the curse of aching joints. A parade of travelers into the interior in the nineteenth century found arthritis and rheumatism to be a frequent problem among the Indians (Raymond 1870-71, 165; Dall 1870, 195; Learnard 1900, 666; Herron 1901, 69).

Traditional methods of treating arthritis and rheumatic pains were legion, another indication of the pervasiveness of the problem in Native society. These methods included the use of heat, medicinal plant and animal substances, piercing and bleeding, and shamanism (e.g., Lantis 1959, 10-11; Ager and Ager 1980; Spencer 1959, 329).

CRIPPLING CONDITIONS

Many early narratives attest that the Alaska Natives suffered from various disabling conditions of the musculoskeletal system. Some of these were the result of genetic tendency or birth injury, while others were acquired later in life from infectious disease, chronic illness, or accident.

The most common deformities seemed to be those of the extremities. Among the possible causes were trauma, surgical amputation, nerve injury, infection, or heredity. Several such crippling conditions of the arm are known from the Aleutians alone in early times. Veniaminov (*in* Black 1984, 178) tells of an Atka boy who was born with one arm. He was cruelly ridiculed by his mother's family, a situation that later blew up into open warfare between the Atkans and Unalaskans. The son of a toyon (chief) of Umnak Island was said to have had a maimed hand that could have been congenital or have been caused by injury (Coxe 1787, 198). Another early account describes a boy from Attu, probably suffering from a broken and infected arm, who was brought to the Russians for baptism in the hope of finding a cure (Black 1984, 67). Finally, as mentioned earlier, an Unalaskan *toyon* was said to have had his hand bitten cleanly off by a sea lion (Hillsen *in* D. Ray 1983, 27).

Reports of congenital anomalies of the extremities are not at all uncommon, examples being clubfoot (Dall 1870, 195), supernumerary digits (Rosse 1883, 26), and congenital dislocation of the hip (Young 1927, 159). One visitor to southeastern Alaska noted that many children had limb deformities (Collis 1890, 104). On St. Lawrence Island, Dr. P. H. J. Lerrigo (1901, 106) saw several cases of webbed fingers and a boy with a badly deformed hand, all of which he related to the high rate of consanguinity among the people.

A couple of early observations are particularly interesting in that they suggest a rare condition known as congenital arthrogryposis, or Kuskokwim disease, which was not described in the medical literature until 1969 (Petajan et al.). The characteristic feature of this disorder is that its victims are born with severe contractures of the major joints, especially the knees, which often forces them to walk on their knees. Captain Cook and several of his officers mention a boy (see fuller discussion below) from Norton Sound whose legs were so contracted that he had to crawl about on his hands and knees (Cook 1967, 3(1):438; 3(2):1439). About a century later Dr. Rosse (1883, 26) observed three cases of "angular ankylosis of the knee joint," two of them in adults and one in a boy.

Missing limbs could result from birth defects and injuries, as we have just seen, or they could be due to surgical amputation. Zagoskin (1967, 92) found a legless old woman near Unalakleet, where a half century later Dr. Call encountered a man whose legs had been amputated at the middle third by his wife as the result of frostbite. Further north at Barrow Call described a twenty-eight-year-old pregnant woman, both of whose legs had been amputated, again for frostbite (*in* [Jarvis] 1899, 115, 121). Others were known to have lost fingers or toes, probably either from frostbite or from trauma (Edmonds 1966, 30; Stoney 1900, 89).

Possible causes of deformities of the spine are infection, birth defect, trauma, paralysis, or the scoliosis of unknown cause sometimes seen in teenagers. Hunchbacks were said to be common among the Kenai Indians in the 1830s (Wrangell 1970, 11), although by this time they had already been in regular contact with the Russians for fifty years. Earlier in terms of outside contact were the reports of Berthold Seemann (1853, 67) and Dall (1870, 195), each of whom saw at least one hunchback among the Seward Peninsula Eskimos and the Koyukon Indians, respectively. Later reports of hunchback are likely to have been due to tuberculosis (*see* Chapter 15).

Paralysis may have several causes, including birth injury, nerve trauma, stroke, or infection, such as poliomyelitis. The earliest record from Alaska comes from the voyage of Portlock (1789, 237), who met a chief in Cook Inlet who was "entirely disabled on one side," probably, he speculated, due to a stroke. A similar report dates from nearly a century later when Capt. W. R. Abercrombie (1900b, 395) described a shaman "paralyzed from an apoplectic seizure" near Yakutat. Among the northern Eskimos, Dr. Rosse (1883, 26) and Jackson (1896b, 88) each described an individual who had become paralyzed as a result of injury. Petroff (1882, 43) mentioned that paralysis was a common affliction of the Eskimos. The Kutchin sometimes used tattooing to "straighten" the deformed face of a person who had suffered paralysis (Osgood 1936, 99).

A remarkable case report comes from the Cook voyage of 1778. While in the vicinity of the present day village of Elim, in Norton Sound, Cook and a party went ashore to collect driftwood. While there a family of four Eskimos approached them, including one, the captain related, "who bore the human shape and that was all, for he was the most deformed cripple I either ever saw or heard of, so much so that I could not even bear to look at him" (Cook 1967, 3(1):438). Lieutenant King, apparently not so squeamish, described the unfortunate individual thus (*in* Cook 1967, 3(2):1439): "He was a young lad, who had a disorder in his face which had already destroy'd one eye, &

the sides were much Swell'd, & one half of his mouth and Nose [were] in a sad condition." He went on to note that the boy had contractures of the legs that prevented him from walking. Dr. Ellis (1782, 2:16) added that he was "a most miserable spectacle, apparently eaten up with disease." Whatever the nature of the disease (or diseases) from which this young man suffered, it is apparent that he had a chronic and crippling condition. The lad was seemingly well taken care of, however, and was probably traveling with his mother.

In the early narratives there are a number of brief allusions to crippling conditions, but without sufficient detail to permit even a reasonable guess at a diagnosis. Among the individual cases, for example, is the "cripple" mentioned by Beechey at Cape Thompson (1831, 1:359), or the "crippled man" who followed Lieutenant Allen (*in* Sherwood 1965b, 112) asking for employment. Murdoch (1892, 40) described a boy with a twisted face, probably from a birth injury. Other early accounts describe the prevalence of crippled individuals in a more collective sense. In southeastern Alaska a missionary found Sitka to be filled with cripples (Willard 1884, 31); another visitor, presumably with some hyperbole, noted that the children for the most part were "blind, deformed in limb, and crippled" (Collis 1890, 104). At St. Michael Dr. Edmonds (1966, 30) found many kinds of malformation, including what he called "ill-shaped bodies." In the interior Dall (1870, 195) found several types of malformation, yet a later explorer felt that the Athapaskans were physically superior to the "coast Indians" (Eskimos) who were "deformed, dwarfed, and more or less diseased" (Learnard 1900, 666).

A final type of crippling disease is not so apparent to the casual observer, or even sometimes to a physician. In recent times several rare genetic disorders have been recognized as having an unusual prevalence in Alaska Natives, probably due to their small and isolated population. These conditions may have few external manifestations, or they may lead, if untreated, to severe disability and early death. Among those that have been recognized among the Yupik Eskimos are serum cholinesterase deficiency, methemoglobinemia, and the salt-losing adrenogenital syndrome (Scott 1972). Kuskokwim disease, mentioned earlier, is yet another example, and there are probably others.

The question of infanticide and senilicide in Native society comes up repeatedly in this regard. There seems to be little doubt that sometimes deformed or crippled individuals were allowed to die because of the greater needs of the community (Weyer 1932, 132). Dr. John Simpson (1855, 927) reported that a child was killed only if afflicted with a "disease of a fatal tendency," whereas Captain Hooper (1881, 57) asserted that the northern Eskimos destroyed all deformed infants at birth. Dr. Edmonds (1966, 30) somewhat later suggested that infants with congenital abnormalities were "quickly disposed of." Likewise, the Eyak Indians were said to cremate immediately the body of a deformed child, along with the placenta, and that failure to observe this custom could be punishable by death (Jacobsen 1977, 210). On the other hand, it is apparent that at least some children with major deformities were allowed to grow up, even in the earliest historical times.

As for the elderly infirm, Beechey (1831, 1:359) observed that the oldest person seen in the vicinity of Cape Thompson was a cripple. Dr. Simpson (1855, 926-27) was particularly impressed with the care the Barrow Eskimos bestowed on their elderly and infirm: "They not only gave them food and clothing, sharing with them every comfort they possess, but on their longest and most fatiguing journeys make provision for their easy conveyance." He observed in one camp of fourteen families one crippled old man, and a blind and helpless old woman, both of whom had been cared for for many years. Later Murdoch (1892, 39) found a local chief described as "a feeble, bowed, tottering old man, very deaf and almost blind," but obviously still respected. Children, especially, were said to be particularly solicitous about the comfort of the elderly (P. Ray 1885, 45). Similar reports come from the Kobuk River (Stoney 1900, 87), St. Lawrence Island (Bruce 1894, 111), and from southeastern Alaska (Krause 1956, 104).

OTHER CHRONIC DISEASES

Atherosclerosis, or hardening of the arteries caused by the deposition of cholesterol-containing plaques on the inner wall of the vessel, has been recognized in autopsies on several fortuitously preserved bodies from earlier times. Dr. Michael R. Zimmerman and his colleagues found a moderate degree of coronary atherosclerosis in the 1600-year-old body of an Eskimo woman from St. Lawrence Island (Zimmerman and Smith 1975, 830), and in a precontact Eskimo woman from Barrow (Zimmerman and Aufderheide 1984, 54). They further described atherosclerotic plaques in the iliac artery, labial artery (Zimmerman et al. 1971, 91), and aorta (Zimmerman et al. 1981, 639) in Aleut mummies. These findings suggest that hardening of the arteries is not simply a product of westernization in Alaska.

The body of a middle-aged Eskimo woman from Barrow revealed a calcified area in the mitral valve of the heart. Although the exact significance of this finding is unclear, it suggests a chronic infection of the heart valves known as bacterial endocarditis (Zimmerman and Aufderheide 1984, 62).

Cancer is another chronic disease for which some paleopathological evidence exists in Alaska. Lagier and his colleagues (1982, 242) examined skull fragments from a burial on St. Lawrence Island and concluded that they showed either multiple myeloma, or more likely a carcinomatous metastasis. Likewise, Lobdell (1980, 65-79) described a skeleton from Kachemak Bay that displayed multiple lesions with many of the characteristics of a malignant hemangioendothelioma, a tumor originating in the blood vessels.

Several chronic conditions of the lung have been described from early human remains, the most common being anthracosis, which has been found not only in all Aleut mummies but in all frozen Eskimos bodies that have been examined (Zimmerman et al. 1971, 99; Zimmerman et al. 1981, 640; Zimmerman and Smith 1975, 830; Zimmerman and Aufderheide 1984, 54, 60). This condition—not strictly speaking a disease—results from the deposition of black pigment in the lungs due to the inhalation of smoke from cooking fires over a period of many years.

Pathologic changes in the lungs and pleurae of these ancient remains were also evident. One Aleut mummy showed changes consistent with moderate emphysema and bronchiectasis, the latter a chronic destructive process of the smaller airways. Furthermore, the patient probably died of pneumonia with sepsis (Zimmerman et al. 1971, 99-100). A second mummy also demonstrated evidence of bronchiectasis, as well as fibrosis of the lungs and pleurae (Zimmerman et al. 1981, 639-40), as did the frozen body of an Eskimo woman from Barrow (Zimmerman and Aufderheide 1984, 54). Similar fibrosis was found in an Eskimo cadaver from St. Lawrence Island (Zimmerman and Smith 1975, 830). Most of these changes suggest either chronic or repeated infection of the lung.

A particularly interesting bit of evidence regarding chronic pulmonary infection comes from northern Alaska, where the study of two frozen Eskimo bodies revealed healed granulomas of the lung and calcified lymph nodes of the chest, secondary to a chronic infectious process such as tuberculosis or histoplasmosis. Despite special tests the investigators were unable to make a final diagnosis, but leaned toward histoplasmosis, a chronic fungous infection of the lung (Zimmerman and Aufderheide 1984, 60-62; Zimmerman and Smith 1975, 831).

It is also notable that two of the five ancient bodies examined in detail in Alaska showed the recovery phase of a condition known as acute tubular necrosis (Zimmerman et al. 1981, 639; Zimmerman and Aufderheide 1984, 62). This entity reflects acute kidney failure, usually secondary to another serious disease or injury.

*   *   *

The four previous chapters have demonstrated that the Alaska Natives in pre-contact times suffered from many types of illness and injury. Some of these threats to health were peculiar to the arctic and subarctic environment, while others were common to the human experience everywhere.

It is worth stressing yet again that the materials presented can easily be misleading. They are based principally on incidental references to health by persons with no specialized knowledge. Moreover, the data are totally random. Anecdotal information is plucked from here and there over a long span of time and can by no means be used to determine the incidence or prevalence of disease. Sometimes it is impossible to conclude with any certainty what disease was being described, much less whether it was aboriginal or introduced.

In spite of these real limitations, however, the information has value in showing, if nothing else, that the Alaska Natives did not enjoy excellent health in precontact times, but rather were plagued by many types of injury, infection, chronic disease, and disability. Unfortunately, many of the details of these health problems and their impact on daily life must remain obscure.

PART II
Health and the Early History of Alaska

Health and disease not only helped to shape Alaskan history, but the very events of history in significant ways determined what the patterns of health and disease would be among the people of Alaska, both Native and newcomer.

The six chapters of this section recount in outline form the highlights of Alaskan history from the earliest explorations by the Russians to the Nome Gold Rush at the end of the nineteenth century. The emphasis is less on political and economic considerations than on the relationships between the Europeans and Americans on the one hand and the Native people on the other. The focus of course is health and disease and the conditions that fostered them both among the established population and those who had recently come from afar. Emphasis also is given to the beginnings and development of health services for the population.

Chapters 5 to 7 cover the period of exploration, the early years of the fur trade in the Aleutians, Kodiak Island, and the North Pacific rim, and the establishment and growth of the Russian-American Company. Special attention is given to the dates and circumstances of early contacts between the Natives and Europeans, and to those whose writings most illuminated contemporary health conditions. Chapter 7 is devoted to the remarkable health care system that the company developed and maintained through the latter years of their administration in Alaska.

Chapters 8 to 10 are concerned with the last third of the nineteenth century, after the purchase of the territory by the United States in 1867. Again, primary emphasis is laid on events and circumstances that bear on health and the spread of disease. Chapter 8 deals with the role of the United States government in the early years of American sovereignty, with special attention to the attempts of several agencies to provide health services or otherwise influence health affairs. The history of commercial interests in Alaska is briefly recounted in Chapter 9, notably the contribution of whalers, traders, commercial fishermen, and miners to the spread of unhygienic living conditions and illness. Chapter 10 deals with one of the few positive forces for health in this period, namely the establishment of missions with their special concern for health, sanitation, sobriety, and education.

5

European Contact, Exploration, and the Early Fur Trade: 1728-1798

THE ALEUTIAN ISLANDS

Vitus Bering and members of the crew of his frail vessel *St. Peter* were the first Europeans to come in contact with the Aleuts, in early September 1741. Bering was hastening home with his men already showing signs of scurvy when a group of islands was sighted to the northward. It was imperative to replenish the fresh water on board and accordingly he sent a boat party ashore, including Georg Wilhelm Steller, the ship's German-born naturalist and surgeon. The shore party in their haste collected brackish water from tidal pools, although Steller had found a much better source further inland. That night a fire was seen from the ship and next morning a party investigated but found only burning embers. A few days later, on September 6, two men in small skin boats paddled out to the ship but would not go on board. Steller, the mate Sven Waxell, and others went ashore and traded with the Natives, even offering them a beaker of gin. When the Russians tried to push off in their boat from the shore the Aleuts held fast to the painter and tried to restrain their interpreter, who was a Chukchi. A musket shot into the air frightened them long enough for the Russians to make their escape. Next day Waxell proposed the capture of a number of kayakers who came out to the ship again, but Bering himself specifically forbade it. Both Waxell and Steller have left accounts of this portentous encounter (Waxell 1962, 89-97; Steller 1988, 97-108), which took place on the Shumagin Islands, named for Nikolai Shumagin, the first of Bering's crew to die of scurvy.

More and more of the sailors developed the telltale signs of scurvy—weakness, depression, joint pains, and swollen gums—as the ship proceeded westward, bucking the heavy seas and whistling winds of fall storms in the Aleutians. Steller had tried to prepare for this contingency by collecting antiscorbutic plants in the Shumagins, but had had neither the time nor the help of others to accomplish the task to his satisfaction. Nearly every day in October there was a burial at sea or further crew members became too disabled to work. Bering himself became ill but Steller shared his personal supply of spoonwort (or scurvy grass: *Cochlearia officinalis*) and soon the captain was able to appear on deck again. By October 18, thirty-two men were unfit for duty. About a week later Steller confided to his journal that "danger and death suddenly got the upper hand on our ship. . . ." (Steller 1988, 119).

Land was sighted a couple of times, but Bering did not dare to send men ashore because they were too weak to weigh the anchor once it was dropped. Finally in early November the ship was beached on what is now called Bering Island in the Commander group. Soon after, Bering and several others succumbed to scurvy, but later fresh meat and new plant growth restored enough of the crew, under Steller's and Waxell's leadership, to build a small vessel and return the following summer to Kamchatka (Steller 1988, 165-69; Waxell 1962, 98-127).

Alexei Chirikov, in command of Bering's other ship, *St. Paul,* also visited the Aleutians on his return voyage from the Alaska mainland in 1741. He had first made landfall in mid-July somewhere in the Panhandle, where he had the misfortune to lose both his boats and seventeen men during an unsuccessful attempt to replenish his water-casks ashore. He and his men were already showing signs of scurvy when they anchored on September 9, probably off Adak Island. As the fog lifted, they saw two men walking on the shore. Soon seven *baidarkas* were paddled out to the ship, but the Aleuts refused to come on board or even to trade until knives were offered. After elaborate attempts to communicate, the Russians finally made it known that they badly needed water, which the Aleuts brought out to the ship in bladders (Chirikov 1922, 1:304-5; Del'Isle de la Croyère 1914, 315-21).

The *St. Paul* then headed west again, its crew gradually weakening from scurvy and thirst. By the time the ship reached Kamchatka on October 10, some twenty men had died, including six from scurvy, among them the astronomer and scientist Louis Del'Isle de la Croyère, who perished as he was being brought ashore. Chirikov himself barely recovered his health following the voyage (Chirikov 1922, 1:309-11; Waxell 1962, 131-32).

Encouraged by Steller's report of countless sea mammals around Bering Island, several independent Siberian fur traders, known as *promyshlenniki,* set off from Kamchatka or Okhotsk in the next few years. Although the captains were skillful navigators, they sailed in small, crudely constructed flat-bottomed vessels known as *shitiki,* which were poorly designed for some of the world's stormiest seas. Several of the early voyages ended ignominiously and tragically in shipwreck, with heavy loss of life due to drowning, exposure, or starvation.

The first of these expeditions to the Aleutians was that of Yakov Chuprov, with Mikhail Nevodchikov as navigator. In September 1745 the *Eudoxia* reached Agattu, where the crew encountered many Aleuts on the beach who seemed eager to trade. When Chuprov and others went ashore for water next day, a misunderstanding led to an Aleut being injured by gunfire (Coxe 1787, 33). The Russians retreated to Attu Island where they captured two Aleuts in a scuffle. Since the captives seemed to be well treated, the Aleuts soon came out of hiding to trade and were persuaded to deliver hostages, a practice that nearly all the early Russian traders insisted upon. The Russians beached their vessel, built shelters of sod and driftwood, adopted Aleut clothing and lived through the winter on Native foods. Violence broke out, however, when a party from the crew provoked a quarrel over women, and in the uneven struggle some fifteen Aleuts were killed (Berkh 1974, 5). Soon the Russians were forcing the Natives to hunt sea otter for them while they themselves lived in comfort with the wives of the hunters. The vessel, laden with furs, finally set sail for home in September 1746 and was later wrecked with a loss of twelve men (Bancroft 1886, 99-107).

Another early trader in the Aleutians was Andreiian Tolstykh, who made several voyages in the 1740s and 1750s. He always treated the Aleut chiefs with respect, and developed harmonious relations with the people wherever he went. His generosity and good sense were usually rewarded by rich cargoes of furs (Berkh 1974, 18; Black 1980, 93).

These two *promyshlenniki,* Chuprov and Tolstykh, were prototypes of the traders who sailed to the islands over the next few decades. Unfortunately for the Aleuts, there were many more in Chuprov's mold than in Tolstykh's. Gradually the Russians pushed eastward along the chain of islands, as the sea otter and other fur-bearing animals became too scarce to be profitable. The Aleuts resisted where they could but were overwhelmed by superior weaponry. They were forced to hunt for the Russians, their good behavior and submission guaranteed by their wives and children held, and often abused, as hostages (Sauer 1802, appendix 56; Okun 1979, 195).

The Russians themselves often suffered during this time because of the frailty of their ships, the incompetence of their crews, or simply because of the unpredictable weather of the north Pacific and Bering Sea. The men who signed on for such voyages were often debt-ridden misfits swept from the streets of the larger Siberian towns. Other crew members were indigenous peoples of the region who had had little experience in the open sea. Some of the captains were inexperienced, and not infrequently subordinated considerations of safety to those of quick profit. Nearly one vessel out of three was lost. Many a Siberian with the gleam of wealth in his eye ended his days with a quick death in icy waters or a lingering one from starvation and exposure on a surf-pounded rocky shore (Brooks 1973, 184; Okun 1979, 175-76; Hulley 1958, 58-59).

By 1760 the Russians had reached the Fox Islands and were intensively hunting around Umnak and Unalaska islands. The Aleuts were beginning to realize that their future was grim indeed unless the hated newcomers could be driven out once and for all. A party of eleven Russians was wiped out on Atka that year as a prelude to a new sense of confrontation (Bancroft 1886, 122). Several armed skirmishes occurred in early 1762, on Unga and Umnak islands, involving the crew of the *Sv. Gavriil*. A number of Aleut women were kidnapped, and, later seeing one of their party murdered, some thirteen jumped into the sea and were drowned. Sergeant Pushkarev in retaliation for this defiance had most of the rest of the women thrown overboard (Berkh 1974, 25-26). Although word of such atrocities was forwarded to the imperial authorities, little was done to prevent them for nearly a decade.

During the winter of 1763-1764, when seven or more Russian vessels were in the eastern Aleutians, a coordinated uprising of the Aleuts occurred. By the following summer four ships wintering on Umnak, Unalaska, and Unimak were destroyed and their crews largely killed by the defiant Aleuts (Black 1980, 94). In a single incident near present-day Nikolski, the Aleuts killed twenty men under Dennis Medvedev and burned his ship. In recent years the archeological remains of this disaster have been identified with certainty. The Aleut oral tradition accords closely with the physical remains (Laughlin 1980, 120-26). A sorry remnant from these bloody encounters was rescued by Stepan Glotov, who was then returning from Kodiak Island (Bancroft 1886, 135-40). These survivors ultimately joined with Ivan Soloviev, nicknamed the "terrible nightingale," to seek their revenge.

Soloviev had independently learned of the Medvedev disaster and was fully prepared when the Aleuts attacked him in force. At the end of the encounter one hundred of them lay dead. He then attacked a village of three hundred, destroying their boats, weapons, and tools, and blowing up their dwellings with bladders filled with gunpowder (Berkh 1974, 41-42; Veniaminov 1984, 251-52). On one occasion he was said to have tied up twelve Aleuts in a line and shot a musket ball through the chest of the first to see how many could be killed with one shot (*in* Shelikhov 1981, 129; see also Golovin 1983, 107). Soloviev and his men systematically destroyed the villages on the islands from Umnak to Akutan Pass, killing hundreds of Aleut warriors. In addition to the loss of able-bodied men, the Aleuts were also deprived of much of their means of subsistence (Black 1980, 94-95). In any event, they were never a serious threat to the Russians again. After 1766 they were a demoralized people and for the next half century were virtually the slaves of the Russians.

In 1764 Catherine II ordered that an official expedition to the Aleutians be organized to make accurate charts of the region and to investigate the activities of the *promyshlenniki*, particularly with regard to the collection of tribute. Captain-Lieutenant Petr Krenitsyn was given command, assisted by Lt. Mikhail Levashov. After many delays, they finally reached the Aleutians in August 1768 and surveyed Umnak, Unalaska, and the so-called Krenitsyn Islands to the east. They also visited Unimak Island and the Alaska Peninsula, both of which were only imperfectly known at that time. Krenitsyn wintered on the eastern part of Unimak Island, where his crew suffered terribly from scurvy. They had very few contacts with the Aleuts, who feared not only the Russians but the Eskimos of the Alaska Peninsula. By May only thirteen could walk. Ultimately thirty-five men died of scurvy, with one account placing the total at sixty-nine (Black 1980, 96). Levashov had wintered on Unalaska Island and was successful in establishing friendly relations with the Aleuts. Despite the relative abundance of food, several of his men became sick. By May, twenty-two men were ill with scurvy. The two ships, their crews decimated by disease, finally rendezvoused in June 1769 and returned with difficulty to Kamchatka, where Krenitsyn drowned. Although the entire expedition was plagued with misfortune, Levashov did succeed in making valuable ethnographic observations on the Aleuts (Glushankov 1973, 204-10; Masterson and Brower 1948, 57-60).

One or two other expeditions deserve brief mention. Captain Cook stopped twice in 1778 in Samganoodha Bay, on Unalaska Island near Unalga Pass. On his return visit he spent over three weeks there repairing his ships, during which time he had a friendly encounter with Gerasim Ismailov, a Russian navigator based at Captain's Harbor at a semi-permanent post established a few years before. John Ledyard, the only American in Cook's crew, was the messenger who went from the ship to the settlement to carry Cook's greetings, and has left a colorful account of his adventure (Ledyard 1963, 90-98). The various diarists of the expedition have much to say about the Aleuts, especially David Samwell, one of the surgeons (Cook 1967, 3(1):265, 460-68; 3(2):1137-52 [Samwell]; Ellis 1782, 1:283-89, 2:45-46).

In June 1786 Gerasim Pribylov of the so-called Lebedev-Lastochkin Company discovered St. George Island and left a crew of hunters for the winter. The following June, on a rare clear day, these hunters discovered the island of St. Paul. Both the islands were unbelievably rich in sea mammals. Within a few years the Russians had imported Aleuts, mostly from Atka and Unalaska, to hunt and live there on a permanent basis (Bancroft 1886, 192-193).

An expedition under Capt. Joseph Billings was sent out by Catherine II to explore, to make scientific observations, to collect tribute, and to investigate allegations of cruelty against the Natives. It was a poorly managed affair from the beginning but also suffered its share of bad luck. In 1790 the *Glory of Russia* sailed to the Aleutians, Kodiak, and Prince William Sound, and then returned to Kamchatka, with scurvy making its appearance among the crew before they reached home (Sauer 1802, 208-9). The following year two ships went to Unalaska and wintered there, with both crews again suffering badly from scurvy (Sauer 1802, 263-76). The narratives of Lt. Gavriil Sarychev (Sarytschew 1807, 2:58-59, 69), Martin Sauer, and especially the physician-naturalist Dr. Merck (1980) contain much of ethnographic and medical interest.

In his report to Catherine II, Billings noted the "abject state of slavery in which these islanders live." The Aleuts were forced to hunt in all kinds of weather and over great distances, and were not even given adequate clothing. While the hunters were gone, the Russians took by force the youngest and most handsome of the women for their "companions." The men who were too weak to go out to hunt were kept "employed in domestic drudgery," while the women were forced to make and mend clothing from inferior material. Any opposition led to cruel punishment or simply murder (Sauer 1802, appendix 55-56; *see also* Chapter 18).

KODIAK AND THE NORTH PACIFIC RIM

Stepan Glotov in 1763 was the first of the *promyshleniki* to reach Kodiak Island, in his eastward search for rich new hunting grounds. The Koniag were ill-disposed to trade and constantly harassed the Russians in their camp. Glotov's men, in fact, suffered greatly from cold, hunger, disease, and hostilities during the winter that followed. Nine perished from scurvy (Coxe 1787, 131).

It is of interest that in the 1840s Holmberg (1985, 57-58) was able to record the recollections of an old man who remembered as a boy of nine or ten this first visit of Europeans to Kodiak. When the Koniag elders were debating whether to trade with the newcomers, an old man wisely counselled: "Who knows what kinds of sickness they may bring us?"

Kodiak Island was left relatively undisturbed thereafter until 1784, when Grigorii Shelikhov, a wealthy and ambitious young merchant of Irkutsk, landed in what he named Three Saints' Bay, with the intention of founding the first permanent Russian settlement in Alaska. Once again the Koniag resented the intrusion and before long a pitched battle occurred, which ended in the deaths of many Natives from cannon fire (Shelikhov 1981, 36-49).

Shelikhov had come to stay and had even brought along his wife. He built storehouses, barracks, and other buildings, and the following spring sent out parties to explore Kodiak Island, Afognak Island, Cook Inlet, and even Prince William Sound. Over the next couple of years he established small posts at Karluk on Kodiak Island (1785), Afognak Island (1786) and Fort Alexandrov, on the Kenai Peninsula (1786) (Fedorova 1973, 136).

The first European in the Prince William Sound area was Bering, whose men visited Kayak Island in July 1741. Steller observed some recent human habitations but no contact was made (Steller 1988, 65-69). Captain Cook arrived at the same location in May 1778 and proceeded northwestward to Hinchinbrook Island and into Prince William Sound. He and his men had several peaceful encounters with the Chugach Eskimos and left valuable descriptions of their appearance and customs (Cook 1967, 3(1):350; 3(2):1111; Rickman 1781, 248-9; Ellis 1782, 2:236-246). During the next few weeks Cook proceeded westward and discovered and explored the inlet (he took it to be a river) that now bears his name. He met Natives, probably Chugach Eskimos, on the west side of the inlet and found them in possession of blue beads and knives doubtless obtained from the Russians.

The following year Ygnacio Arteaga commanded a small Spanish vessel that reached Prince William Sound and the entrance to Cook Inlet before being forced to turn back because of scurvy. His report also contains a few ethnographic observations on the Chugach (Arteaga n.d., 96).

In 1783 the first Russians penetrated Prince William Sound, led by Potap Zaikov, who was based at Unalaska. With three ships and a large contingent of Russians and Aleut hunters, Zaikov stopped first at Kayak Island and then moved his base to Nuchek, on Hinchinbrook Island, where Cook and Arteaga had also stopped. The Russians treated the local Natives in a highhanded manner, as they had been treating the Aleuts for decades, and the Chugach Eskimos answered these indignities with a shower of spears and arrows. The Russians had sent their small hunting and exploring parties in various directions and several of these small detachments were wiped out by the aggressive Eskimos. The survivors established winter quarters on Montague Island, where they passed a grim winter with insufficient food to sustain them. Nearly half of the remaining men died of scurvy before spring (Berkh 1974, 62-63; Masterson and Brower 1948, 91; Bancroft 1886, 186-90).

A somewhat similar fate awaited an English adventurer, John Meares, who reached Prince William Sound in 1786 after a brief sojourn in Cook Inlet. He had spent the summer trading for furs, but in his enthusiasm remained so long he found himself compelled to winter in the sound, near the present village of Tatitlek. The vessel was ill-prepared for such an extended stay, and many members of the crew suffered severely from scurvy, the ship's surgeon being one of the first to die. The Chugach did not attack but instead seemed to be waiting for nature to take its course. At last in May of the following spring a boat from another English vessel, commanded by Captain George Dixon, rescued the wretched survivors. Twenty-three out of a ship's company of forty-seven had perished that winter (Meares 1790, xi-xxxvi; Dixon 1789, 155).

Captains Nathaniel Portlock and George Dixon had sailed to the north Pacific coast for the first time the previous year. After a month of trading in Cook Inlet they had been forced by contrary weather to return to Hawaii. In 1787 they returned north, arriving in April in Prince William Sound. Portlock spent a couple of months at Nuchek and sent smaller boat crews to Cook Inlet and around the sound to trade. Dixon sojourned only briefly in Prince William Sound before moving to Yakutat Bay. The accounts of both voyages give valuable ethnographic information on the Chugaches (Portlock 1789, 248-49; Dixon 1789, 68).

A Spanish expedition under Estaban José Martínez and Gonzalo López de Haro visited the sound in 1788, traded peacefully with the Natives, with the latter even visiting the Russians at Three Saints' Bay and Unalaska (Archer 1980, 136). That same summer the Russians themselves sent Gerasim Izmailov and Dmitrii Bocharov from Kodiak to Prince William Sound to consolidate their claims to the area. Once more the Russians suffered hunger and found themselves in armed conflict with the Chugaches (*in* Shelikhov 1981, 90, 104).

Shelikhov had departed from Three Saints' Bay in 1786, leaving Konstantin Samoilov in charge, but three years later, since the colony seemed to be stagnating, he appointed the Greek Evstrat Delarov as manager. During the latter's tenure Martin Sauer (1802, 171-73) from the Billings Expedition visited the settlement, which he described in 1790 as having fifty Russians and five houses, plus barracks, storehouses, a smithy, and a special building where about three hundred Koniag hostages were housed. Some six hundred skin boats were used for hunting, each with two or three men. The women were employed in curing and drying fish, collecting useful plants, and making clothing.

In 1790 the post of manager of Shelikhov's establishment was given to Aleksandr Baranov, who arrived the following year after suffering shipwreck at Unalaska (Khlebnikov 1973, 2-5). One of the first of his reforms was to move the settlement from Three Saints' Bay, where flooding was becoming a serious problem, to a new site called Pavlovsk, or St. Paul's, Harbor, a more protected area where wood for building and for fuel was available (Bancroft 1886, 324).

In the summer of 1792 Baranov made an exploratory trip to Prince William Sound, where he had a hostile encounter with a Tlingit war party looking for their Chugach enemies near Nuchek (Khlebnikov 1973, 8-9). The next year he established a shipbuilding site, called Voskresenskaia Gavan, near present-day Seward. It was around this time that he took in hand the problem of the company of a rival fur trader Lebedev-Lastochkin, who had established a post called St. George in upper Cook Inlet (Kasilof) in 1786, a second fortified one called Nikolaevsk (Kenai) in 1791, and in 1793 a fort called Fort Constantine and Elena near Nuchek in Prince William Sound (Fedorova 1973, 136). These posts were specifically intended to squeeze out the Shelikhov-Golikov Company, and when Baranov saw his own interests threatened, he highhandedly arrested the manager of the Nikolaevsk post and sent him under guard to Okhotsk (Bancroft 1886, 342; Okun 1979, 35; Tikhmenev 1978, 35).

When Shelikhov was trying to get support for his commercial enterprise from the empress herself, he had written in glowing (and exaggerated) terms about his efforts to convert the Natives in America to the Orthodox faith. He requested that missionaries be sent, and to his surprise Catherine agreed and arranged to send to Kodiak in 1794 no fewer than ten clerics, including Father Ioasaf, the Archimandrite from the Valaam monastery near St.

Petersburg. This contingent of churchmen, who seemed totally unprepared for life in the wild, were thrust, to Baranov's dismay, on the new colony at St. Paul's, where no quarters and no church were available. After much initial friction and mutual antagonism between Baranov and Father Ioasaf (*see* Tikhmenev 1979, 79-82), the missionaries later fanned out to various sites in the colonies, opened schools, and no doubt did much to prevent abuses of the Native people by the fur traders. They also tried to demonstrate that some Russians, at least, were not there simply to exploit them. One of the missionaries, Hieromonk Iuvenalii (or Juvenal) was thought for many years to have been murdered by the Natives near Iliamna Lake in 1796 (Tikhmenev 1978, 47), but more recent evidence suggests that his death occurred at the hands of the Yupik Eskimos near present-day Quinhagak (Oleksa 1987, 14-15).

At the same time, the empress acceded to Shelikhov's repeated requests to send exiled convicts from Siberia to serve as permanent farmers and artisans in the colonies. Some fifty-one persons from twenty-seven families were dispatched from Irkutsk and also arrived at Kodiak in 1794. Most of these died over the next two decades from hunger, overwork, and sickness. In 1823 four survivors and some of their dependents were finally permitted to return to Russia (Sarafian 1977a).

SOUTHEASTERN ALASKA

On July 17, 1741, Abram Dementiev, mate of Chirikov's vessel the *St. Paul,* became perhaps the first European to set foot on the coast of southeastern Alaska. Although the exact location is uncertain, it appears to have been near Salisbury Sound, between Chicagof and Kruzof Islands (although others say further south). Unfortunately, Dementiev did not return to tell the tale, for his entire boat crew and another sent to fetch him disappeared without a trace, victims either of treacherous currents or, more likely, of the local Tlingit Indians (Chirikov 1922, 1:315-17).

The next European ship came a full generation later, in 1775. That year the Spaniard Lt. Juan Francisco de la Bodega y Quadra explored the coast in a tiny vessel as far north as Cross Sound, where a severe outbreak of scurvy in his crew forced him to turn back. Bodega made at least one landing in Alaska, where he had a friendly encounter with the Indians (Moore 1986, 162-169; Mourelle 1920, 47, 51-53).

Captain Cook sailed by southeastern Alaska in May 1778 on his way north but made no landings, though he did name several landmarks, including Mt. Edgecumbe. The following year Bodega reached Alaska again, this time under the command of Lt. Ygnacio Arteaga. The two Spanish vessels, *Favorita* and *Princesa,* respectively, spent several weeks in Bucareli Bay, near present-day Craig. While there the crews began to show signs of sickness and a small hospital had to be set up on shore to accommodate them. At least one victim died (Bodega y Quadra n.d., 15-16). Although relations with the Indians were friendly at first, they became increasingly strained and nearly reached the stage of hostilities. The ships later sailed for Prince William Sound where the men were seriously plagued by scurvy (Arteaga n.d., 75, 97; Tero 1973).

The French joined the quest for furs in 1786 with the voyage of Capt. J. F. G. de La Pérouse. Trending southward from his landfall at Cape St. Elias he entered a natural harbor now known as Lituya Bay. There he remained for nearly a month engaged in trading, exploring, and making scientific observations. Tragedy struck on one occasion when twenty-one officers and men were drowned as their small boats capsized in the perilous currents of the harbor entrance. The report of this expedition contains much interesting ethnographic information on the Tlingit, including some of medical interest (La Pérouse 1799, 2:357-64; Fortuine 1984a, 60-61).

Around this time a number of British and American ships were also trading these waters but left few published records. An exception is Captain Dixon, who in 1787 spent two weeks in Yakutat Bay at a site he called Port Mulgrave. From there he headed southward, pausing briefly for trade near Sitka Sound. His observations on the Tlingit are of special value in this period (Dixon 1789, 172-87). His commanding officer Capt. Nathaniel Portlock also visited this coast in 1787 and remained for two weeks to trade with the Indians at Portlock Harbor, some sixty miles south of Cross Sound (Portlock 1789, 248-49).

The Russian navigators Izmailov and Bocharov sailed from Kodiak in the spring of 1788, arriving at Yakutat Bay in June. There they traded successfully with a large contingent of Chilkat Tlingit and then explored the coast southward as far as Lituya Bay (Tikhmenev 1978, 25; Bancroft 1886, 268-70).

In 1791 a French ship under Etienne Marchand traded in Sitka Bay for nearly two weeks (Fleurieu 1801, 1:189-258) and a Spanish vessel under Alejandro Malaspina visited Yakutat Bay, where they were received in a friendly manner (Cutter 1972, 42-49). Robert Gray, a merchant from Boston, also traded extensively in southeastern Alaska that year (Krause 1956, 22). Then George Vancouver spent the greater part of the summers of 1793 and 1794 charting in detail the bays, inlets, and harbors of the Alexander Archipelago (Vancouver 1798, 2:307-424; 3:216-264). Of these voyages, only that of Marchand has much of medical or even ethnographic value (Fleurieu 1801, 2:217-91).

Baranov first encountered the Tlingit in 1792, when he and his Aleut hunters beat off an attack from them at Nuchek. In 1794 he sent a large expedition of *baidarkas* under Igor Purtov to trade for furs at Yakutat, where he met one of Vancouver's vessels. Negotiations with the Indians there were carried on with considerable suspicion and maneuvering on both sides, but after the exchange of hostages Purtov got away safely with a cargo of furs (Tikhmenev 1979, 50). The next year Zaikov arrived at Yakutat to follow up the trade agreement. Mutual trouble was averted only when relations were interrupted by what was said to be an outbreak of smallpox in two Aleuts (Bancroft 1886, 347-50).

A favorite dream of Shelikhov's was to found an agricultural colony in Russian America, and to this end he requested from the empress the privilege of buying serfs. The summer of 1794 saw the arrival at Kodiak of some thirty families of serfs, together with the large band of exiles and missionaries previously mentioned. Baranov knew that such a colony at Yakutat was impractical, yet he felt obligated to carry out Shelikhov's pledge to the empress. Accordingly, the following summer the serfs and exiles were dutifully taken to Yakutat. Little progress seems to have been accomplished on the colony that year and in 1796 a new manager named Ivan Polomoshnoi accompanied additional settlers. Baranov himself came later that summer with more settlers and workers to help construct fortifications and other buildings. The colony suffered misfortune from the very beginning. Of eighty settlers and hunters, close to a third died of scurvy during the first winter (Tikhmenev 1978, 42-44; Khlebnikov 1973, 20; *see also* Hanable 1973, 78).

THE BERING SEA AND NORTHWARD

In the late summer of 1728 Vitus Bering was sailing northward in his tiny vessel *St. Gabriel* to determine whether the continents of Asia and America were joined. Rounding Cape Chukotski, he sighted an island on August 11 to which he gave the name of St. Lawrence—the first European glimpse of what is now Alaska. One of his men was sent ashore to find Natives but saw only empty huts. The ship continued north, passing through what is now known as Bering Strait on the western side. On the return trip Bering sighted and named one of the Diomede Islands, but fog veiled the American shore (Golder 1914, 145-46).

Credit for the first European sighting of the northern mainland of Alaska must go to an obscure Russian surveyor named Mikhail Gvozdev. In August 1732 he sailed northeast from Cape Chukotski and reached the Diomede Islands. Attempts to land on the larger island were met with a shower of arrows, and musket fire was offered in return. After a landing elsewhere they met other Natives, but all refused to pay the requested tribute. From the island they were able to see the "Large Country," the mainland of Alaska. After attempting a landing on Little Diomede, and meeting a hostile reception there as well, Gvozdev sailed for the mainland on August 21, passing close enough to the shore, probably near Wales, to see the Native huts. Without attempting to land there they sailed southwest and on August 22 sighted what was probably King Island, where a man dressed in a shirt of whale intestines paddled out in a skin boat and talked with them (I. Skurikhin *in* Dmytryshyn and Crownhart-Vaughan 1986, 132-34; Gvozdev *in* Golder 1914, 160-62; D. Ray 1975, 22-26).

Captain Cook left Unalaska in July 1778 and sailed along the north coast of the Alaska Peninsula to Bristol Bay, rounded Cape Newenham and found himself in the shoaling waters of Kuskokwim Bay, where his crew met several Eskimos. Thereafter he stood out to sea and next sighted land at Sledge Island, near Nome, where his men landed but found no Natives. Continuing northward, he sighted (and named) King Island and Cape Prince of Wales before ultimately being stopped by sea ice near Icy Cape. On his return trip Cook passed St. Lawrence Island and entered Norton Sound, which he explored in some detail. During this phase of the voyage, Cook and his men met several groups of Eskimos whom they described at length (Cook 1967, 3(1):403, 438; 3(2): 1439-40; Ellis 1782, 1:330-31, 2:12-16).

In 1779 a Cossack named Ivan Kobelev was sent from Siberia to visit the Diomede Islands, which he did in July of that year. There he found a large village on Big Diomede and a smaller one of about 160 persons on Little Diomede (D. Ray 1975, 33-34).

The next visitors to leave a record of the northern Natives were from the Billings Expedition in July 1791. The *Glory of Russia* spent four days near Cook's Cape Rodney, where the men traded in a friendly manner with the Eskimos. Some valuable ethnographic accounts, with a few medical observations, resulted from these encounters (Sarytschew 1807, 2:45; Merck 1980, 190).

Kobelev, this time accompanied by Nikolai Daurkin, returned to the Diomede Islands in 1791 and had peaceful trade with the Eskimos there for several days. On June 11 he visited the mainland village of Kigigmen (Wales) but found it deserted, possibly because of a famine but more likely because of fear of a Chukchi attack. The two Russians passed along the coast, noting many small deserted settlements, and finally put out to sea once more. They visited King Island, where they were hospitably received, before returning to Siberia (D. Ray 1975, 52-55).

THE EIGHTEENTH CENTURY IN RETROSPECT

The keynotes of eighteenth century Alaskan history might be listed as courage, greed, violence, and hardship. These qualities were particularly evident in the contacts and relationships between the Russians and the Aleuts, but to a lesser extent they may be traced throughout the first seventy years of recorded history in Alaska. Certainly explorers such as Bering and Cook, or the *promyshlenniki* such as Tolstykh or even the bloody Soloviev, did not lack courage in facing the unknown. And the nameless but brave Aleuts, Koniag, Chugach, and Tlingit, who fought to the death with inadequate weapons to save their lives and families, were equally endowed with courage. Greed was of course a prominent motive among the Russian *promyshlenniki,* but it equally well motivated the English, Spanish, and French who sailed the coasts looking for the sea otter and other valuable mammals. The Native people were not without greed themselves in their willingness to trade their abundant furs for the tools and trinkets of a different culture. Violence marked a distressing number of encounters between the Natives and the newcomers, some of it pure aggression, some of it self-defense, and some of it simply wanton cruelty perpetrated by the stronger on the weaker. Finally, countless individuals suffered hardship on both sides, not only as a direct result of violent encounters with each other, but also from disease, hunger, exposure, and the loss of friends and loved ones.

What are the health implications of these eighteenth-century events? The principal recurrent themes are trauma and hunger. Both Europeans and Natives found themselves exposed to many new kinds of danger. The Europeans, for example, had little experience with the capricious but violent weather of the high latitudes both at sea and on land, and many victims of drowning and cold injury were the result. The Natives of course were faced for the first time with firearms ranging from muskets to cannons. Scurvy was a problem that affected primarily the Europeans, who tried to subsist for long periods on salt meat and ship's biscuit, usually with disastrous results. The Native people, with their regular use of plant food and fresh meat, rarely developed scurvy (Fortuine 1988a, 35-39), but families often suffered hunger and even starvation as a result of the death or enforced long absence of the father and other hunters.

By the close of the century there had been few epidemics recorded in Alaska except for smallpox in southeastern Alaska and a couple other small outbreaks of disease. It is likely that syphilis and probably tuberculosis had already been introduced to the Native peoples by the Russians. Alcohol abuse was a problem primarily of the Russians, not the Natives.

In 1798 the Aleuts were by and large a subject race, as were the Koniag and probably the Chugach. The original numbers of each had greatly decreased due to violence, starvation, and disease. By 1798 the lives of very few of these peoples were untouched by the Russians. Although the Indians of southeastern Alaska had had many brief encounters, some of them violent, with the Russians and other Europeans, they were able to maintain their traditional life and values intact. At this time the Eskimos north of the Alaska Peninsula and the Athapaskans of the interior were virtually untouched culturally except for the gradual acquisition of new technology through trade.

6

The Years of the Russian-American Company: 1799-1867

SITKA AND SOUTHEASTERN ALASKA

The year 1799 was pivotal in the history of Alaska. In July Tsar Paul I granted a charter to the new Russian-American Company, which was to have exclusive trading privileges in the colonies for a period of twenty years. Baranov was appointed chief manager of the new company, which amalgamated the Shelikhov-Golikov Company with several of its rivals. That same year Baranov had undertaken to move his base of operations from Kodiak to southeastern Alaska, where he saw the future of the fur trade to lie, but calamity repeatedly dogged his efforts. In the spring Baranov set out with twenty-two Russians in two small vessels, accompanied by a fleet of several hundred *baidarkas* with Native hunters. The flotilla made its way to Prince William Sound, where it was joined by an additional 250 *baidarkas* that had wintered at Nuchek (Bancroft 1886, 386; Hulley 1958, 123; Andrews 1945, 50).

As they left the sound, however, thirty *baidarkas* were swamped in heavy seas, with the loss of sixty persons. Stopping that night on a beach, the party was attacked by the Tlingit. Moving on to the post at Yakutat, Baranov found the settlers in a wretched, quarrelsome, and starving condition. When the expedition finally reached Sitka Sound, work had already begun on a fort called St. Michael Redoubt about six miles north of present-day Sitka. Building continued through the summer, and by the end Baranov felt he could send a substantial number of Aleuts back to Kodiak. As the large fleet of skin boats headed north, they stopped for the night at the site now known as Peril Strait, where at least a hundred Aleuts died from eating poisoned mussels (*see* Chapter 2). A small party, including Baranov, wintered over at the fort to finish the buildings.

This forlorn group suffered from cold, hunger, and scurvy. To compound their troubles they heard that an epidemic of respiratory disease had occurred at Yakutat, with further loss of life. Baranov himself left for Kodiak late in 1800, finding his outposts in Prince William Sound, Cook Inlet, and the Aleutians short of provisions and threatened by hostile Natives (Tikhmenev 1978, 63; Andrews 1945, 50).

The fledgling colony at St. Michael thus had an uneasy start, further endangered by the many American and British ships bartering guns and liquor for furs among the surrounding Indians. In June 1802 the ultimate disaster struck the settlement. While many Aleut hunters were away, the Tlingit staged a surprise attack on the fort, killing all the twenty or so males and carrying away over thirty women and children as slaves (Tikhmenev 1979, 134-39). A few frightened survivors watched the fort burn from the woods, where luckily they had been at the time of the attack, and later they were able to attract the attention of some foreign vessels nearby. By deception a British captain named Henry Barber managed to capture the Tlingit leaders, whom he exchanged for the Russian and Aleut survivors. He then sailed for Kodiak, where he blackmailed Baranov with an exorbitant ransom demand for the return of the Russians and Aleuts (Schuhmacher 1979). Other stragglers were killed by the Tlingit or ultimately made their way to Yakutat, where Indians also attacked that year (Tikhmenev 1978, 65-66; Tikhmenev 1979, 151, 174).

In 1804 Baranov returned to Sitka in force and burning for revenge. A Russian warship, the *Neva,* commanded by Captain Lisianskii, had already arrived, and once forces were joined the ship's cannons bombarded and destroyed the Tlingit village and fort. On the same site, the new and stronger fort known as New Archangel, or Sitka, was built (Lisiansky 1814, 149-68, 235-44; Tikhmenev 1979, 149).

The following August Count Nikolai Rezanov, the High Chamberlain of the Tsar, arrived in Sitka together with his personal physician, the German naturalist Georg H. von Langsdorff. (*See* Figure 8.) The winter that followed was bleak, stormy, and offered the specter of starvation to the some two hundred Russians and Creoles at the fort. Heavy gales caused several company vessels bringing supplies to founder and also wiped out half the *baidarka* fleet, with heavy loss of life. To darken the Russians' spirits further, word was received that their settlement at Yakutat was wiped out by the Tlingit (Hanable 1973, 79). Native rebellion spread to Prince William Sound and even to Cook Inlet but was effectively checked before serious harm resulted. A party of two hundred Aleut hunters returning to Kodiak around this time perished at sea because of their unwillingness to land when they had received word of the disaster at Yakutat (Gedeon *in* Pierce 1978, 143; Bancroft 1886, 455-56).

Meanwhile conditions became increasingly serious at New Archangel. Because of the weather and the hostility of the Tlingit, hunting and fishing

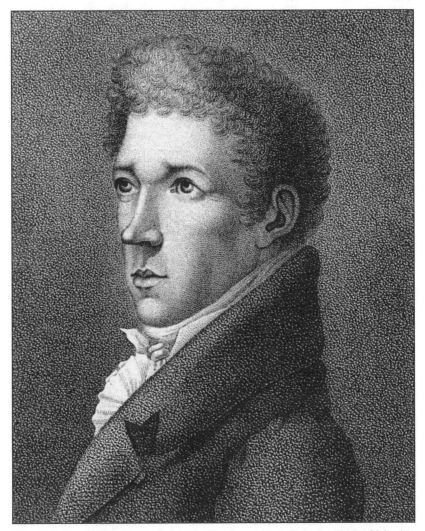

Figure 8. Dr. Georg H. von Langsdorff, who visited Sitka in 1805-1806 with Rezanov. (Langsdorff 1814.)

were out of the question. Scurvy broke out in January, killing eight and incapacitating sixty, despite the fact that Baranov had purchased an American ship *Juno* and her cargo of foodstuffs in the fall (D'Wolf 1861, 52-54). As an act of desperation, Rezanov took most of the able men who remained and sailed to the California coast in the *Juno* to purchase food from the Spanish colonies. Returning in June 1806, he found the contingent at Sitka beginning to recover by taking advantage of a good spring herring run and by purchasing some food from visiting American trading vessels (Rezanov 1926, 5-8, 68-69). Rezanov left for home in September and died while crossing Siberia, but not before he had sent a series of reports to the tsar and the board of directors, including recommendations for the future of the colony (Tikhmenev 1979, 149-151, 153-227). Langsdorff (1814, 2:93-96) also wrote an account of his experiences in Russian America, including a detailed description of the terrible living conditions of squalor and scurvy suffered by the Russian and Creole workers at Sitka (*see* Chapter 18).

After these recurrent and demoralizing misfortunes, conditions began to improve gradually in the colony. Baranov made New Archangel his permanent headquarters after several further sojourns in Kodiak. He continued trading arrangements with American ships, despite official displeasure that they continued to sell firearms and alcohol to the Indians. As a way of assuring a future food supply for the colony, Baranov in 1812 also established a post called Fort Ross on the northern California coast (Tikhmenev 1979, 133-42). For the same reason the chief manager wished to expand trade relations with Hawaii. In 1815 he sent there a German physician named Georg Schäffer, who had arrived the previous year in Sitka on the naval vessel *Suvorov,* but the doctor exceeded his instructions by attempting to annex the islands for Russia, thereby causing considerable official embarrassment (Pierce 1967, 71-82).

Partly as a result of Rezanov's recommendations, regular supply ships began to come from Russia, either via Okhotsk or by the circumnavigation route. Some of these vessels also brought inspectors from the government or company headquarters at St. Petersburg. Baranov around this time was physically and emotionally exhausted and frequently requested a replacement to be sent from Russia (Tikhmenev 1979, 144, 187; Berkh 1979, 43; Khlebnikov 1973, 85). At least two men chosen for the job died before reaching Sitka, one in Okhotsk, and one on the wreck of the *Neva* in 1813, almost within sight of Sitka (Khlebnikov 1976, 15; Berkh 1979, 37). Baranov kept his post until 1818, when he was somewhat unceremoniously removed and replaced by Captain-Lieutenant L. A. Hagemeister, who himself left within one year because of poor health (Pierce 1984, 128, 151). Baranov, who had almost become a legend in Alaska, died the following year en route to Russia. Virtually all subsequent chief managers were naval officers detailed to the Russian-American Company.

Under the second charter, which ran from 1821 to 1841, the company was governed on a far more formal basis, with greater attention to discipline, and guided by detailed regulations covering every aspect of life. Many rules specifically safeguarded the rights and privileges of the workers, including Creoles and Natives. Conditions in the lonely outposts also improved, with the beginnings of schools, missions, and even hospitals (Sarafian 1971).

In 1821 the tsar tried to exclude all foreign vessels from within a hundred miles of the Alaskan coast, but the United States and Great Britain immediately protested. Formal agreements with both of these countries a few years later essentially restored free trade, and defined the boundaries of Russian America (Hulley 1958, 147-151). Both of these conventions had expired by 1835 and Russia declined to renew them. By this time the Hudson's Bay Company had entered into competition in the Stikine River area, causing the Russians to build Fort Dionysius in 1833 near present-day Wrangell. In 1839 the coastal strip from Cross Sound southward was leased to the Hudson's Bay Company. Fort Dionysius and another post taken over by the British in southeastern Alaska had several hostile encounters with the Indians (Hulley 1958, 160-64; Tikhmenev 1978, 169-73).

Under the third charter, which ran from 1841 to 1861, the governors were again largely naval officers. By mutual agreement with the Hudson's Bay Company, no liquor or firearms could be sold to the Natives; in fact liquor was forbidden to be sold anywhere in the colonies. Economic conditions remained marginal, as the fur trade continued to decline. The Russian-American Company became increasingly involved in alternative economic activities, such as shipbuilding, whaling, and the tea trade with the Orient. Two new sources of income were the outgrowth of the California Gold Rush in 1849, namely the virtual emptying of company warehouses to supply the needs of the miners and the shipment of ice from Alaska to San Francisco, this latter trade lasting right up to 1867 (Bancroft 1886, 568-69; Hulley 1958, 174-78).

The round of daily life at Sitka evolved considerably over the early nineteenth century. The first years of the settlement were marked by hunger, disease, and the constant threat of Indian attack. Life was bad, with little relief except boredom from the daily drudgery of work. Alcohol flowed freely, including the locally fermented concoction known as *kvass*. The

Russian workers were a crude, unlettered lot, often from the dregs of Siberian society, not a few of them former convicts. They drank hard, worked as little as possible, and were often surly and sometimes even mutinous. They were paid in company shares and most were hopelessly in debt (Okun 1979, 175-77).

Many of the men took Aleut or Koniag concubines or wives, Baranov himself having lived for years with a Kenaitze chief's daughter who bore him several children. The children of their unions, who were Creoles, had a special status in the colony and many showed considerable talent and leadership ability in the next generation of the company. Among them were noted explorers, priests, traders, navigators, and *feldshers*, the latter trained medical practitioners most closely comparable to modern physician's assistants (Barbara Smith 1980, 6; Khlebnikov 1976, 95).

The company employed as hunters at Sitka hundreds of Aleuts and Koniag, nearly all of them having made the long journey by water in their own small skin boats. These Natives were the lifeblood of the company's business, yet they were treated harshly and unfairly, often being made to go to sea in dangerous weather to hunt while the women were forced to gather food, sew clothing, and serve the whims of the Russians at the fort. Also at the fort were Tlingit hostages, frequently sons of the local headmen, who were to guarantee the peace (Tikhmenev 1978, 154-55). These hostages were treated reasonably well but kept under close guard. Sometimes in return the Russians gave a few Creoles as hostages to the Tlingit.

Throughout the years of the Russian-American Company the Tlingit maintained a sullen hostility toward the Russians, who were forced to be constantly on their guard. Trading was only permitted under careful surveillance and no more than a few Indians were permitted into the fort at one time. The most serious encounter took place as late as 1855, and resulted in two Russians dead and seventeen wounded, with the Tlingit suffering some sixty casualties (Tikhmenev 1978, 353; Okun 1979, 209).

Health conditions in the early period were poor because of the dangerous life, damp weather, crowded housing, and periodic food shortages. The commonest disorders were sores, scurvy, colic, eye diseases, and, among the Tlingit, smallpox (Tikhmenev 1978, 83).

During the 1820s and 1830s the quality of life at Sitka improved somewhat. The new administration enforced discipline to a much greater extent, including the control of alcohol consumption and the prohibition of abuse of the Natives. Some of the officers brought their wives and children to Alaska and refurbished their homes with some of the elegance they were used to in St. Petersburg. The governor's residence on the headland overlooking the harbor became the social center of the colony. Among the ruling elite, the evenings were spent in masked balls, concerts, and whist, with French the language of the drawing room.

Sitka's first church was built in 1816 but was rather inactive in the earlier years. Father Ivan Veniaminov, the Russian Orthodox missionary who had served in Unalaska for ten years, came to New Archangel in 1834, but despite his genius and hard work, he was unable to make much progress in converting the Tlingit until a disastrous smallpox epidemic in 1835-1837 demonstrated the powerlessness of their shamans (*see* Chapter 13).

The lives of the Russians and Creoles gradually improved over the years. The old share system was finally concerted to a cash salary, but many employees remained so heavily in debt they could not leave the colony. Medical services had become available in 1820 and were constantly improving. The prohibition of alcohol probably distressed them but it no doubt improved their health and productivity.

In the last twenty-five years of the Russian-American Company, life at New Archangel, at least for the officers, took on a certain air of imperial decadence. The wives of the governors entertained in elegant and lavish style (Hulley 1958, 177-80; Golovin 1983, 91, 114). Music was readily available and only the finest champagnes and liqueurs were served. In describing a farewell dinner in 1842, Sir George Simpson, chief factor of the Hudson's Bay Company, wrote, "The glass, the plate, and the appointments in general were very costly; the viands were excellent; and Governor Etolin played the part of the host to perfection" (*in* Brooks 1973, 217). At this time the town supported a bishop, assisted by several priests, deacons, and followers. There was even a Lutheran church, which served many of the Finnish seamen and other foreign employees. Two important church buildings were begun in 1844—the cathedral of St. Michael Archangel, which was dedicated in 1848, and another substantial building that was to serve as a seminary (Bensin n.d., 51, 53). This latter structure was later to be converted to a hospital.

After 1844 there were two mission schools, one for boys and one for girls, each with about thirty to forty students, mostly Creoles. The boys, if they did well in school, went on to attend the Colonial Academy, which provided technical training in the natural sciences, mathematics, and languages. These graduates were obligated to serve the company for ten to fifteen years, which some of them did with considerable distinction. The girls learned needlework, languages, geography, history, and other knowledge thought at the time to be proper for their sex (Tikhmenev 1978, 387-89; Hulley 1953, 178-79).

Although life for the ordinary worker had gradually improved, it was hardly enviable. Starvation was no longer a threat, although the ample food could be monotonous. Both the workers and their wives were often drunk, and Sir George Simpson (1847, 2:190) thought that the majority looked sallow and unhealthy. The principal diseases treated at the hospital, according to him, were "typhus and continued fevers, pulmonary complaints, syphilis, affections of the eye, and haemoptysis."

By the end of the Russian administration New Archangel had a population of about 2500 persons, many of them children. Dominating the fine harbor facilities were the large refurbished governor's residence, later known as "Baranov's Castle," and the Cathedral of St. Michael Archangel, the former the workplace of a prince and the latter of a bishop. Public facilities had continued to increase over the years and now included two other Orthodox and the Lutheran church, several schools, a library, a theater, and a forty-bed hospital. For the officers life was increasingly genteel, but for the employees it was disciplined, with required church attendance, uniforms, and many regulations, including strict ones governing relations with the Natives, and—perhaps even tougher—limiting drinking to only two rations of liquor per week. By the 1850s more and more of the middle-level jobs of the company were held by Creoles, who had been born and educated in the company's service (Tikhmenev 1978, 422, 446).

KODIAK, THE ALEUTIANS, AND THE PACIFIC RIM

When Baranov left his settlement of St. Paul's on Kodiak Island in 1799, accompanied by a huge fleet of *baidarkas,* he had probably already made up his mind to transfer his base of operations to southeastern Alaska permanently. The succession of major disasters must have given him pause, but by 1808 the new settlement was on a firm footing and New Archangel had become the capital of Russian America. Thereafter, the relative importance of Kodiak declined, not least because of the great loss of lives, many of them Koniag, associated with the founding of the new capital. Throughout the remaining years of the Russian-American Company, however, Kodiak, because of its location and resources, maintained its place as a seaport, shipbuilding site, and trade and administrative center for the small posts in the Kodiak Island group, Cook Inlet, Alaska Peninsula, and Prince William Sound.

When Count Rezanov stopped at St. Paul's Harbor for several weeks in 1805 he was greatly disappointed with what he saw. The buildings were drafty and badly constructed, and trade goods were of poor quality. Despite the promises of Shelikhov a decade before, church work had made relatively little progress and the school consisted of the older children teaching the younger (Tikhmenev 1978, 83). During his short stay, however, Rezanov established a proper school, to be run by the missionaries, and pretentiously called it the "Imperial Academy of Science in Russian America." To equip the school's library he donated many fine books that he had brought from halfway around the world (Bancroft 1886, 449). He also arranged that ten people, usually Creoles, should be sent on each transport ship to Russia for higher education, including navigation and medicine. Rezanov made clear that these students were first to be vaccinated against smallpox (Tikhmenev 1978, 92). That this precaution was not always followed is shown by a report about a decade later of a promising student who had died of smallpox on the way to St. Petersburg (University of Alaska 1936-1938, 4:142).

Rezanov went on to establish a school for Creole girls, a local court for handling abuses, including quarrels between Natives and Russians, and even planned to set up a hospital for the use of both the company employees and the Natives (Tikhmenev 1978, 93). It may have been Rezanov's influence that caused Dr. Karl Mordgorst, surgeon of the *Neva*, to be temporarily posted to Kodiak in 1807-1808 (*see* Chapter 7). In his recommendations to the directors of the company, the count urged that more attention be paid to selecting for employment men in good health. He further recommended that the administration give more attention to the morals of their employees, and that they be restrained from drunkenness (Tikhmenev 1978, 94-95).

The first missionaries who had arrived at St. Paul's Harbor in 1794 had had no church and a rather hostile environment in which to work. By 1796 they had built a church and begun to fan out to other parts of Kodiak Island, the Alaska Peninsula, the Aleutians, Kenai Peninsula, and eastward as far as Yakutat. Life was by no means easy. Father Iuvenalii, as previously noted, headed westward over the Alaska Peninsula and met his death at the hands of the Natives within a year. Father Makarii was witness to many abuses of the Aleuts and had his life threatened by the *promyshlenniki*. Archimandrite Ioasaf was sent to Irkutsk to be consecrated as bishop in 1799 but was shipwrecked and drowned during his return trip to Kodiak. Throughout, the churchmen railed against the drunken and immoral life of the fur traders in general and Baranov in particular. Hieromonk Gedeon (or Gideon) was sent by the Holy Synod to investigate clerical abuses in the colonies and in 1804 arrived in Kodiak with Captain Lisianskii on the *Neva*. While there he also established schools, appointed Father Herman (or German) as head of the mission and incidentally left a detailed and extremely valuable ethnographic account, including an analysis of traditional Koniag medical practices (Black 1977, 94-99; Pierce 1978, 127-36). The subsequent history of the Orthodox Church in Russian America was dominated by three men: Father Herman, Father Veniaminov and Father Netsvetov (Bensin n.d.).

Father Herman had arrived with the original missionaries in 1794, and until his death in 1837 labored quietly as a hermit and teacher on Spruce Island, where he built a school and orphanage. During a terrible epidemic at Kodiak in 1819 he rendered special services to the sick and was even credited with miraculous cures. He predicted that an epidemic would occur at the time of his death, which in fact took place during the great smallpox epidemic (Pierce 1978, 69-70; *see also* Chapter 11). This humble worker was canonized by the Orthodox Church of America in 1970 as St. Herman of Alaska.

Father Ivan Veniaminov arrived in Alaska in 1824 as missionary to the Aleuts. He spent ten years at Unalaska, during which time he had a profound effect on the region and its people. Not only did he build a church, a school, and a weather observatory, largely with his own hands, but also plunged enthusiastically into a study of the language, history, and culture of the Aleuts. He compiled an Aleut-Russian dictionary and gave the Aleuts their first written language—still in use today in liturgical services. There was no aspect of Aleut life that escaped his notice or his sympathetic interest, including much of what is known about early Aleut medical practices (Veniaminov 1984, 290-293). Father Veniaminov was transferred to Sitka in 1834 and in 1840 became Archimandrite Innokentii and the first Bishop of Kamchatka, the Kuriles, and the Aleutians. In 1868 the former Alaskan missionary was appointed Metropolitan of Moscow, the highest position in the Russian Orthodox Church. On October 6, 1977, he was also canonized, as St. Innocent of Alaska (Veniaminov 1984, vi-xiv).

Father Iakov Netsvetov in a way represented the future of the Orthodox Church in Alaska. He was a Creole trained at the seminary in Irkutsk, where Veniaminov had studied. Netsvetov was assigned in 1828 to the Atka District, where he ministered to the people of the surrounding islands for nearly sixteen years. In 1845 he was transferred to the new outpost known as the Kwikpak Mission at Ikogmiut on the lower Yukon, serving there another seventeen years (Barbara Smith 1980, 5-6). He was an inveterate diarist and his journals have been recently published, giving much insight into life in the Aleutians and in southwestern Alaska during this period (Netsvetov 1980; 1984). In the Unalaska and Atka districts the posts were small, lonely, and stormy. There were only a few permanent settlements, such as Captain's Bay (Iliuliuk) on Unalaska and Korovin Bay on Atka, in both of which a church, small school, and clinic were built, but which afforded few other comforts of civilization.

St. Paul's Harbor (Kodiak), on the other hand, was not only larger, but also enjoyed a more favorable location, climate, and soil. Wood for shipbuilding, for example, was abundant near the settlement. The perennial problem of food supply in the colonies prompted several agricultural experiments around the Kodiak District. After the predictable failure of the agricultural project at Yakutat, attempts were made to grow grain and garden vegetables in small plots around Kodiak. Even tobacco was grown, although it did not go to seed (Tikhmenev 1978, 84). Small-scale farming was also tried in other parts of Kodiak and the other districts but with little success, except for turnips, radishes, potatoes, and a few other vegetables. Although agriculture was basically a failure, some success in raising livestock was achieved. On Kodiak and on some of the Aleutian Islands, cattle, pigs, and chickens were kept and provided some variety to the otherwise monotonous diet of *iukola,* or dried fish (Gibson 1976, 93-97).

Although home-grown and Native foods supplied much of the provisions necessary for maintenance of the colonies, the Russians also depended heavily on supply ships from Okhotsk or even St. Petersburg. These ships brought out flour, butter, beef, and other commodities and returned with a load of furs (Gibson 1976, 82). It was the uncertainty of these voyages, some of which ended in shipwreck, that prompted the search for alternative and closer sources of food, such as the Fort Ross colony in California and trade relations with Hawaii.

Life for the Russians and Creoles was often hard, but it was nothing compared to that of the Koniag, Aleuts, Chugach, and Kenaitze that lived in proximity to the Russian settlements and outposts. Most overt abuses had been officially prohibited since the eighteenth century, but the Natives still often suffered at the hands of cruel foremen, especially in the smaller, more isolated posts. Dr. Langsdorff (1814, 2:70) reported that he personally observed some Aleuts (Koniag?) being tortured to death by *promyshlenniki* in 1805. Rezanov the same year shipped a Russian hunter in irons from Atka to Irkutsk for having beaten an Aleut woman and her infant son to death. It seems apparent that abuses continued for many years, including the forcible abduction of women, despite vigorous company policies to the contrary (Langsdorff 1814, 2:91; Sarafian 1971, 181-87; *see also* Chapter 18).

Besides physical abuse, many Native people suffered hardship simply by the loss of their freedom to live as independent families in their traditional cultural milieu. Native hunters, especially Aleuts and Koniag, were forced to go to sea in their skin boats repeatedly in all kinds of weather and were under continual pressure to produce results. Their wives and children, although perhaps no longer technically hostages as in earlier times, were left at home alone for months and even years, especially if sons or husbands were sent to faraway places such as Sitka, Fort Ross, or the Pribilofs (Okun 1979, 194-95). Without the means to hunt or fish themselves in the traditional manner, the women and their residual families became more and more dependent on European food, which frequently was insufficient in supply and quality.

Health patterns were also changing. Introduced diseases such as syphilis and tuberculosis, plus epidemic plagues, particularly smallpox, broke the health of these once proud peoples. Demoralization resulting from the loss of cultural pride also played a role in the progressive decline in population. Although some effort was made by the company to reverse these trends, the attitude in St. Petersburg seemed to be that the gradual extinction of the Natives was an act of God (Sarafian 1971, 196).

By the first years of the nineteenth century most of the coastal regions of the northern Pacific rim had been explored, although much hydrographic work remained to be done. In the constant search for new fur resources, however, some attention began to be directed toward going beyond the coast and into the vast interior along the major waterways. These expeditions led to some of the first European contacts with the Athapaskan tribes.

The Copper River had been first ascended in 1783 by Leontii Nagaev, who was one of those who sailed with Zaikov that year from Unalaska. Nagaev himself apparently met only Chugach Eskimos, although he heard of the Copper River Natives, presumably Ahtna (or possibly Eyak Indians), who lived further upriver (Bancroft 1886, 191). Other early attempts were made to ascend the river, including that of Konstantin Samoilov, who was killed by the Ahtna in 1796, and the *promyshlennik* Potochkin, who wintered along the river in 1798-1799. In 1803 a Russian named Bazhenov ascended the river for two hundred miles but on a subsequent journey he also was killed by the Indians.

In 1818 the trading agent A. I. Klimovskii, a Creole, reached the confluence of the Copper and Chitina rivers (perhaps as far as the mouth of the Gulkana River), and on his return journey built a cabin on the east bank of the Copper. By 1822 the company had established a trading post there, but it was apparently soon abandoned. In 1843 Grigoriev, setting off from Nuchek, reached Tazlina Lake in the Copper River. Four years later Ens. R. Serebrennikov and a party of ten Creoles ascended the Copper River, wintered at Taral, then reached Tazlina Lake the following spring. After further travels in the vicinity, the entire party was wiped out by the Ahtna (Hanable 1982, 24-28).

The Susitna River, emptying into northern Cook Inlet, was apparently not the object of systematic exploration until relatively late, although the Russians had maintained permanent trading posts on Cook Inlet since the 1780s. The only explorer of record appears to be a certain Malakhov, who ascended the river in 1834 and then extended his explorations a decade later. Although he undoubtedly met Tanaina Indians, no narrative of his journey seems to have survived (Brooks 1973, 235).

BRISTOL BAY TO NORTON SOUND

Baranov, in one of his last acts as chief manager, sent out an expedition under Petr Korsakovskii in 1818 to explore the land around Nushagak Bay, and to establish a fort and trading post there. The party crossed the Alaska Peninsula to Lake Iliamna, then descended the Kvichak River to Bristol Bay. After exploring Nushagak Bay they proceeded westward and even rounded Cape Newenham before turning back (Tikhmenev 1978, 158-159). The following summer Korsakovskii led another expedition into Bristol Bay and that year established a trading post at the mouth of the Nushagak River (Vanstone 1988, 8). A talented Creole named Fedor Kolmakov, who was left in charge of the new Alexandrov Redoubt, established friendly trade relations with the surrounding Eskimos and even converted some of them to Christianity (Tikhmenev 1978, 180). The post never achieved great importance because of the indifference to trade of the local Eskimos. It included a manager, some twenty employees, and an Orthodox mission. Tobacco was one of the trade items in greatest demand (Tikhmenev 1978, 425).

In 1821 two vessels, under the command of V. S. Khromchenko and Arvid Adolf Etholin, explored the western part of Bristol Bay, Kuskokwim Bay, Nunivak Island, and parts of Norton Sound. Khromchenko left some interesting ethnographic and medical observations of the Eskimos in these regions, including his belief that syphilis occurred among them

(Khromchenko 1973). The following summer both Khromchenko and Etholin continued their explorations in this area.

In 1829 Ens. Ivan Ya. Vasilev led an exploring party up the Nushagak River and westward over to the Upper Tikchik Lakes. Later that summer he also explored the Wood River and Alegnagik Lake. The following year he succeeded in reaching the Kuskokwim River, via the Holitna River, and descended it to its mouth (VanStone 1988, 77-109). Accompanying Vasilev on this memorable journey were Kolmakov and another Creole named Semen Lukin, who later returned to the Kuskokwim to establish a post first on the Holitna River in 1832 and the following year on the Kuskokwim. A third post became known as Fort Kolmakov in 1841 and remained the center of Russian trade and influence on the Kuskokwim (VanStone 1967, 11; Oswalt 1980). From their new base on the Kuskokwim, Lukin and others ranged widely, trading with the Eskimos and Indians of the interior.

Kolmakov Redoubt was located on the south bank of the Kuskokwim a few miles above the present town of Aniak. The site has been thoroughly excavated in recent years (Oswalt 1980). In 1841 the population at the fort was forty-two, of whom fifteen were adult men and the rest women and children. About half of the men were Creoles and the remainder of the workers were Eskimos who received their pay in trade goods. Although this was the only post serving a large area, it was never a profitable one because of the difficulties in reaching it (Zagoskin 1967, 252-54). It was finally abandoned in 1866 (Oswalt 1980).

In 1833 Lt. Mikhail Tebenkov, a talented navigator and later governor of the colonies, built a post called St. Michael on an island near the northern mouth of the Yukon. This station soon became the focus of all Russian trading activity in the northern sector, including the lower Yukon River. Because of its strategic position, it controlled trade both on the Yukon and along the shores of Norton Sound. The fort also later gained importance as ships, particularly whalers, increased their numbers in the Bering Sea. In 1845 the post included a house for the manager, barracks for the workers, warehouses, a bathhouse, kitchen, and other buildings surrounded by a log palisade with watchtowers equipped with six small cannon. Such fortifications were felt to be necessary after a concerted attack on the fort by the Eskimos in 1836. Although there were originally two Native villages on the island, one of them was decimated by the smallpox epidemic in 1838-1839. In 1842 an Orthodox chapel was built and in 1845 a church was established outside the walls of the fort (Zagoskin 1967, 96-100).

The same winter the post was built, the Creole Andrei Glazunov left St. Michael with a small party, crossed the eastern shore of Norton Sound, and descended the Anvik River to the Yukon, where in a half-starved condition they were assisted by the Athapaskan Indians. Glazunov continued downriver, portaged to the Kuskokwim, where he met Lukin, and ascended to the mouth of the Stony River. From there, despite advice to the contrary, he attempted to cross to Cook Inlet by ascending the Stony River but was forced to turn back, finally reaching the Kuskokwim River completely out of provisions and close to starvation (VanStone 1959, 37-47).

Another Creole named P. V. Malakhov left St. Michael in February 1838, portaged to the Yukon from near Unalakleet, and ascended on the ice to the Koyukuk, returning that summer down the Yukon by boat. He left some men to build a post at Nulato, but they had to abandon the site in the winter for lack of provisions, leaving the Indians to plunder and burn the buildings. A small trading post was established at Unalakleet in 1842 and later that year a more permanent one at Nulato. From both these posts traders ranged into the surrounding country, trading both with Eskimos and Athapaskan Indians (Hulley 1958, 156; Bancroft 1886, 552-553).

Life at these northern posts was very simple and austere. The three largest of them, namely Alexandrov, Kolmakov, and St. Michael, were called redoubts and included log fortifications, whereas smaller outposts such as Ikogmiut, Nulato, and Unalakleet had only one or two Russians or Creoles and a few primitive buildings. More than once such stations were destroyed by the Natives.

The great smallpox epidemic (*see* Chapter 13) reached the Yukon-Kuskokwim Delta area in 1838 and spread rapidly up the Yukon and along the southern shores of Norton Sound that year and the next, finally coming to an end in 1840. Mortality was appallingly high and the population never fully recovered. When Zagoskin (1967, 204, 243, 281) traveled through the area a few years later he found many abandoned village sites resulting from the epidemic.

The Russian Orthodox Church gained a foothold in this region as early as 1819 when Kolmakov baptized some of the Eskimos near Alexandrov Redoubt. Father Veniaminov himself visited the fort in 1829 and again in 1832 and converted more to his faith (Tikhmenev 1978, 194-95). By 1842 the church had established a chapel at Kolmakov Redoubt and in 1845 a mission on the lower Yukon at Ikogmiut, now called Russian Mission. Two eminent churchmen served at the latter station: Father Netsvetov, already mentioned, and Father Illarion, who arrived in 1862. Both kept journals which mention epidemic diseases and starvation, and which describe their slow struggle against the shamans (Netsvetov 1984; Oswalt 1960, 102-14). Netsvetov, while ordering medicines from his bishop in 1847, noted that the principal diseases were intestinal, skin, and respiratory disorders, the latter including the spitting of blood (*in* University of Alaska 1936-1938, 1:369).

NORTH TO THE ARCTIC

In July 1816 Lt. Otto von Kotzebue set out from Kamchatka on a leg of his round-the-world voyage in the Russian brig *Riurik.* After stopping briefly on St. Lawrence Island, he sailed through the Bering Strait, landed several times on the northern coast of the Seward Peninsula, and over the following month explored the southern and eastern reaches of the sound that bears his name. Several detailed reports of this voyage contain ethnographic and scattered medical observations, including those of Kotzebue himself (Kotzebue 1821, 1:190-253), the artist Louis Choris (VanStone 1960, 146-58) and the naturalist Adelbert von Chamisso (1986). The ship's surgeon, Dr. Friedrich Eschscholtz (1821, 2:317-47), left many valuable notes on the health of the crew during the voyage (*see also* Fortuine 1984b, 118-19).

Other Russian voyages under Gleb Shishmarev and Mikhail Vasilev continued explorations of Kotzebue Sound in 1820, pushing as far north as Icy Cape, as Cook had done. Shishmarev returned north the following year, stopping at St. Lawrence Island and the coast north of Kotzebue Sound. Vasilev that year cruised in Norton Sound, then northward through the strait to the Diomedes and as far as Cape Lisburne. Khromchenko, already mentioned, explored the northern shore of Norton Sound in 1821 and 1822 (D. Ray 1975, 66-70).

In 1826 the Russians for the first time since Cook's voyage met foreign competition in the Arctic. The British, as part of their continuing efforts to discover the Northwest Passage, had sent John Franklin overland from the eastward and Lt. Frederick Beechey by ship from the westward with the hope that they could rendezvous somewhere on the north coast of Alaska. Franklin descended the Mackenzie River and pushed westward along the northern coast of Alaska. Meanwhile, Beechey was forced to turn back because of unfavorable ice conditions near Icy Cape, but sent ahead his smaller boat under the command of Sailing Master Thomas Elson in the hope of meeting Franklin's party. Elson carefully worked his boat northeastward through the shore ice all the way to Point Barrow, which he reached nine days after Franklin had turned back at Return Point, some 150 miles to the eastward. At Barrow Elson sensed hostility on the part of the Eskimos and for that reason spent little time there (*in* Beechey 1831, 1:417-42). The following summer Beechey again tried to reach Barrow, but was prevented by ice far short of his goal and had to content himself with a survey of Hotham Inlet and the northern and western portions of the Seward Peninsula. Beechey had many encounters, some definitely unfriendly, with the northern Eskimos, but he himself was a keen and sympathetic observer of their life and customs (Beechey 1831, 1:332-93; 2: 303-5).

In 1830 Etholin explored much of the north coast of Norton Sound as far as the Bering Strait, including Sledge Island and King Island. Three years later Tebenkov retraced much of the same route, making careful navigational charts (D. Ray 1975, 122).

In 1837 Thomas Simpson of the Hudson's Bay Company became the first to explore the north coast from Return Island to Barrow. There he was impressed by an "immense" cemetery which suggested to him that a recent epidemic had struck the people (T. Simpson 1843, 153-54). The following summer a Russian party under the leadership of a Koniag Creole named Aleksandr Kashevarov, traveling eastward in large skin boats called *bairdaras,* reached a point thirty-five miles beyond Point Barrow, although their passage was under constant hostile pressure from the Eskimos (Kashevarov 1977).

The year 1848 marked a turning point in relations between Europeans and the northern Eskimos. Prior to this time contacts had been brief and relatively infrequent, mainly by the officers and crew of tightly disciplined naval ships or vessels of the Russian-American Company. In 1848, however, the first American whaling vessel passed the Bering Strait and the arctic regions were changed forever (*see* Chapter 9).

Yet another significant event in 1848 was the arrival in the Arctic of the first two of a number of ships of the British Royal Navy engaged in the search for Franklin's last expedition, which had disappeared in the central Canadian Arctic a few years before. From 1848 to 1854 no fewer than eight ships and a private yacht sailed these seas either in search of Franklin himself, or in support of the effort by others. Among the more important ships were the *Herald,* under Capt. Henry Kellett, and the *Plover* under Comdr. T. E. L. Moore, both of which arrived in 1848, and the *Enterprise* and *Investigator,* under Capt. Richard Collinson and Comdr. Robert McClure, respectively, which entered the Bering Sea in 1850. One or more of four supply ships were also in the region of the Bering Strait through these years (D. Ray 1975, 141). These voyages contributed much to an understanding and knowledge of the northern parts of Alaska and their people.

Among all these stalwart vessels it was the *Plover,* first under the command of Moore and later under Rochefort Maguire, that most deserves notice. This hardy ship spent no fewer than six consecutive winters in the north, including one in Siberia, one on Chamisso Island, two in Port Clarence and two in Point Barrow. During this period, members of her crew made long overland journeys and had many contacts with the Eskimos. Dr. John Simpson (1855), the surgeon of the *Plover,* is credited with writing the first important ethnography of the Point Barrow Eskimos (D. Ray 1975, 141-42).

Before the curtain fell on the Russian-American Company in 1867, a final burst of activity in exploration occurred as a result of plans to build a telegraph line, known as the Collins Overland Line, to connect North America and Asia across the Bering Strait. From 1865 to 1869 surveys for the proposed route added much to our knowledge of the Alaskan interior and its people (Sherwood 1965b, 15-35).

The Russian-American portion of the survey was under the direction of a young American scientist named Robert Kennicott, who had already spent the winter of 1860-1861 at Fort Yukon collecting specimens for the Smithsonian Institution. He was assisted by several notable American scientists, including William Healy Dall, Henry W. Elliott, and Henry M. Bannister, each of whom made a name for himself in later years. Once in Alaska the party had serious problems of supply and morale, not least because of the increasing mental illness of Kennicott, who finally died unexpectedly at Nulato in May in 1866 at the age of thirty (James 1942).

Work went on, however, and in 1866 Frank Ketchum and Michael Lebarge, accompanied by the Creole Ivan Lukin, son of Semen, ascended the Yukon by boat all the way to Fort Yukon, a feat which Lukin alone had performed three years before. The following winter the same group once more visited Fort Yukon, this time overland, and then the next summer followed the Great River to its headwaters in the Yukon Territory (Sherwood 1965b, 25-30; Brooks 1973, 243). Dall, who became scientific chief of the expedition, portaged to the Yukon on November 1867 and ascended to Nulato, accompanied by an English artist, Frederick Whymper. The following year they also reached Fort Yukon and returned with Ketchum and Lebarge. Another party under Baron Otto von Bendeleben explored the southern Seward Peninsula and even discovered evidences of placer gold.

Others explored the Yukon Delta and the area west of the Koyukuk. Although the Telegraph Expedition was suddenly abandoned when word was received of the successful laying of the Atlantic cable, the work was not in vain, for many areas of the territory were examined for the first time. There were unfortunately few published narratives of the expedition. Dall himself (1870) wrote by far the most important book, which has much ethnographic information, especially on the Athapaskan Indians but also the Eskimos and Aleuts. His companion Whymper (1868) wrote a popular account of his travels, as did George Adams (1982).

7

The Health Care System
of the Russian-American
Company

THE MEDICAL ESTABLISHMENT AT THE CAPITAL

In 1810, Lt. V. M. Golovnin of the Russian naval sloop *Diana*, while visiting Baranov in his residence at New Archangel, expressed admiration for the paintings that had been sent out from St. Petersburg to adorn the walls of the chief manager's home. Baranov with a smile replied that, instead of pictures, "it would have been wiser to send out physicians, as there was not one in the colonies, nor even a surgeon or apothecary." His guest expressed surprise that the directors of the company had not seen fit to send surgeons to a country with such an unhealthy climate, and where wounds were a constant threat, to which Baranov replied, "I do not know whether the directors trouble themselves to think about it; but we doctor ourselves a little, and if a man is wounded, so as to require an operation, he must die" (Bancroft 1886, 467-68).

The chief manager had long recognized the need for medical care, even during his earlier days with the Shelikhov-Golikov Company. In 1795, while still at Kodiak, he had petitioned for a company pharmacy to make available drugs to treat the workers' illnesses, noting that he had freely given out his own stock for this purpose (*in* Pierce 1976, 105). Beginning in 1804 the home office of the Russian-American Company sent a supply of drugs to the colonies, but for the most part no one had the knowledge to use them properly (Sarafian 1971, 102).

Count Rezanov pointedly observed in his report that the absence of medical care discouraged applicants for jobs with the company and demoralized those already working (Sarafian 1971, 103-4). He also felt that a hospital could be used for any Natives that might apply to the Russians for medical aid (Tikhmenev 1978, 93). Golovnin (1985/86, 64-65), who returned to Sitka on an inspection tour in 1818, accused the company in his report "of poor maintenance and meager provisioning of its employees and of not supplying any kind of aid to those suffering from diseases." He went on to comment (1985/86, 65-70) on "the lack of medical care and decent provision for the sick, due to which one only somewhat dangerously ill is most likely as good as dead." In his general account of the voyage (1979, 125) he further noted that the wet, raw climate of the capital caused many diseases among the employees, especially scurvy, which in numerous cases had been fatal.

During this period Russian naval vessels regularly visited the capital, usually with a physician on board, some of whom spent a few months ashore (Ivashintsov 1980, 136-37). The first doctor to stay for an extended period was the previously mentioned Georg Schäffer, who arrived in the colonies on the *Suvorov* in November 1814. After a dispute with the captain Schäffer decided to leave the ship and stay on at Sitka, where he remained until in October 1815 he was sent by Baranov on his disastrous mission to the Hawaiian Islands (Pierce 1967). In July 1817 the *Suvorov* returned to Sitka, this time with Vasilii Bervi on board as physician. Bervi remained at the capital until November 1818, when he sailed with Hagemeister on the *Kutuzov*. While in Russian America Dr. Bervi had several adventures and was rewarded on his departure by the chief manager with a sea otter pelt "of medium quality" (Pierce 1984, 139-40). In September 1818 Hagemeister requested Anton Novitskii, staff surgeon on Golovnin's sloop *Kamchatka*, to perform a "fitness for duty" examination for him so that he could return to Russia (Pierce 1984, 127-28).

According to Sarafian (1971, 104-5) a twenty-bed hospital was built at New Archangel between 1818 and 1820. As early as February 1818 Chief Manager Hagemeister mentioned a hospital at the capital and gave instructions for the care of patients there. Later he also requested that medical instruments left at Kodiak by the *Neva* be shipped to New Archangel because they were expensive items and no one at Kodiak knew how to use them. That year Simeon Ianovskii, Hagemeister's successor, ordered various drugs from Canton, China, and requested that medicinal herbs be collected at Bodega Bay, near Fort Ross. In November 1818 the chief manager commended a Creole named Nikolai Eranskoi for zeal in his work at the hospital (Pierce 1984, 22, 36, 151, 154, 175).

The hospital, it would seem, was not staffed by a physician at the beginning. In March 1817 the board of directors of the company promised Baranov a physician, while at the same time they urged him to send a few bright young men to St. Petersburg to study medicine or pharmacy (University of Alaska 1936-1938, 4:140, 142). But it was not until the administration of a later manager, Matvei Muraviev, that a surgeon named Volkov was finally assigned to the colonies. In March 1820 he was already en route. The board cautioned the manager about assigning the work of the new medical officer. Noting the absence till then of a "regularly maintained hospital," the chief manager was instructed to organize "this useful institution." He was also reminded that Volkov was required by his contract to train young Creoles in the healing arts (University of Alaska 1936-1938, 4: 205-6).

Under Chief Manager Muraviev each hospitalized employee was charged seventy-five kopecks a day in order to offset the cost of the hospital and doctor, but by 1821 this practice had been abandoned and care was rendered free of charge, probably as an inducement for employment (Sarafian 1971, 105). The medical services were instead financed by deducting one-half percent from profits, and to a lesser extent through the sale of confiscated furs and a five percent tax on auctions held on property left behind when officials departed the colonies (Khlebnikov 1976, 95).

New Archangel was no doubt considered a hardship post by the doctors and pharmacists sent there. Staff turnover was high (Khlebnikov 1976, 95) and it is possible the highest quality professionals did not volunteer. Within a year of his arrival Surgeon Volkov had a debt problem that had to be investigated (University of Alaska 1936-1938, 4:219). Some years later a pharmacist with chronic alcoholism had to have his salary cut off to get him home (Golovin 1979, 66). In 1830 Chief Manager Ferdinand Wrangell found a physician named Dr. Simon unfit for duty (probably because of alcoholism) and returned him to Russia via the next ship (Pierce 1986, 13).

Few descriptions of the first hospital at New Archangel are known. An early resident of the capital wrote that since 1825 "three good rooms" had been set aside for the pharmacy and the medical staff who worked there. The infirmary itself was a large separate room with eight beds for seriously ill patients, whereas other patients stayed in their own quarters and came to receive medications each morning. The facility was well equipped for its time and comparable to that of a good-sized Russian town. Drugs were of good quality and sent out annually in adequate supply from St. Petersburg. Surgical instruments were said to be of excellent workmanship. Patients admitted to the hospital were given fresh food, tea, and sugar without cost (Khlebnikov 1976, 95).

When Captain Litke visited Sitka in 1827 (1987, 46, 51), he reported that the hospital building housed eight beds, the pharmacy, and a clinic for outpatient care of minor illnesses. He described the facility as very clean and amply furnished, and provided with a good stock of drugs. The inpatients were well fed, not only with fresh fish but with potatoes from the local gardens. At the time of his visit, four Creole medical students were receiving training at the hospital.

According to an account by one of the doctors in the 1830s, there were in fact two hospitals, the main one for men and a smaller facility for women. The larger building, now with twenty-four beds, measured fifty-four by forty-eight feet and had two stories. On the main floor were a kitchen, pharmacy, consulting room, waiting room, and three rooms for patients. At one end of a long portico were latrines which were washed by the incoming tide. Also on the main floor were small storage rooms for bandages and provisions. The upper floor was used for the storage of medications and linens, and contained a place for hanging dried herbs. The woman's hospital was apparently made necessary by the smallpox epidemic that had devastated Sitka and the surrounding area at this time. It was a part of a damp, chilly dwelling and the number of beds never exceeded four (Blaschke 1842, 79-80). A map of Sitka dating from 1838 shows the men's hospital located on what was then a peninsula near the site of the present-day Franklin building at the corner of Harbor Drive and Maksoutoff Street. The smaller women's facility was originally situated behind the old St. Michael's church (R. Maschin *in* Blaschke 1842). (*See* Figure 9.)

The British naval officer Capt. Edward Belcher visited New Archangel in 1837, not long after the smallpox epidemic. In a tour of the hospital and school he found "much to admire." In the hospital he was particularly impressed by the practice of putting the patient's name, date of admission, and diagnosis on a plaque over each bed so that visitors would be given timely warning of any contagion (Belcher and Simpkinson 1979, 22).

In the early 1840s the hospital at the capital was enlarged to forty beds (Sarafian 1971, 108). An eminent and always articulate visitor who arrived in 1842 around the time of the opening of the new hospital was Sir George Simpson, chief factor of the Hudson's Bay Company. He was impressed with what he saw although he felt the expense of maintaining the hospital must have been very heavy. "In its wards," he concluded grandly, "and, in short, in all the requisite appointments, the institution in question would do no disgrace to England" (G. Simpson 1847, 2:190).

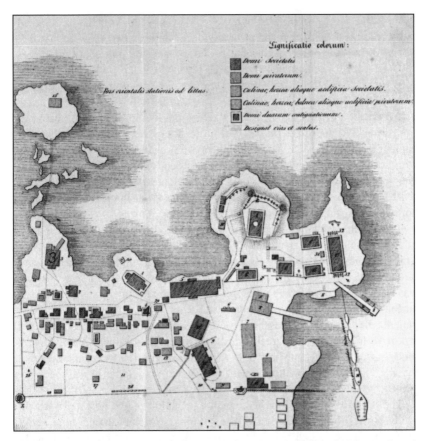

Figure 9. A view of Sitka in 1838, by R. Maschin. Men's hospital is no. 3 and women's hospital is no. 4. (A portion of *Oppidi, Novi-Archangelscensis, in* Blaschke 1842, appendix, Rare Book Collection, Archives, Alaska and Polar Regions Dept., University of Alaska Fairbanks.)

Probably in 1858 the hospital was transferred to a new location, a large building formerly housing the seminary. This two-story log structure had been built between 1844 and 1847 and, when the school moved to Yakutsk in 1858, was turned over to the Russian-American Company. Located next to the bishop's house (which still stands today), the substantial building was converted to a hospital soon afterward (Blee [1986], 24).

In 1862 P. N. Golovin (1979, 65) described it as "fairly large, and there is fresh air in the rooms whose windows face the sea, but the air is damp and stuffy in the rooms on the northwest side." A few years later it was depicted by a visitor as a "very neat and clean building" (Whymper 1868, 75). In 1872 a U.S. Army doctor wrote that the hospital faced the bay about eight feet above sea level. Constructed of squared logs, it was covered on the outside with boards and inside with boards or canvas. The building measured eighty-five by forty-one feet in size (Brooke 1875, 480-81).

According to Golovin (1979, 66) the hospital had its share of problems at this time. The hospital linens, although adequate in supply, were not laundered often enough. The bedclothes were changed only on Saturdays, with hospital gowns replaced on Wednesdays and Saturdays—not enough in view of the "slovenly" habits of the patients. Generally, he found the hospital could not boast of cleanliness, probably because it was too expensive to hire housekeepers and laundry workers.

There were also complaints about the hospital diet, especially the shortage of fresh food, particularly meat. The usual hospital diet was a soup made from salt meat or dried fish. In summer fresh fish might be available but rarely fresh meat. Golovin (1979, 66) recommended that when wild game was available, a portion should be set aside for the hospital patients. Further, he felt that chickens might be purchased from time to time for the sickest patients, or some of the preserved foods used from the warehouses. Another report from this period agreed that hospital patients rarely received fresh food, but noted that their basic diet of salt meat and fish was supplemented by rice, barley soup, white or black bread, tea, and sugar (Sarafian 1971, 108-9).

The report of a recent archeological excavation of the hospital trash pit sheds further light on the diet of the patients. Probably dating from about 1860, the pit contained bones from cows, deer, and wild birds, but usually the more undesirable cuts. These findings suggest that although the best food went to others, the monotonous diet of the patients at the hospital was sometimes broken by meat, perhaps on holidays or weekends. It is also of interest that the trash pit yielded up a number of medical artifacts of the time, including medicine bottles, evaporating dishes, mortars and pestles, and a graduated vessel (Blee [1986], 199, 407).

In the 1830s the sole physician was assisted by an experienced naval surgeon, who often doubled as a pharmacist, and by a senior Creole *feldsher* and five or six Creole apprentices serving as general hospital workers. In addition the hospital had a cook, housekeeper, and two servants, not to mention a midwife and her assistant, and three washerwomen and a maid for the women's hospital (Blaschke 1842, 80).

The new hospital at New Archangel had a medical staff of one, two, or sometimes three physicians, depending on availability. The normal complement was two, one of whom supervised the hospital patients and the other of whom took care of employees in their own quarters. This second, or perhaps third, physician was also in charge of supervising the work of the many *feldshers* who worked at outlying company posts. At New Archangel itself the physician staff in later years was supplemented by three or more *feldshers*, a pharmacist, one or more midwives, and up to six apprentices, who were usually Creole (Golovin 1979, 66).

The apprentices, or students, were an important part of the program from the very beginning. Volkov, the first physician, had been instructed specifically to train young Creoles in preparing simple medicines, treating simple injuries, and rendering first aid (University of Alaska 1936-1938, 4:206). At an early date it was hoped that such young men, knowing the local language and making their home permanently in the colonies, would be able to provide medical services at the smaller outlying posts (Khlebnikov 1976, 95). In 1860-1861 four apprentices were stationed at New Archangel, and five more at Kodiak, probably reflecting the latter's proximity to most of the small company posts (Sarafian 1971, 107). In addition, the midwives at New Archangel and Kodiak, who were employed to assist Russian and Creole women in childbirth, also trained Creole women to take over this function. Golovin (1979, 67-68), in fact, proposed that the traditional Aleut midwives be retrained, to avoid the tragic obstetrical outcomes often seen among the Natives.

The names of a number of the physicians serving at New Archangel during this period are known. Several have German names, reflecting the fact that many physicians, scientists, and technicians in the Russian service at this time were ethnic Germans. Perhaps the best known medical officer was Dr. Eduard Blaschke, who led the smallpox control efforts during the terrible epidemic of the late 1830s, and who later wrote an extensive geographical, climatological, and medical description of Sitka (Blaschke 1842). (*See* Figure 10.) Two other doctors of some significance were Aleksandr Romanovskii, who served from about 1840 to 1845 and Alexander Frankenhaeuser, who was in New Archangel from about 1841 to 1848. Both left an account of their experiences published in St. Petersburg in 1849 (*in* Pierce 1974; see also Ivashintsov 1980, 121, 148). More recently a series of medical articles by Dr. Z. Govorlivyi (n.d.), who worked at Sitka in the the 1850s, has been made available in translation.

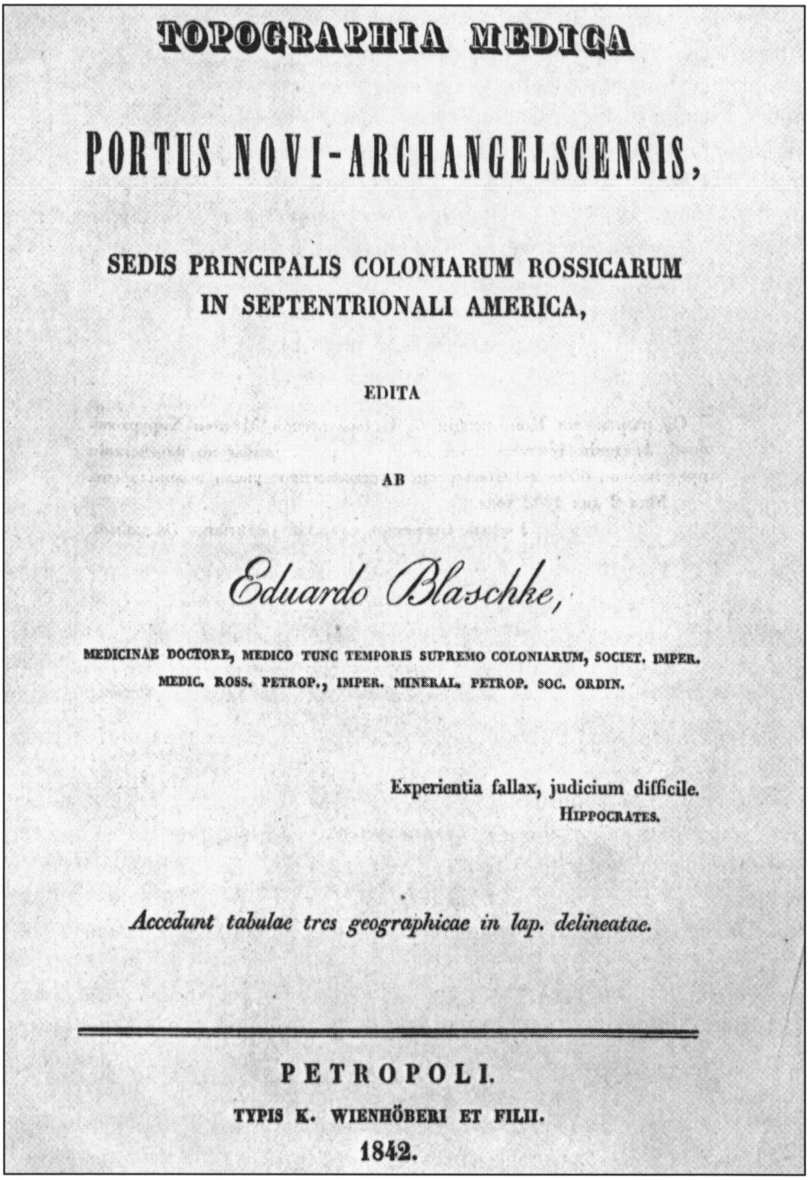

TOPOGRAPHIA MEDICA

PORTUS NOVI-ARCHANGELSCENSIS,

SEDIS PRINCIPALIS COLONIARUM ROSSICARUM
IN SEPTENTRIONALI AMERICA,

EDITA

AB

Eduardo Blaschke,

MEDICINAE DOCTORE, MEDICO TUNC TEMPORIS SUPREMO COLONIARUM, SOCIET. IMPER.
MEDIC. ROSS. PETROP., IMPER. MINERAL. PETROP. SOC. ORDIN.

Experientia fallax, judicium difficile.
HIPPOCRATES.

Accedunt tabulae tres geographicae in lap. delineatae.

PETROPOLI.

TYPIS K. WIENHÖBERI ET FILII.

1842.

Figure 10. The first medical treatise on Alaska, by Dr. Eduard Blaschke, medical officer at New Archangel. (V. Lada-Mocarski, 1969.)

Workload figures for the hospital at New Archangel are known through the reports of Romanovskii and Frankenhaeuser for the 1840s and later from the reports of Golovin and others in the 1860s. In evaluating these reports it is well to keep in mind that the hospital primarily served lower level employees, either Russian or Creole, who were those with the most significant health problems. Officers and other officials were cared for in their own homes. Women also were treated at home, except for a few Tlingit women infected with syphilis, for whom a special room was set aside in the hospital. Besides the inpatients, an outpatient clinic was held every morning at seven o'clock, for the benefit of those who had "some slight external or internal problem" (Golovin 1979, 65-66).

In 1845-1846 some 590 persons were treated at the hospital, of whom only 16 (2.7 percent) died. In those same years 51 deaths were recorded at Sitka, indicating that more than two-thirds of the deaths occurred outside the hospital. In a summary of hospital workload over a four-year period between 1843 and 1848, a total of 2383 patients were admitted, an average of 1.6 per day. The average hospital census was 26, for an occupancy of 66 percent on the basis of forty available beds. The average length of stay was approximately sixteen days. During the four-year period only 56 patients died in the hospital, a mere 2.3 percent of the total number admitted (Frankenhaeuser *in* Pierce 1974, 26, 30-31).

In 1860 the total number of inpatients and outpatients was 1400, of whom 1328, or 95 percent, were listed as cured. Only 22 patients died that year, for a fatality rate of 1.6 percent, and 50 were still hospitalized at the end of the reporting period (Golovin 1979, 67), suggesting that an epidemic was in progress. A couple of years later the average hospital census was only ten, the marked decline being attributed to the decline of syphilis and scurvy (Rosse 1883, 17).

As Simpson had suggested, the costs of maintaining the hospital were very high. By 1860 the annual cost of salaries and supplies for the New Archangel facility alone was 45,000 paper rubles (Golovin 1979, 67).

HEALING HOT SPRINGS

The Alaska Natives long ago discovered the soothing and healing properties of the warm springs which are found in many parts of Alaska. These springs, heated by volcanic action, often contain a high mineral content thought to be helpful not only externally but internally for many kinds of illness. Whenever such springs were found, the Russians seized upon them with alacrity to try to remove the chill from their bones. Some were already familiar with such healing springs from the great "spas" of Europe, such as Vichy, Baden-Baden, and Karlsbad, which enjoyed high renown in the eighteenth and nineteenth centuries.

Only a short while after moving his headquarters to Sitka Sound, Baranov, who in the past had suffered several painful and slow-healing injuries (Tikhmenev 1979, 96, 142), must have learned of the volcanic springs about twelve miles to the south, and used for years by the Tlingit. Lisianskii spent about ten days there in August 1805 with members of his crew who were suffering from various illnesses. He described the springs as flowing into a man-made basin about three hundred yards from shore. The waters were said to be 151° Fahrenheit at the spring and about 100° Fahrenheit in the pool. The water itself was impregnated with sulfur and also contained salt and magnesia (Lisiansky 1814, 231-32). Captain D'Wolf (1861, 59), an American trader, also visited the site around this time, and left this poetic description: "Situated in a beautiful, romantic place, the water runs down from the foot of a high mountain, in a small serpentine rivulet, for several hundred yards, and empties into a broad basin." In Khlebnikov's account (1976, 34) of Russian America from 1817 to 1832, he noted that the Tlingit had used the hot springs for a long time to treat various illnesses. He went on:

Today many persons use them as a cure. They heal wounds quickly and cure arthritis and scurvy. . . . At the source the water is very hot, but it can be drunk. At first the taste is unpleasant, but once one becomes accustomed to it, the smell is not repulsive when it is hot. No one can bathe in it for more than 15 minutes; after that length of time one experiences a great lassitude and the head begins to spin.

Dr. Blaschke (1842, 29-30) seemed skeptical of the healing powers of the waters, although he noted that many people used them for various ailments, including ulcerous skin conditions, constipation, scrofula, and rheumatism. According to him, the temperature of the springs ranged between 50° and 52° Réaumur (about 144.5° to 149° Fahrenheit), and contained, as a colleague reported, a heavy load of minerals, ninety-seven percent of which was sulfur.

By the 1840s nearly every visitor to the capital made the refreshing trip to the springs, as did many of the residents of the town. The popularity of the site led to the construction of a facility which in translation was called "sheltered curative hot springs" (Caldwell 1986, 188). There in a twelve-month period, according to a medical report (Frankenhaeuser *in* Pierce 1974,

31), some thirty sick persons from the colony used the waters, of whom twelve were cured and six showed improvement. Sir George Simpson (1847, 2:194) described the scene in 1842:

> The establishment in the neighbourhood consisted of three snug cottages, being kept in order by an old fellow, of a Russian and his daughter, both of whom, whether from choice or by way of example, took a plunge every day for half an hour at a time. The damsel's rosy cheeks seemed to speak volumes in favour of the waters, though, perhaps, they were merely the result of being cooked every forenoon. . . . The buildings are pleasantly situated on the sloping face of a bank. . . . There springs up a luxuriant verdure, in consequence of the genial warmth diffused by the waters, which send up a column of vapour to mark the spot from a considerable distance.

He went on to remark that the establishment was used as a hospital for invalids from Sitka. The waters were said to be used externally for rheumatism, fevers, and syphilis, and internally (sic) for skin diseases. Two separate bathing pools were fed by the springs, one for Whites and one for Indians, the latter continuing to use the springs as they had for generations.

Within a decade of Simpson's visit, however, a party of Stikine Indians destroyed the facilities as an act of revenge for being treacherously attacked by the local Sitka Tlingit under the very eyes of the Russians (Krause 1956, 45). According to Golovin (1979, 68), no permanent structures had been rebuilt at the site by 1862 and the springs had reverted to the sole use of the Indians, who lived there in small huts made from tree branches. The chief manager that year proposed to construct a new clinic the following spring, to consist of a building reinforced against attack for the Russians and a separate building some distance away for the Indians. It was not until well into the American period that a new facility was in fact built, later to be known as Goddard Hot Springs (Caldwell 1986, 191-93).

Hot springs were known elsewhere in Russian America and used for healing purposes, especially in the Aleutians. As early as 1762, several Russians were killed by Aleuts while bathing in warm springs near Unalaska (Berkh 1974, 24-25). A number of these hot springs were known on the island of Unalaska (Bancroft 1886, 124n; Chamisso 1986, 57). Father Veniaminov (1984, 214), who lived at Unalaska for ten years, said the Aleuts often used these springs for bathing, considering them "very healthy."

The most detailed record of healing hot springs in the Aleutians is the diary of Father Netsvetov (1980, 228), the Creole priest who was based for sixteen years on the island of Atka. Netsvetov repeatedly resorted to the springs about six miles away from his home for the treatment of a chronic but unspecified illness. He would often spend several days there, perhaps more as a respite from his demanding work than for any true healing properties of the waters. It is interesting to note that Father Netsvetov found the waters to be less effective in the early summer, possibly because they were diluted by the spring snow melt. In 1873 Dall found some very hot natural springs on Atka with the ruins of bathhouses nearby (Bancroft 1886, 712-713n).

Warm springs are found in many other places in Alaska. Manley Hot Springs and Chena Hot Springs are two well-known sites in the interior. Serpentine Hot Springs, located 160 miles north of Nome, has been used at least in recent years for Native healing (Book et al. 1983). Other hot springs may be found on the Buckland River, on a tributary of the Kobuk, and near the headwaters of the Selawik River (E. S. Burch, Jr. 1986, personal communication). Although undoubtedly the local Natives knew about these springs and probably used them, there is no record that the Russians did. Of course they had their own cultural institution, the steambath, which they could set up almost anywhere to soothe their aching joints.

KODIAK AND THE OUTPOSTS

The need for medical care in the smaller company posts, as well as in New Archangel, was recognized by the directors from the very beginning, as their provision for the medical training of Creole boys attests. After Baranov moved his base to Sitka Sound in the early 1800s, the settlement of St. Paul's Harbor, or Kodiak, declined somewhat in importance. Many ships continued to stop there, however, almost all of them Russian, and from time to time the ship's surgeon (if there was one) would provide some medical care. As mentioned earlier, Lieutenant Hagemeister of the *Neva* left his surgeon Karl Mordgorst at Kodiak for the winter of 1807-1808 while he himself went on to Sitka. There the doctor apparently set up a small hospital, for during the winter he rather unskillfully amputated both feet and several fingers of the Scottish seaman Archibald Campbell, who had suffered shipwreck and severe frostbite. When Dr. Mordgorst (whom Campbell calls "Nordgoorst") had to return to Russia in the late spring of 1808, he left his patient under the care of an "Assistant Surgeon." The latter may in fact have been an apprentice trained by Mordgorst, for the doctor had rather pretentiously named his makeshift hospital the "Chief District College of Counsellor and Chevalier Baranov" (Campbell 1819, 69, 189-91).

Sarafian (1971, 105) states that a small ten-bed facility was built between 1818 and 1820 at Kodiak, around the same time the main hospital at New Archangel was built. Captain Litke (1987, 46), however, specifically noted that in 1827 the only hospital in the colonies was at the capital. By the time of Wrangell's tenure as chief manager (1830-1835) the hospital at Kodiak was definitely established (Wrangell 1980, 14). This hospital was never under the immediate direction of a physician but rather of an experienced *feldsher*. In 1862 this was a man named Petrov, who had been recruited from the local staff and was said to have a wide knowledge of local diseases. At that time Petrov was assisted by two other *feldshers*, five apprentices, and perhaps a midwife (Tikhmenev 1978, 371; Golovin 1979, 67). During the summer months or under special circumstances, such as an epidemic, one of the medical officers from New Archangel would visit. Likewise, the regular Kodiak staff often visited the smaller outposts in the district (Golovin 1979, 67).

One of the earlier references to the Kodiak hospital comes from the report of Dr. Romanovskii, who in 1840 sent many syphilitic Chugach he found in Prince William Sound to Kodiak for treatment (*in* Pierce 1974, 16-17). His colleague Dr. Frankenhaeuser (*in* Pierce 1974, 22-23, 28) gives statistics for the hospital in 1844 and again in 1846. In the two years 730 patients were treated, of whom 26, or 3.6 percent, died. The commonest diagnoses were abscesses, minor wounds, and catarrhal diseases. In the early 1860s comparable statistics were reported, although the case fatality by then had fallen to approximately two percent (Golovin 1979, 67).

Other small health facilities were built by the Russian-American Company in the outlying districts but none attained the status of Kodiak and most were staffed by a single *feldsher* or even an apprentice. A ten-bed facility was established in 1827 at Unalaska and at the same time a similar facility at Fort Ross, the Russian outpost in California. Two years later the company built an eight-bed facility at Atka (Sarafian 1971, 107), but these may have been little more than clean temporary quarters for the sick. Golovin (1979, 67) reported that in 1862 there were *feldshers* stationed at Unalaska, Atka, the mining site at Kenai, and at St. Michael.

Contemporary references to these small facilities are few. Father Veniaminov (1984, 91) speaks of an eight-bed facility in his description of Unalaska in 1834. Father Netsvetov (1980, 64, 226, 236, 240) repeatedly mentions in his diary the hospital facility at Atka and his relations with at least two different Creole *feldshers*, one of whom doubled as a teacher. Each of these small facilities was supplied with surgical instruments and drugs sent out from New Archangel. Smallpox vaccine was also made available from time to time and the *feldshers* and others were expected to administer it (Golovin 1979, 67). Occasionally they would receive a visit from a visiting senior *feldsher,* or even a physician, from New Archangel, Kodiak, or a company ship.

At the smaller posts the medical responsibility was placed on the shoulders of the managers or priests, some of whom accepted this mantle reluctantly. Each was supplied with the *feldsher's* kit, a few drugs, and smallpox vaccine. These workers had very little supervision, since the traveling medical officers and the surgeons on board the larger company ships rarely visited such small outposts.

The ships, in fact, were another problem. The small coastal vessels had neither doctor nor *feldsher,* yet their crews were constantly exposed to danger. To deal with this problem the captain was given a *feldsher's* kit and a few essential medications, together with instructions for their use. Golovin (1979, 67) recognized these measures as inadequate but noted that costs precluded another solution.

A HEALTH CARE SYSTEM

In many ways the organization of the medical program of the Russian-American Company in the nineteenth century is akin to that of a model health care system of today. The company seems to have recognized at an early date and quite clearly the need for good health care both as an employment incentive and as a means to increase productivity. The system that evolved over the next four decades had many problems, caused by logistics, high costs, bureaucratic inertia, and abuse by the workers, but it also demonstrated some admirable qualities, especially in comparison to the lack of direction in health care that followed the transfer of Alaska to the United States a few years later.

To recapitulate, the company system toward the close of the Russian period consisted of a central hospital in Sitka, where physician care was available and most supplies, drugs, and equipment for the colonies were stored. The physicians there were responsible for all medical care in the colonies, and therefore directly or indirectly supervised other health facilities and workers. The principal satellite was Kodiak, under an experienced *feldsher,* but there were other smaller units that were also directly dependent

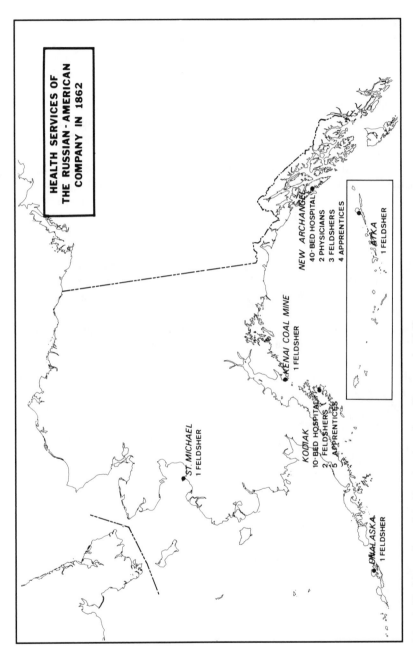

Map 1. Health services of the Russian-American Company in 1862.

on the central hospital. The small stations without a *feldsher* were regularly visited by the district *feldsher* and the outlying districts themselves were visited periodically by the medical officers from New Archangel. (*See* Map 1.)

Much emphasis throughout the system was placed on training at all levels. At New Archangel the physicians no doubt trained the *feldshers* as well as the apprentices, while the midwives trained their own assistants. In Kodiak and probably elsewhere the senior *feldshers* trained the apprentices. Both physicians and *feldshers* used their periodic visits to teach the health workers in the smaller posts.

Another strikingly modern feature is the emphasis laid on prevention, which in the nineteenth century had not reached a very high level of sophistication in medicine. As will be seen in Chapters 14 and 15 of this book, considerable thought and effort were given by the members of the company medical staff to the prevention and control of disease, especially smallpox and syphilis.

The mounting costs of the system also seem authentically modern. By 1860 the total costs of the medical program were estimated at over 67,000 paper rubles, with two-thirds of the total being spent at New Archangel (Golovin 1979, 67). It was apparent that the system was becoming a strain on company resources, yet it seemed to be effective, and officials must have been well aware that any cuts in benefits would be unpopular.

As a final note, it should be restated that the health program was designed for the employees of the company. Many employees were Alaska Native, or at least Creoles, and they of course received care, but by and large the Native people were not affected one way or the other by the presence of hospitals, physicians, or *feldshers* in their midst. Notable exceptions to the rule were the forced treatment of syphilitic women in New Archangel and Kodiak in the 1840s and 1850s and the smallpox vaccinations imposed on the Alaska Natives living in proximity to Russian posts in the late 1830s (*see* Chapters 13 and 14). In both cases, of course, it was largely self-interest, not altruism, that dictated policy.

8

Health Care and the
United States Govenment

The raising of the American flag over Sitka (as the capital was henceforth called) took place on October 18, 1867. It was appropriately a military ceremony, for the U.S. Army was to rule Alaska for the next decade. Congress established a Military District and a Customs District for Alaska. Perhaps the Army was selected to rule because it was a mobile unit of government that could set up an administrative structure quickly in a remote place; perhaps also there were lingering fears that Alaska was inhabited by "uncivilized" and perhaps hostile Indians. Army garrisons were established at six posts over the next two years: Sitka, Wrangell, and Tongass in southeastern Alaska, plus Kodiak, Kenai, and the Pribilofs. By 1869 there were about five hundred soldiers in Alaska, about half of them at Sitka. In 1871 all the posts were evacuated with the exception of Sitka and Wrangell (Brooks 1973, 267).

One of the first army doctors of whom we have a record was a Dr. Chismore, who was posted to Fort Tongass, close to the entrance to Portland Inlet. Dr. Emil Teichmann (1963, 123-25), who visited the station in 1868, reported that the army surgeon there enjoyed a respect not common among the Indians, who came great distances to consult him.

At Fort Wrangell, situated to guard the mouth of the Stikine River, a small medical facility burned to the ground with all its stores in November 1868, and was probably not rebuilt (U.S. Army Alaska 1962, 12).

At Sitka the Army took over the old Russian hospital. According to Assistant Surgeon John Brooke (1875, 480-81):

> The chief entrance is by a double door in the front, which opens into a wide hall, and from this hall an open staircase leads to the second story, while in the rear of the staircase is a room which serves as a

post-mortem room. The portion of the first floor which is on the east side of the hall is divided into five rooms of reasonable size, and is used as quarters by the medical officer at the hospital.

On the opposite side of the hall were five more rooms, used for an office, steward's quarters, dispensary, messroom, and kitchen. Upstairs was a wide hall, from the rear end of which was a door leading to an outside stairway giving access to the watercloset. One upstairs room by that time was set aside for the use of Indian patients. The west end of the second floor included an L-shaped ward, which at least in 1872 had an average of only six patients at a time. Opening into the ward, which was heated by a woodstove, were an attendants' room and a bathroom, the latter equipped with a washbasin, bathtub, and watercloset (then not in use). There were two commodes in the hospital and "an ordinary pit, housed over, a few yards behind the building." (*See* Figure 11.)

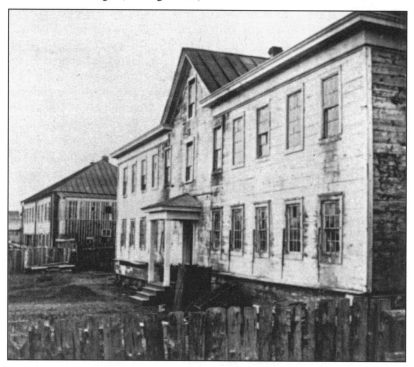

Figure 11. The last Russian hospital (foreground) at Sitka, later taken over by the U.S. Army. (Photograph courtesy The Bancroft Library, Berkeley, California.)

Initially, Indians were not accepted for treatment, but a street confrontation in 1868 led to an abrupt change in policy. One day Vincent Colyer, sent as a U.S. Indian agent to Alaska in 1868 to determine whether the new territory should be declared "Indian Country," saw a crowd around an Indian girl who was moaning as if in great pain. Gen. Jefferson C. Davis, the commander of the Alaska District, happened to pass by at that moment and Colyer persuaded him to accept the child for treatment at the hospital. She was put into a wretched tumbledown part of the building, but the precedent was at least set. Next day General Davis detailed Dr. J. G. Tonner to act as surgeon to the Indians living near the town (Colyer 1869, 981).

Dr. Tonner was exhorted to fulfill his charge "in a true Christian spirit" and to report weekly on his progress. In his first report he pointed out rather defensively that the post surgeons had been giving medical assistance to the Indians even before the general's order and that in fact they had put a great deal of effort into the task without compensation. For the sick ones he felt hospital care was necessary, but "there being no provisions for feeding or nursing such, I am unable to take them in. There are two rooms at the post hospital which by a little labor could soon be arranged comfortably for them; then the authority to issue a ration to each patient, and provisions made for the payment of a nurse. . . ." (*in* Colyer 1869, 1023-24).

The hospital thus began, with some reluctance, to give limited medical care to Indians. Before long, as the only source of medical care in the town in the first few years, it was also taking members of the general population. This included former employees of the Russian-American Company, who felt entitled to care by the new government (R. White 1880, 37).

One of the best accounts of Sitka and its hospital under army rule was that of the niece of Lady Jane Franklin, Sophia Cracroft (1981, 16, 69), who visited with her aunt in 1870. Miss Cracroft was a lively young woman and immediately attracted the attentions of several of the young medical officers. Dr. W. H. Ensign seemed especially prominent in her account and earned her praise for having converted the dirty, miserable old hospital to one where "all was airy and beautifully clean, with ample space." When Lady Franklin left Sitka, Dr. Ensign made up a prescription for her at the hospital.

Beyond their occasional medical treatment of Indians and their gentlemanly behavior toward visiting ladies, the Army did not make a good impression on those with whom they came in contact in Alaska. By and large the soldiers were a crude, violent, and drunken lot, many of whom had seen combat in the Civil War or on the western frontier. General Davis saw his principal function as keeping the peace and enforcing the ban on the importation of liquor. In neither task was he particularly successful. Some of the worst violence and drunkenness reported from that period were by the men of his command. For example, an Indian in Wrangell was beaten to near death by drunken soldiers (Colyer 1869, 999) and in Sitka a twenty-three-year-old Creole girl was beaten so badly by a soldier that she suffered permanent brain damage (University of Alaska 1936-1938, 3:4). The officers were certainly not above reproach either, and several incidents show violence and other inappropriate behavior on their part while under the influence of alcohol (Sherwood 1965a, 312).

A few quarrels had a tragic outcome on a grander scale. In 1868 a sentry at Sitka, due to a misunderstanding, had fired on a Tlingit canoe carrying men visiting from the village of Kake. When the Indians failed to receive the compensation they expected for the death of their men, they killed two White traders in retaliation. General Davis thereupon decided that an unequivocal lesson was appropriate and ordered the village of Kake itself to be burned. Twenty-nine houses and a number of boats were accordingly destroyed by an army detachment in January 1869 (Sherwood 1965a, 308-9). Another serious incident occurred at Wrangell in 1869. The wife of an army sergeant rescued a Stikine Indian women from being beaten by her drunken husband, and was rewarded by having her third finger bitten off. During the attempt to arrest the Indian some soldiers unintentionally shot and killed one Stikine and wounded another, whereupon the Indians exacted their revenge by killing a local trader. Soon the soldiers and the Tlingit were exchanging barrages of gunfire until finally the murderer of the trader was yielded up for trial by a court-martial and ultimate execution (Sherwood 1965a, 309-10).

Nor were the Army and the Tlingit the only problems. Sitka at this time was also host for a great influx of adventurers, profiteers, speculators, and ladies of easy virtue, most of them coming from the cities of the west coast. The capital had a boom town mentality, with all that term implies. Lawlessness, brawling, and drunkenness were the order of the day. As early as 1867 a group of responsible citizens had gotten together to form a city council, elect a mayor, and even appoint a health officer. Little resulted from their worthy efforts, however, because the new city government lacked enforcement powers or tax authority. To compound the law and order problem further, the Army abruptly withdrew all its troops from Alaska in 1877 to help quell an Indian uprising in the continental United States (Hulley 1958, 205-6, 211).

During the 1880s the Army to some extent redeemed itself by sponsoring several explorations of note. In 1884 Capt. William R. Abercrombie (1900b) led an important expedition to explore the Copper River. An even more noteworthy exploit was the extraordinary journey of 1500 miles in 1885 led by Lt. Henry Allen (1887), who ascended the Copper River and then explored the valleys of the Tanana, Yukon, and Koyukuk rivers. Also in 1885 Lt. Frederick Schwatka (1885), who was a physician by training, traveled from Sitka through the Chilkoot Pass and then by raft and boat down the entire length of the Yukon River to St. Michael. None of these expeditions had significant medical implications, except for a few scattered observations on the health of the Athapaskan Indians who were encountered.

Just before the turn of the century the Army was called in to assist with relief efforts for miners who were trying to reach the Yukon via Valdez and the Copper River valley. According to reports reaching San Francisco, hundreds of miners were dying of scurvy, frostbite, and starvation. Captain Abercrombie, who was already familiar with the area, was asked to organize the rescue operation. He arrived at Valdez in April 1899 and immediately arranged for the rental of suitable buildings for a hospital and cookhouse (Abercrombie 1900a, 40). The makeshift hospital was moved two months later to Savanport, across Valdez Arm, where firewood was more readily available. Within a few months most of the sickest miners had recovered or had been shipped on to Seattle. Only those remained who required amputation from frostbite or more intensive care for scurvy. During the few months of the hospital's existence it had extended medical or food relief to nearly five hundred persons (Abercrombie 1900a, 19-20). Medical relief to suffering miners was also freely rendered around this time by the Army in the upper Yukon, for example at Rampart and Fort Yukon (Richardson 1900, 504-5).

During the terrible influenza and measles epidemic of 1900, when thousands of Alaska Natives died, army medical officers gave freely of their time, skills, and resources at St. Michael (Brady 1900, 50), Nome (Jenness 1962, 31), Tanana (Stuck 1920, 166), and no doubt elsewhere.

THE U.S. NAVY

When the U.S. Army pulled its troops out of Alaska in June 1877, it left the territory without a government. The senior federal official was the collector of customs, who himself shortly afterward left Alaska because of illness. The people of Sitka became alarmed at the increasing hostility on the part of the Tlingit, whose passions were often inflamed by illicit alcohol. Storehouses were being looted and pillaged and many people feared for their lives. Even the hospital building was stripped of useful furnishings (Sherwood 1965a, 323). Before his departure the customs collector had urgently requested that a revenue cutter be sent to Alaskan waters to keep the peace, but the calls went unheeded. The Treasury Department, the parent agency of the customs, felt unequal to the task of governing the sprawling territory and in fact was not even paying the salaries of its collectors (Gruening 1954, 38-39). It did finally send a small revenue cutter, the *Wolcott,* for a brief visit in October, but the vessel was lightly armed with only three borrowed twelve-pounders (U.S. Senate 1880, 18). Captain Selden of the Revenue Cutter Service agreed that the local populace seemed to be in some danger from the Indians.

In 1878 the situation worsened in both Sitka and Wrangell, most of the ugly incidents continuing to involve drunkenness and claims for compensation. In early 1879 two further episodes, each again having to do with the Tlingits' differing ideas of justice, engendered much hostility. On the night of February 6 a band of armed intoxicated Tlingit tried to enter the town of Sitka, but fortunately the tense situation was defused by a friendly Indian leader. The next day the frightened citizens formed a committee of safety and prepared to offer armed resistance to any further forays. Since they had not been successful in obtaining help from the U.S. Government, they sent an urgent appeal to the British Government to dispatch a warship then stationed at Esquimalt, on Vancouver Island. After an exchange of diplomatic courtesies with Washington, the H.M.S. *Osprey,* armed with six heavy guns and 141 men, sailed for Sitka (A'Court 1976). The warship, soon joined by the puny *Wolcott,* remained at Sitka for a little more than a month before returning to British Columbia. Embarrassed by all the negative publicity attendant on the event, the U.S. Navy sent to Sitka the corvette U.S.S. *Alaska,* which remained there until relieved by the U.S.S. *Jamestown,* under the command of L. A. Beardslee, on June 14. Over the next five years Alaska was ruled from the deck of a vessel of the U.S. Navy (Sherwood 1965a, 328-31; Hanable 1978).

When Beardslee arrived in Sitka, he became convinced that the community had narrowly missed a massacre, which had been averted only by the help of a few friendly Indians. Within a month of his arrival, he ordered a raid on houses known to contain stills, a foray resulting in the destruction of forty-one stills and 150 gallons of liquor. He then enlisted twenty-three Indians who agreed to help him seek out and destroy stills wherever they could be found. He encouraged a peaceful frame of mind among the Tlingit by anchoring the *Jamestown* opposite the settlement with its guns trained on the village. During his tenure Beardslee also freed some Tlingit slaves and prevented several women from being executed as "witches," or sorcerers (Beardslee 1882; Hanable 1978, 322-23).

In September 1880 Comdr. Henry Glass replaced Beardslee as captain of the *Jamestown,* which remained in Alaskan waters for another full year. Glass continued efforts to suppress the liquor trade but found his ship too unwieldy to chase the smugglers in the small bays and inlets of the Alexander Archipelago. In January 1881, however, he was successful in causing the destruction of no less than two hundred stills in the Tlingit village. In March he contributed to the health of the village further by organizing a clean-up campaign, including the construction of drainage ditches. And just like his predecessor, Glass found it necessary to free some Indian slaves and save some accused of sorcery from a grisly death (U.S. House of Representatives 1882, 10, 28, 30). When violence threatened in May 1881 at the mining camp later to become Juneau, Glass declared the territory to be under martial law (U.S. House of Representatives 1882, 36; Hanable 1978, 324-25).

The hospital in Sitka apparently lay abandoned for two years until the Navy took over the building in 1879. Having little shore-based activity and with medical officers on board their ships, the Navy had little use for the structure, which had recently been used as a stable (Jackson 1881, 7). In March 1881 Commander Glass (U.S. House of Representatives 1882, 10-11) requested the Navy Department for authority to spend two hundred dollars to refurbish one room of the building as a hospital for Natives. This facility was needed, he went on, because of the many requests for medical services that could not be properly cared for in the homes. What the department's reaction was to this project is uncertain, but only two months later Glass assigned a crew to rehabilitate the rotting building before turning it over to the Presbyterian mission for use as a school (U.S. House of Representatives 1882, 30; Hanable 1978, 325; *see also* Chapter 10).

Commander Glass and the *Jamestown* left Alaska in August 1881 and were replaced by the U.S.S. *Wachusett,* the first of several steam-powered vessels that had the capacity to give chase to smugglers. After September 1882 the U.S.S. *Adams* took charge, followed by the U.S.S. *Pinta,* whose skipper turned over the reins of government to the first civilian governor in September 1884. (*See* Figure 12.)

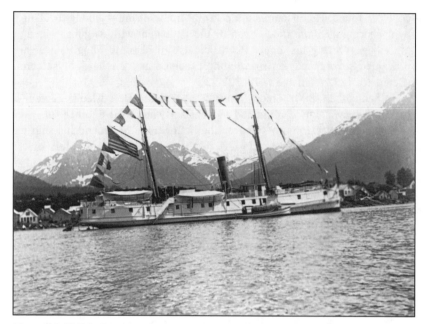

Figure 12. U.S.S. *Pinta*, a naval ship that cruised Alaskan waters in the 1880s and 1890s with a medical officer on board. (Rufus Rose Collection, Archives, Alaska and Polar Regions Dept., University of Alaska Fairbanks.)

Naval vessels remained in Alaskan waters until the turn of the century. The *Pinta* itself was posted to Alaska at least until 1895 and the reports of its medical officers are valuable sources of information on diseases in the Native population. One of them, Dr. H. B. Fitts, was extensively quoted in the governor's report to the U.S. Department of the Interior in 1890 (Knapp 1890, 24). The *Thetis* was another notable naval ship in Alaskan waters during the 1880s (Noble and Strobridge 1979).

Before leaving the Navy's role in the history of medicine in Alaska, it would be well to mention briefly the names of a few naval officers who made significant contributions to ethnology and exploration. Lt. George M. Stoney (1900) went to the Arctic on the Revenue Marine Ship *Corwin* in 1883 and during that summer and the following one he explored Hotham Inlet and the Kobuk River. In 1885-1886 he returned to the area with a much larger party and wintered in the Kobuk region, this time under naval auspices. His report of these expeditions, published some years later, is an important source of medical information on the Eskimos of the region

(Stoney 1900; Sherwood 1965b, 119-32). In southeastern Alaska, an area more familiar to the Navy, two naval officers, Ens. Albert P. Niblack (1888) and Lt. G. F. Emmons (1905), spent considerable time and effort collecting ethnological materials on the Tlingit and Haida for the Smithsonian Institution. Niblack's report in particular is an important review of the regional Indian culture, including matters of health.

THE DEPARTMENT OF THE TREASURY

Since in the early days of American sovereignty the customs laws were virtually the only ones governing Alaska, the Department of the Treasury was deeply involved in the affairs of the territory. Three separate agencies played a part: the Customs Service, the Revenue Cutter (or Marine) Service (which later evolved into the Coast Guard), and the Marine Hospital Service (which ultimately became the Public Health Service). All three worked together closely in their tasks. Although the primary goal of the Treasury Department was to collect customs duties and to stop the illicit trade in alcohol and firearms, members of the three agencies found themselves involved in civil government, rendering judicial decisions, rescuing shipwrecked sailors, lending humanitarian aid to the sick and injured, carrying famous passengers northward, supplying schools and missions, exploring new country, and even transporting reindeer from Siberia.

In July 1868 Congress had extended to Alaska the laws regarding customs, commerce, and navigation. William Sumner Dodge, posted to Alaska as a special agent of the Treasury Department, was also elected the town's first mayor. In his federal capacity, he was overwhelmed by appeals for justice in personal quarrels and many other affairs needing a civilian authority. With few resources for enforcement of customs regulations, whiskey and gun traders flourished and thereby led to an increase in the very violence and quarrels he was trying to suppress in his other capacities (Hinckley 1984).

The first revenue cutter to reach Alaska had carried a scientific party in 1867. The following year the *Wayanda* cruised from the southern tip of Alaska to the Bering Sea with Dr. Thomas T. Minor on board as surgeon. Minor had been charged by the Smithsonian Institution to collect natural history specimens and evaluate the territory's resources (Sherwood 1965b, 120). In these early years the revenue cutters made other patrols, including the first one north of the Bering Strait, by the *Reliance* in 1870 (D. Ray 1975,

190). For the most part, however, they assisted in the collection of customs and in suppression of the liquor trade, primarily in the Panhandle.

As pointed out earlier, matters reached a crisis in 1877 when the then collector, M. P. Berry, was left as the only federal official in the territory during a time of great fear and unrest. A special agent of the Treasury Department, William Gouverneur Morris, was commissioned to investigate the Alaska situation, and his report (1879) gave dramatic examples of the situation at this time. The Revenue Cutters *Walcott* and *Richard A. Rush* had made brief stops at Sitka around this time, but neither was authorized to remain there to patrol the region.

The first extended voyage of which we have a detailed medical account was that of the *Richard A. Rush,* which made the trip north in 1879 under Capt. George W. Bailey. Both Bailey and the medical officer, Assistant Surgeon Robert White, left interesting narratives of the voyage. Dr. White's report (1880) is replete with medical information on the people all the way from Fort Simpson, B.C., to the Pribilofs, where he remained for two months while the ship went north with the physician employed at St. Paul by the Alaska Commercial Company (Bailey 1880, 19). After stops in the Panhandle, Kodiak, the Aleutians, and the Pribilofs, the *Rush* sailed north to the Bering Strait, where Bailey (1880, 26) noted much evidence of illicit whiskey trading.

White (1880, 41-47) felt he had two main functions, which were to become familiar to all doctors on the revenue cutters: to provide medical care to the crew and passengers, and to render "professional assistance" and medicines to the Native and White inhabitants of the settlements the ships visited. This second function, he emphasized, was "with the concurrence of the commanding officer." He (1880, 40) must have spent a great deal of time in medical care activities ashore, for his report has much to say on disease prevalence, Native customs, traditional medicine, and general social conditions for nearly every port of call. In the Aleutians, particularly, he left in each village "a small supply of safe and harmless remedies, which could do little injury if improperly administered."

The following summer the cutter *Thomas A. Corwin* made the first of several memorable voyages to the Arctic under the command of Capt. C. L. Hooper. (*See* Figure 13.) One of the principal results of this trip was the news that hundreds of St. Lawrence Island Eskimos had died of starvation the previous year (Hooper 1881, 10-11; *see* Chapter 18). In the summer of 1881 the *Corwin* returned to the Arctic, this time carrying the famous naturalist John Muir, who wrote a book about the voyage (1917), and the noted ethnographer and naturalist Edward W. Nelson, who in the immediate prior years had been based at St. Michael as an army weather observer. The ship again stopped at St. Lawrence Island, where important ethnographic materials, including human skulls, were collected for the U.S. National Museum.

The medical officer on this voyage was Dr. Irving C. Rosse of the Marine Hospital Service, who wrote a detailed appendix to Captain Hooper's report. This account is rich in medical observations on the Native people and on life as a ship's doctor. He cites many contemporary authorities, including a long passage from Father Veniaminov. Though a useful source for this period, the writing is marred by a pedantic and pompous style (Rosse 1883).

Captain Michael A. Healy, who became the best known of the revenue cutter officers, took the *Corwin* north for several years, notably 1884 and 1885, following which Congress published his full reports (Healy 1889; Healy 1887). Dr. H. W. Yemans was the medical officer on both voyages and provided much direct care to sick and injured whalers, shipwrecked sailors,

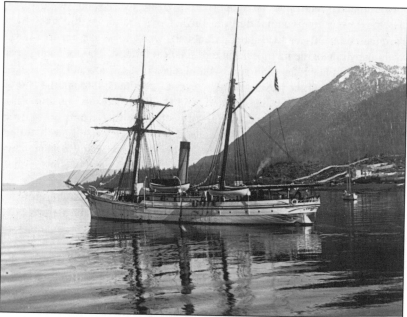

Figure 13. U.S. Revenue Cutter *Corwin*, whose medical officer regularly provided assistance to whalers and the people of western Alaska. (Rufus Rose Collection, Archives, Alaska and Polar Regions Dept., University of Alaska Fairbanks.)

miners, and the Natives in their villages. He also provided a description of the eruption of Bogoslof volcano (Healy 1889, 19). In his account of the 1885 voyage Healy wrote (1887, 17), "The value of the services of a medical officer in the Arctic cannot be too highly estimated. . . . When the *Corwin* first went north the Indians had a great repugnance to receiving medical attendance from a doctor, but would resort to their shaman to cure all their ailments. Now, however, the doctor is sought by them in all their ills. . . ."

The overriding concern of the revenue cutters, however, was to suppress the liquor traffic. Healy became almost a legendary figure for his pursuit of this quest. In 1884 (1889, 17) he wrote with evident pride that the general health and social conditions were much improved now that "the whiskey traffic in northern Alaska has almost entirely ceased." It is ironic that Healy himself later succumbed to alcoholism (*see* Chapter 17).

The voyages of the *Corwin* also contributed to the exploration of Alaska. As mentioned earlier Lieutenant Stoney of the Navy, while assigned to the ship, carried out his initial explorations of the Kobuk River in 1883 with encouragement and material support from Healy (Sherwood 1965b, 124). The next year Healy supported the further exploration of the river by a revenue cutter officer Lt. John C. Cantwell, who prepared a report (1889) with many ethnographic notes, some of medical interest. The following year Cantwell continued his explorations and wrote a further account (1887).

The voyages of the Revenue Cutter Service continued through the end of the century and beyond, but detailed published accounts are generally not available. Nearly all ships carried a physician, either from the Marine Hospital Service or from the Revenue Cutter Service itself, who found himself one of the busiest members of the ship's company. During this period there are records of doctors performing amputations, treating serious injuries on board ship or ashore, fighting epidemics in the villages as well as outbreaks on board, and dealing with advanced cases of tuberculosis, syphilis, and starvation. In one incident the doctor treated some shipwrecked and marooned sailors who had eaten the body of one of their shipmates to stay alive (James White 1894; Jackson 1897a, 1455).

In the late 1880s the *Bear* replaced the *Corwin* as the flagship of the Bering Sea Patrol, as the annual trips north had come to be known. The *Bear* was already justly famous as the rescue ship of the A. W. Greeley Expedition, which had come to grief some years before on Ellesmere Island in the Canadian Arctic. The best-known Alaskan exploit of the ship was the relief of the whaling fleet unexpectedly caught in the ice near Barrow in 1897-1898. The ship had already returned to Seattle when an urgent plea came that hundreds of whaling crew members would starve before spring unless food could be provided. The *Bear,* then under the command of Capt. Francis Tuttle, sailed in late November and, after some anxious moments in the stormy Bering Sea, reached Nelson Island in mid-December. There a party of four men were selected, led by Lt. D. H. Jarvis and including Dr. Samuel J. Call, a physician with already a long experience in Alaska (Cocke 1974). Jarvis purchased dogs, sleds, and supplies at the village and then mushed northward toward St. Michael assisted by a local trader as guide. Undergoing severe hardships, the Overland Relief Expedition, as it came to be known, ultimately reached Port Clarence, near Bering Strait, on January 10.

For the next three weeks they collected domesticated reindeer from the herds of the Seward Peninsula. Finally on February 3, 1898, the party, now augmented by several herdsmen driving no less than 438 reindeer, set off toward the stranded ships. Passing over the ice of Kotzebue Sound and along the Arctic Coast, the group, after many hardships, reached the first whaling ship on March 25 and Barrow a few days later (Boyd 1972). Many of the whalers were living in their icebound ships and others had moved ashore. They were filthy, hungry, and demoralized and not a few were sick with scurvy and other illnesses. Dr. H. Richmond Marsh, a missionary-teacher, had been on hand through the winter to take care of the most serious problems, but when Dr. Call arrived he took charge of the medical service, no doubt creating some tension in the process. Once the immediate problems of food shortage and medical care were taken care of, Dr. Call had time on his hands until the *Bear* returned to pick them up in the late summer. He used the opportunity to study the health situation among the Barrow Eskimos and left an account containing useful medical observations (*in* [Jarvis] 1899, 114-25). (*See* Figure 14.)

The Revenue Cutter Service and its physicians also distinguished themselves in the terrible influenza and measles epidemic in western Alaska in 1900. The ships brought medical supplies, drugs, and physician services to many stricken communities during this time. Perhaps the most detailed account of the epidemic was published by a Revenue Cutter Service physician aboard a Yukon River steamer that summer (J. White 1902). The epidemic and its consequences are discussed in detail in Chapter 12.

All in all, the doctors of the Revenue Cutter Service, some of whom, especially after 1888, were detailed from the Marine Hospital Service, made an invaluable contribution to the health and well-being of Alaskans in the latter third of the nineteenth century. The medical care was of course

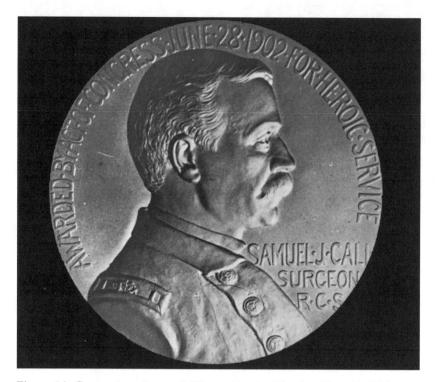

Figure 14. Commemorative medallion authorized by President McKinley to recognize Dr. Samuel J. Call for his part in the rescue of stranded whalers at Point Barrow in 1897-98. (S. J. Call Collection, Archives, Alaska and Polar Regions Dept., University of Alaska Fairbanks.)

episodic in nature, but sometimes lifesaving at sea for the men of the whaling fleets, and on land for the traders, missionaries, teachers, and Alaska Natives. Beyond direct medical care, the doctors provided advice and assistance in the control of epidemics and helped supply remote trading posts and missions with drugs and essential supplies. Perhaps the most useful health service the Revenue Cutter Service performed was its primary one—the suppression of the liquor trade that was causing untold harm to the Native communities along the coast. The writings of the captains and their medical officers also must not be discounted in evaluating their influence; for example, the reports of Captains Hooper and Healy, of Doctors White, Rosse, and Call were eloquent in describing the needs of this area for members of Congress, government officials, and the public at large.

Before leaving the Treasury Department, a brief note is appropriate about the special situation at Unalaska, which enjoyed the status of "Gateway to the Bering Sea." This community had always been a convenient stopping place for the hundreds of ships sailing from the north Pacific to the Bering Sea and beyond. As early as 1879 Captain Bailey of the *Rush* reported that the local trader and priest had joined efforts to raise money to build a small hospital, after which they planned to petition the government for a physician. Bailey (1880, 24) thought it a "worthy charity" to station a Marine Hospital Service physician there, but his recommendation was not acted on until two decades later, when hundreds of ships were passing through the Aleutians en route to the gold fields at Nome. In 1894 a visiting sea-captain mentioned that a navy surgeon was stationed at Unalaska (West 1965, 51), but the doctor may have simply been on temporary duty from a naval vessel such as the *Pinta*. In 1900 the Marine Hospital Service leased a building from the Alaska Commercial Company at Dutch Harbor and established a twenty-bed hospital, with two wards, an operating room, dispensary, and office. The staff consisted of two commissioned officers, including Dr. Dunlop Moore as officer-in-charge, a steward, and three attendants. The hospital lasted only a brief time, during the peak years of the Gold Rush (Brady 1900, 36, 61).

THE REINDEER SERVICE

An unusual and somewhat controversial item of Alaskan history was the introduction of domesticated reindeer into northwestern Alaska beginning in 1891. This idea was first proposed by Dr. Charles Townsend, naturalist on the 1885 voyage of the *Corwin*. During the voyage of the *Bear* in 1890, Captain Healy mentioned it to Dr. Sheldon Jackson, a former Presbyterian missionary then serving as U.S. General Agent for Education in Alaska. Jackson was making his first trip to the Arctic to inspect missions and schools for the government. As he gazed at the bleak tundra and scattered villages of the Eskimos he became convinced that the people were rapidly dying out, due to the baneful influences of whiskey and the decline of food resources (D. Ray 1975, 226). He seized on Healy's suggestion that the importation of Siberian reindeer could lead to a new source of food and a new industry.

Jackson made a proposal to the Interior Department in his report that year but action in Congress failed in 1891 and again in 1892. Undaunted, he raised enough private funds in 1891 to purchase sixteen reindeer in Siberia and with the help of Healy and the *Bear* to bring them back to Alaska. These initial animals were landed in the Aleutian Islands and all died of starvation before the winter was out. The following year Healy, on questionable authority, made five trips to the Siberian coast to purchase 171 additional head, which were landed near Port Clarence at a spot later called Teller Reindeer Station. When an appropriation finally passed Congress in 1893, the herd was already growing. Initially four Chukchi were brought in to teach the Eskimos herding techniques. In 1894, however, the Siberians returned home and six Norwegian Lapps arrived to take over the teaching and herd management duties. Between 1891 and 1902 a total of 1280 reindeer were imported and landed, largely at Teller. During this period animals were loaned to various missions, where Eskimos were involved in their care and were paid for their services by animals of their own. Only the surplus males could be slaughtered for profit (Brickey and Brickey 1975, 17).

This project is of medical interest for two reasons. Jackson's justification for it in the first place was to save the Eskimos from starvation. His premise was probably wrong, as evidenced by the fact that the Eskimos were actually increasing in number around this time on the Seward Peninsula (D. Ray 1975, 226). In any event the whole basis for the program changed within a few years from the purpose of "saving the Eskimos" to the establishment of a new and profitable industry, all of this with the apparent blessing of Jackson (D. Ray 1975, 237).

The second aspect of medical interest is that at least two of the staff in the 1890s were physicians. The superintendent at Teller Station noted in his report of 1895 that, although the local Lutheran missionary and schoolteacher Tollef L. Brevig had a supply of medicines at his home, physicians needed to be assigned because the fifty or so employees were uncomfortable with the absence of medical care. The Lapps, he said, also were clamoring for a doctor and the Eskimos needed one as well (although they apparently hadn't asked), so that it would be unnecessary for them to resort to "witches." As further justification he noted that Port Clarence was the only deep-water harbor in the area and that whalers often stopped for the purpose of seeking medical help (Jackson 1896b, 82, 88-89).

The 1897 report indicated that a physician, Dr. A. N. Kittelsen, had been hired and had attended sixty-six cases of illness the previous year, of whom one died—the wife of a Laplander. He had also provided medical care to the Swedish Covenant missionaries in Golovin and, most encouraging of all, had attended over 250 cases of illness among the Eskimos, some of whom had come from as far as two hundred miles. The superintendent felt vindicated for recommending a physician, since more and more the shamans seemed to be losing the confidence of their people (Jackson 1898c, 56). For a short period Dr. Kittelsen also served as superintendent of the station (D. Ray 1975, 238).

In December 1897 the headquarters of the reindeer project were moved from Teller Station to a new site called Eaton Station on the Unalakleet River some distance up from the village of Unalakleet. Dr. Kittelsen also served there as temporary superintendent, but in a few months resigned from the project to prospect for gold (Jackson 1899, 1774). The teacher selected for the new site was another physician, Dr. Francis H. Gambell of Iowa, who also performed the necessary medical work. Dr. Gambell was a man of considerable talent and energy. In addition to serving as physician and teacher at the station, he also soon assumed the duties of acting superintendent. As if those responsibilities were insufficient to occupy his time, he undertook an evening school to teach English to the adults of the community. During his first year he was described as grubbing a patch of ground for a vegetable garden, prospecting in Golovnin Bay, traveling by boat to St. Michael for the mail, and regularly skating the ten or so miles down the river to Unalakleet, usually to attend the sick. At Eaton Station he provided care not only to the sick employees, including the imported Lapp herders, but also to the sick reindeer. Native patients came to consult him from as far away as the middle Yukon, King Island, the Diomedes, and the Bering coast. Many sick miners also found their way to Eaton Station for treatment. In 1898-1899 he listed the diagnoses and clinical outcomes of 106 patients he treated, omitting "minor cases, such as headaches, constipation, sprains, etc. . . ." (F. Gambell 1900, 69-71; Jackson 1901b, 11). (*See* Figure 15.)

THE PLEA FOR GOVERNMENT NATIVE HOSPITALS

The need for hospitals to care for the Native people became increasingly apparent to many during the last decades of the nineteenth century. Nearly everyone recognized that health conditions were deteriorating, principally from the destructive effects of tuberculosis and alcohol. There was general recognition as well that the federal government would ultimately have to assume the burden of providing health care. The military services had made some reluctant efforts in this direction, as we have seen, and the Treasury Department had done even more. Only after civil government came to Alaska in 1884, however, did the medical care of the Natives become an issue of responsibility, although little or nothing was actually accomplished for at least two more decades.

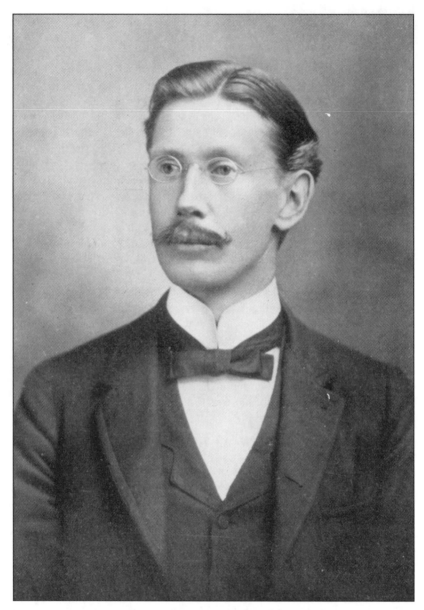

Figure 15. Dr. Francis H. Gambell, superintendent of Eaton Reindeer Station. (Jackson 1900.)

In 1886 the second appointed governor, Alfred Swineford, made the earliest appeals, noting that "despotic Russia" had seen fit to provide hospitals at Sitka, Kodiak, Unalaska, and Hot Springs at an annual cost of $10,000 but that the United States had abandoned them. If it was the desire of the government to save the Native people from extinction, then in his view a hospital was "absolutely indispensable." "The appeals from these people are incessant," he went on, "and I see them dying almost daily for the want of the medical care and attention which, it seems to me, a humane government ought not to hesitate to provide them." He closed his appeals to Washington: "That we cannot successfully minister to a mind diseased is not more true than that we cannot hope for the complete mental regeneration of a people whom we abandon to physical decay" (Swineford 1886, 28-29).

The appeal was taken up three years later by his successor Gov. Lyman E. Knapp (1889, 22), although in more modest terms: "But I do feel strongly in favor of the establishment of governmental hospitals in places of convenient access in the Territory. . . . It would seem that this much is due the natives. . . ." These hospitals he saw as the only way to eliminate tuberculosis and syphilis, for example, and cherished the hope that such facilities could even act as an "educating influence toward personal cleanliness and a higher civilization" (Knapp 1889, 22). In his report the following year, Governor Knapp (1890, 24) pressed his case again, this time adducing in support the testimony of several missionaries, military officers, and physicians.

In his last appeal as governor, Knapp (1892, 58) summed up his growing conviction:

I am profoundly impressed with the idea that, as a nation, we owe it to ourselves and to the natives of Alaska that we build, equip, and support hospitals in various parts of the Territory for the care of the sick and the chronically diseased. Humanity demands it, treaty obligations require it, and self-interest ought to prompt it. . . . Leave alone all our expensive explorations and scientific investigations if you must, omit all appropriations for schools if our great and rich nation cannot afford to educate its wards, withdraw missions and other civilizing influences if it becomes a necessary alternative, but do not fail to afford relief to suffering humanity.

Other voices were heard. Dr. P. H. J. Lerrigo (1901, 105), a missionary teacher on St. Lawrence Island, suggested that private philanthropy might be willing to found a Native hospital. But it was Dr. Carroll Fox (1902, 1616) of the Marine Hospital Service who wrote most prophetically. After investigating the prevalence of tuberculosis in southeastern Alaska, he wrote the surgeon general that such a matter, since it dealt with sanitation and hygiene, was a proper task for the Marine Hospital Service. He proposed stationing a medical officer in the territory to supervise health work in the Native villages, including vaccination. "I would even go so far as to suggest," he concluded, "the establishment of a hospital for the care and isolation of tubercular patients." A decade or so later the first federal hospital for Natives opened in Juneau, under the Bureau of Education of the Department of the Interior. More than a half century later, however, it was the U.S. Public Health Service, the direct descendant of the Marine Hospital Service, that took over the operation of all federal hospitals for Alaska Natives in the territory, including several that were devoted to the care of tuberculosis (Fortuine 1975a, 19-20).

9

Whalers, Traders, Fishermen, and Prospectors

WHALERS

Although the beginnings of commercial whaling in the Bering Sea and Arctic Ocean fall well within the period of the Russian-American Company, the subject is treated in this chapter because most of the ships were American and the pursuit of whales probably reached its peak during the early years of American sovereignty.

As early as 1840 New England whaling ships had discovered the abundance of whales in the Gulf of Alaska. Word spread rapidly and before long many other ships from New England ports were hunting south of the Alaska Peninsula and Aleutians. In 1845 the first ships entered the Bering Sea and only three years later a New York whaler, the *Superior*, under Captain Thomas Roys, ventured through the Bering Strait. The following year no fewer than fifty whalers, forty-six of them American, sailed through the strait. At first they were phenomenally successful, but within a few years their initial high hopes were tempered by considerably smaller catches. By 1854, acting on a tip from Captain Collinson of the British Royal Navy, five whalers reached Barrow and hunted for the first time in the Beaufort Sea (Bockstoce 1986, 93-98). In the 1860s the whaling fleet suffered major setbacks as a result of the depredations of the Confederate raider *Shenandoah*, which destroyed thirty-four Yankee whalers and took some 1053 prisoners. Much of the damage, ironically, came after the end of the Civil War but before the news had reached the warship (Bockstoce 1986, 125).

The 1870s were marked by ups and downs in the whaling industry, although mostly the latter. Some catches were notably successful, especially once walrus as well as whales began to be hunted. A substantial setback occurred in 1871, however, when in the late summer the greater part of the northern fleet was caught in severe ice conditions near Point Belcher. In all thirty-three ships were lost, their crews being rescued by seven ships that had lagged behind near Icy Cape. Other bad years followed, notably 1876, when eleven ships were wrecked, this time with some loss of life as well (Bockstoce 1986, 151-59; 171).

What motivated the whaling captains to keep trying in the face of these appalling losses and a steep decline in the price of whale oil was the new demand for whalebone, or baleen, which was used mainly for corset stays. New technology was required to keep whaling profitable, however, and in 1880 the American ship *Mary and Helen,* the first steam-powered whaler, passed the Bering Strait and later returned with a very valuable cargo (Bockstoce 1986, 208-10). Such ships had of course much more power and maneuverability in the ice and thus were able to push eastward beyond Point Barrow to Herschel Island, which later became an important rendezvous and overwintering site.

Beginning in 1884 a few shore stations were established, first at Corwin Coal Mine (near Cape Lisburne) and Point Barrow, and a few years later at Point Hope. There whaling crews spent the winter and, using small shore-based boats like the Eskimos, could take advantage of the spring whale migration (Bockstoce 1986, 233-36). In 1889 whaling ships themselves began spending the winter in the Arctic, usually near Barrow, Herschel Island, or at the mouth of the Mackenzie River, so that they could get an earlier start the following season. During the winter months the crew often lived ashore and hunted caribou for food or traded with the Eskimos for provisions. (*See* Figure 16.)

The great number of ships coming north each year inevitably had a significant impact on the lives of the Eskimos, especially in certain villages. For example, many vessels awaiting favorable ice conditions congregated each year at Port Clarence, just south of the Bering Strait, because it was the only protected harbor in the vicinity. The villages of Point Hope and Barrow, both of which were sites of major shore stations, were also particularly susceptible to the baneful influence of the whalers.

According to Don C. Foote (1964, 17) there were at least six ways in which the whaling crews interacted with the Eskimos. First, crewmen from the ships went ashore at the site of a Native village in order to trade or simply to sightsee. Second, Eskimos often came out to the ships lying at anchor, usually out of curiosity, or for purposes of trade in ivory, whalebone, or crafts. Both of these types of contacts were brief and usually innocuous, except for the trade in liquor. The third type of contact was through shipwreck, when the survivors might live through the winter in a village until rescued the following season by another whaling ship or by the Revenue Marine Service. The fourth type was voluntary overwintering, when the ship allowed itself to be frozen in the ice. The crew usually lived ashore for the winter, and had intensive and often intimate relations with the Natives. Deserters were the fifth type of contact. Conditions were so hard on board whaling ships that even a remote arctic village seemed preferable to life in the "fo'c's'le." Finally, many of the whaling ships, particularly those that overwintered, recruited Eskimo crew members, who were hardy, knowledgeable, and skilled in the hunt. Each of these types of contact could have been responsible for the spread of disease from the whalers to the Eskimos and perhaps in the opposite direction as well.

Life on board a whaling ship was harsh and hazardous in the extreme. Voyages often lasted up to four years, and most of that time was spent in the

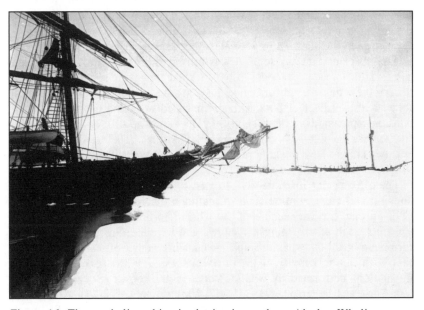

Figure 16. Three whaling ships in the ice in northern Alaska. Whaling crews sometimes traded alcohol and often inadvertently introduced diseases to the Eskimos. (Willoughby Collection, Archives, Alaska and Polar Regions Dept., University of Alaska Fairbanks.)

stormy arctic seas. Chasing the great bowhead whale in a longboat was not only exhausting but fraught with great dangers if the whale put up a fight. Life at sea otherwise was a combination of utter boredom and all the strenuous and repetitive tasks necessary to keep a ship under sail. The crews were largely drawn from the dregs of society on the New Bedford waterfront. Many were criminals or alcoholics, and not a few suffered from syphilis, gonorrhea, tuberculosis, rheumatism, or other chronic diseases (Rosse 1883, 15), including mental disorders (Healy 1887, 7).

Some idea of the conditions that prevailed on whaling ships of this period may be gained from the account of Captain Ellsworth West (1965, 8-9), a New England whaleman who spent many years cruising Alaskan waters. On his first voyage as a seaman in 1882 he passed the first day queasy from seasickness before turning in to sleep on a bunk "as hard and narrow as a coffin." He was soon awakened by a pricking sensation to find his blanket alive with bedbugs. An older shipmate suggested that cockroaches were the answer to bedbugs. A quick trip to the galley, where they were "thick as fleas," produced more than enough for their needs. Soon the bedbugs were gone but the bunk was overrun with roaches. The quarters were small, bilgy, and dark, the only light coming through an overhead scuttle that could be slid open in good weather. During a gale water seeped in everywhere and the blankets became "wet as sop." It was fully two months before the young sailor could stomach the food. For breakfast the men were served hardtack, a chicory brew that passed for coffee, and "scouse," a concoction of potatoes boiled with salt beef or pork. Dinner consisted of boiled potatoes in their skins, accompanied by more salt beef. The pea soup offered from time to time to vary the diet was "likely to be full of worms." The evening meal was usually a kind of hash made from unappetizing leftovers. The only fresh food was bread baked twice a week.

The officers not infrequently resorted to cruel punishments, including flogging and close confinement, to maintain discipline (Bockstoce 1986, 229). Further, the very nature of the whaler's work assured many serious accidents, such as drownings, fractures, and frostbite. Since there were no doctors on board the whaling ships, the captain or other officer had to do his best with a small medical kit or even less. Several records of limb amputations performed by whaling captains are known (Bockstoce 1986, 260; Cook and Pederson 1937, 114-17; [Jarvis] 1899, 122-23). After 1880 the Revenue Marine Service ships carried a surgeon on board who spent much of his time caring for the crews of whaling ships (Healy 1889, 19).

Shipwreck accounted for the loss of a few vessels each summer, quite aside from the major disaster years. Some were crushed in the shifting sea ice and others were driven ashore, where the half-frozen crew, if lucky, found the nearest Eskimo village. The reception ashore was not always hospitable. Charles Brower (1960, 24-25) tells of three men who deserted a whaler near Cape Lisburne. Two of them died of exposure and the third, rescued by the Eskimos, developed pneumonia and was taken outside and killed, on the advice of the shaman, to prevent him from dying in the house and thus making it unfit for further use.

Especially in the later years of the nineteenth century, when whales and walrus were becoming scarce, the whaling crews became responsible for at least some of the brisk trade in liquor and guns that became such a curse to the Eskimos from Port Clarence to Herschel Island (*see* Chapter 17). Some captains—perhaps even the majority—were in fact opposed to trading liquor, but their men were able to trade contraband alcohol surreptitiously (Jackson 1894a, 874; Aldrich 1889, 115). Many others, however, found a few drinks of whiskey encouraged the Eskimos to give a better price for their baleen, ivory, jade, and furs. After 1880 the intensive policing effort of the U.S. Revenue Marine ships led to a rapid decline in these trading abuses by the whalers (Healy 1887, 17), but much of the damage was already done. Both guns and liquor led to serious disruptions of traditional life. The guns contributed to depletion of the animals hunted for food, while abuse of liquor often led not only to violence (Jenness 1957, 164) but also to a failure to hunt, with resulting starvation (Benjamin 1898, 860).

The men who came north on whaling ships from 1848 to 1900 suffered many hardships and privations, often losing their health and even their lives in the arctic regions. Many were already afflicted with chronic diseases, some of which, such as tuberculosis and syphilis, were infectious to others. The influences of the whalers on the Native people were profound. They greatly depleted the numbers of whales and walrus that were essential to the Eskimos' livelihood. They traded guns and liquor, with many adverse consequences for the Natives. Finally, they inadvertently brought new infectious diseases to a susceptible and vulnerable population (*see* Chapters 12, 14, and 15).

TRADERS AND COMMERCIAL INTERESTS

American ships, mostly from New England, were a well-known source of irritation to the Russians as early as the late eighteenth century; in fact, one of Baranov's compelling reasons for establishing a base in southeastern

Alaska was to demonstrate sovereignty and to discourage what they considered to be poaching on their domains. These "Boston ships," as they were called, engaged in independent trade with the Tlingit, buying up sea otter and other pelts for a cargo of guns, ammunition, and liquor, and then proceeding to China, where they received handsome prices for the peltry. By 1806, seventy-two American voyages had been made to the coast. Not only did the Russians resent the loss of revenue from furs they considered rightfully theirs, but the trade in guns and liquor posed a serious threat to their security, as many hostile encounters with the Indians demonstrated (Gibson 1976, 155-60). It is also certainly possible that these early New England traders introduced disease, particularly syphilis (Romanovskii *in* Pierce 1974).

Despite an official policy discouraging outside contact, the fledgling colony at New Archangel was saved from starvation more than once in the early years of the nineteenth century by the timely arrival of an American trading ship. Baranov, even from his Kodiak days, had maintained friendly relations with certain American captains, notably Joseph O'Cain and John D'Wolf, who brought provision to the colonies more dependably than ships from far-off St. Petersburg or even Okhotsk (Gibson 1976, 154). Trade with American ships continued after the departure of Baranov, but on a diminished scale because of the company's greater ability to safeguard its interests, especially in southeastern Alaska.

American traders had ventured to the Aleutians and apparently even as far north as Kotzebue Sound by 1820, offering liquor (Corney 1965, 140) and guns (D. Ray 1975, 67-69, 92-94) in exchange for furs and other items. Other trade items, such as knives, kettles, hatchets, needles, and even tobacco, were less sought after. By the time the first whalers reached the Bering Strait in 1848, the Eskimos were already well acquainted with rum, presumably from trading vessels (Bockstoce 1986, 182). Most of these ships were American, but rather than sailing from Boston, as in earlier years, many were based in San Francisco, Fort Simpson, B.C., the Hawaiian Islands, or even Hong Kong. Their principal stock-in-trade was hard liquor, such as rum or whiskey, breech-loading rifles, and ammunition, all of which were illegal for trade with the Native people. In addition, they dealt in tobacco, molasses (for making homebrew), and a variety of useful iron implements such as knives, axes, and other tools and utensils.

The trading ships ventured north very early in the season, preferably before the arrival of the revenue steamers. They tended to congregate at Port

Clarence, Wales, and Kotzebue Sound, all of which were traditional Eskimo trading centers. As late as 1878 there were eleven trading vessels in Kotzebue Sound, many of them offloading liquor by the barrel. The following year Captain Bailey (1880, 17, 19) of the Revenue Marine Steamer *Rush* investigated the wreck of a trading brig from Honolulu, which had on board a cargo of tobacco, guns, muzzle- and breech-loading rifles, ammunition, and no less than one hundred barrels of rum. Much of this liquor was shipped in bond destined for Siberian communities such as Plover Bay and East Cape and then resold piecemeal in Alaska across the Bering Strait. With price mark-ups and dilution of the rum the trader made a profit of about six hundred percent. Sometimes a wealthy Eskimo purchased a large stock and then sold it by the drink to the members of his community (H. Otis *in* Bailey 1880, 43-44; *see also* Chapter 17).

The presence of liquor often led to drunken violence, or at the least, to an inability of the people to hunt or fish for subsistence. The village of Wales, which was easily accessible to any whaler or trader passing the Bering Strait, was one of those particularly cursed by the availability of alcohol. The teacher-missionary H. L. Thornton (1931, 52), who was later murdered at the village, wrote in lurid detail of the drunken orgies that occurred there. Both Thornton's murder and another violent episode known as the Gilley affair are described in Chapter 18.

In southeastern Alaska, meanwhile, illegal traders were also active, they too trading principally in liquor, guns, and ammunition. Because of the many narrow inlets and hidden harbors it was nearly impossible to ferret them out, despite the presence at Sitka of one or more navy or revenue marine ships. In a letter Captain J. M. Selden of the Revenue Marine Service wrote that sailing vessels were "of no earthly use in these waters" and that what was needed rather were small, fast steam launches to patrol the inland waterways against smugglers (*in* Colyer 1869, 1020). None were forthcoming and the smugglers continued to thrive through most of the nineteenth century, supplying Indians with liquor and other contraband goods.

A similar situation prevailed in the Aleutians (Colyer 1869, 1022), although here the isolated and sparsely populated villages made the trade relatively unprofitable. On the Pribilofs the importation of liquor was expressly forbidden (and carefully monitored), but the Aleuts were able to bring in the ingredients for their homebrew called *kvass* (H. Elliott 1875, 25).

Besides the independent sea-going traders there were scattered land-based independent traders in some coastal villages and towns and in the interior, chiefly along the major rivers. Most of these were engaged to some extent in the fur trade, buying up furs in exchange for basic supplies. Few if any traders in the interior dealt in liquor, however, for they recognized all too clearly its destructive effects on their own livelihood. These traders of the forest are probably underrated in history, for some were men of great fortitude and humanity who learned the Native languages, often married Native women, and acted generally as intermediaries between disparate and clashing cultures. They were frequently called upon to help in times of illness or injury and freely extended credit in times of scarcity and hunger (Hinckley 1972, 93).

Many such traders were affiliated more or less with a larger company, notably the sprawling Alaska Commercial Company. This began in 1867 as the Hutchinson, Kohl and Company, when a San Francisco merchant named Hutchinson succeeded in purchasing all the assets, including buildings, ships, and warehouse stocks, of the Russian-American Company. Two years later the Alaska Commercial Company was incorporated and the following year was granted by Congress a twenty-year exclusive lease on the Pribilof Islands. The company also developed several of the old Russian posts, especially Unalaska and St. Michael, into bases for a far-flung empire of small trading establishments. As a matter of policy (and economics), it decided not to operate in southeastern Alaska (Hulley 1958, 207-8).

On the Pribilofs the company created, according to the terms of its lease, a kind of combination welfare state and plantation economy. On the positive side (at least on paper), the company provided schools, support for widows and orphans, new houses, and a physician on each island for the Aleuts. According to Henry W. Elliott (1880, 20, 108), who sometimes viewed the Pribilofs as an Eden in the Bering Sea, there was a hospital on St. Paul "with a complete stock of drugs, and skilled physicians on both islands to take care of the people, free of cost." The physicians, he said, "have already, by their efforts, seconded by the example of the other white residents, induced greater cleanliness and a more healthful mode of living among the natives."

Although these health facilities and services were more than any other Alaska Natives enjoyed at this time, they by no means guaranteed health. As Elliott himself pointed out elsewhere (1886, 238), the Aleuts when ill seemed so despondent and resigned to their fate that they made no effort to live. The major cause of death was tuberculosis, and despite the prohibition of alcohol on the island, many succumbed to the effects of homebrew, or *kvass*.

These observations demonstrate that the Pribilof Aleuts were not living in a healthy environment, either physical or mental. In effect they had lost their economic and social freedom, and with it their will and motivation. They had become serfs bound not to the soil but to the beaches and tundra of their stormy islands (Torrey 1978, 73-85). This process had begun under the Russians and, although sweetened by more material goods, continued to develop under American rule.

On the mainland, the Alaska Commercial Company operated in a different manner. Utilizing to the full both knowledgeable Creoles who had been with the Russian-American Company and semi-independent fur traders and prospectors with an intimate knowledge of the country, it soon developed a wide network of stations from Prince William Sound to their major northern post, which in the earlier years was St. Michael. The latter served as headquarters for many small stations along the Yukon River and its tributaries as far as Fort Yukon, an old Hudson's Bay Company post that had been proven in 1869 to be in U.S. territory (Raymond 1870-71; Lain 1977). The Alaska Commercial Company had its own ships, including river steamers, its own rudimentary medical system (Dr. Call of the Overland Relief Expedition was once a company doctor at Unalaska), and worked in harmony with the Russian Orthodox Church. The company was an important force in the economic development of Alaska. Although it certainly hastened cultural change among the Natives, sometimes for the worse, it generally treated them fairly, often offering credit and even medical care when it was available. There were other trading companies in Alaska, notably the North American Trading and Transportation Company, founded by John J. Healy, which primarily served the prospectors of the upper reaches of the Yukon River (Burlingame 1978). None, however, had the impact of the Alaska Commercial Company.

The Alaska canned-salmon industry began early in the American period with the establishment of a saltery at Klawock in 1868. Ten years later a cannery was built there and another near the site of old Sitka (Hulley 1958, 217-18). In five more years, a large saltery and cannery opened at Loring on Naha Bay north of Ketchikan (Roppel 1975). In 1883 the first cannery was established at Nushagak (VanStone 1972) and in 1890 at Naknek in the Bristol Bay region. By 1898 there were some fifty-five canneries operating each summer on the coasts of Alaska (Hulley 1958, 218).

In the early years, the salmon packers employed few Alaskans either in the canneries or on their fishing boats, except in southeastern Alaska. Large numbers of local workers, first of all, were not available at the isolated cannery sites for a short season, and in any event the industrialists felt that the Natives were unreliable and inefficient workers (VanStone 1967, 73). For the most part Chinese laborers were employed on the factory lines while Caucasians from the Pacific coast of the United States operated the fishing boats (Roppel 1975). The work was hectic and exhausting during the short season, and with the crude machinery of the period and the absence of safety inspections, it is likely that many injuries resulted. The Chinese, who were often afflicted with tuberculosis and other diseases, lived in cramped, poorly ventilated barracks that fostered the spread of disease. They also used alcohol, tobacco, and opium—habits they often encouraged among the local Natives (VanStone 1967, 76-77).

PROSPECTORS AND MINERS

The last five years of nineteenth-century Alaskan history were dominated by rapid change brought about by the influx of thousands of hopeful gold seekers who poured into the territory at Skagway and Dyea in southeastern Alaska, at Valdez in Prince William Sound, and at St. Michael and Nome in northwestern Alaska. These men and women, from all over the United States and in fact from many foreign countries as well, had only one goal: to get rich quickly, either by mining gold themselves or by profiting from those that did, and then leaving for home to enjoy the fruits of their hardship. This massive migration left Alaska and its people no longer what they were before. Communities grew, flourished, and died within a few years, blank areas on the map were rapidly filled in, and traditional life was greatly disrupted by new and intense trading and other contact with the Natives. The health implications were also significant, not only for the migrants, who suffered much hardship and disease, but also for the Natives, who were exposed more intensely than ever before to acute and chronic infectious diseases to which they had little prior exposure.

Gold had been discovered in Alaska as early as 1849 when the Russian-American Company sent a mining engineer, Petr Doroshin, to the Kenai Peninsula. Doroshin was successful in finding "color" on the Kenai River but not in profitable amounts. He did suggest the development of several coal deposits, such as the one at Port Graham, which was worked from 1855 to 1860 (Golder 1916; Pierce 1975).

In 1871 gold was discovered in the Cassiar district of British Columbia and thousands of prospectors flooded into the country (Brooks 1973, 299). Fort Wrangell, which controlled the approach to the Stikine River valley, suddenly became the first of Alaska's boom towns, complete with saloons, gambling halls, outfitters, and houses of prostitution. The town catered, as so many others in the next few decades, to the needs of both those eager souls on the way to the gold fields, and to those returning in jubilation or sadness (Hinckley 1972, 70).

In that same year two Sitka prospectors, Richard Harris and Joseph Juneau, found rich placer gold deposits near the present site of Juneau. Shortly after a major quartz lode formation was discovered across the Gastineau Channel at present-day Douglas, which became the site of the huge Treadwell Mine. This operation soon expanded to include a giant pit known as the "Glory Hole," whose sides enclosed thirteen acres (Brooks 1973, 302-5). The Treadwell complex grew rapidly, from an original five-stamp mill to 880 stamps and 450 employees about a decade later. Since the demand for mine and mill labor could not be satisfied initially with local residents, nor with Indians, who abhorred the noise and regimentation, Treadwell imported Chinese workers in large numbers. These immigrants worked long hours for low pay under hazardous and unhealthful conditions. Yet that was not the sum of their troubles. In 1886 a gang of Juneau "toughs" undertook to drive out the Chinese with dynamite, guns, and muscle. Governor Swineford hastened up from Sitka to restore order but not before the Chinese had been herded aboard two schooners and shipped south (Hinckley 1972, 169-70).

Prior to the establishment of civil government in Alaska in 1884, no person could legally own land in Alaska, nor was there any effective legal means to settle disputes or punish crimes. In the Juneau mining district the miners evolved their own form of representative government called the miners' meeting, which served as jury and judge in many disputes. In 1881 some White men were killed by the Tlingit and the miners took matters into their own hands by capturing and hanging the supposed perpetrators. The miners went on to organize militia companies to protect themselves and to maintain order (Brooks 1973, 307). In later years these miners' meetings continued to exist in isolated parts of the territory, far beyond the reach of the primitive judicial system. Since prison was usually not an option, the miners not infrequently imposed fines, banishment, and even capital punishment for theft or murder.

In 1873 L. N. "Jack" McQuesten and Arthur Harper entered the upper reaches of the Yukon via Canada and spent the greater part of the rest of their lives prospecting the Yukon River and its tributaries while serving as agents for the Alaska Commercial Company. In 1878 Harper was the first to explore the upper section of the Tanana River and to find evidence of gold on the Fortymile, near the Canadian border. McQuesten devoted himself primarily to the fur trade and to serving the needs of the increasing numbers of prospectors and traders who came into the Yukon country. Many of the latter were arriving over the Chilkoot Pass, which had been reluctantly opened by the Chilkats in 1880 after negotiations with one of Captain Beardslee's officers (Brooks 1973, 321-24).

During the 1880s prospecting continued in the lower reaches of the Yukon, the Koyukuk, and on the Kuskokwim. The big find, however, was coarse gold in the river bars of the Fortymile and Franklin rivers in 1886, on the Alaska side of the boundary. One of the miners, Tom Williams, died of pneumonia after crossing the Chilkoot Pass in winter to bring the news out, so that additional supplies could be brought in with the first boat (De Armond 1973).

In 1893 two Creoles discovered gold in significant quantities in the Birch Creek area. Within three years the town of Circle City had sprouted up, with a population of one thousand, including many women, and facilities such as a sawmill, hospital, and even an opera house (Hinckley 1972, 215-16; Brooks 1973, 333). This region continued as the largest concentration of miners on the Yukon until the discovery of the riches of the Klondike in 1896. Gold was also discovered near Rampart in 1893 and a boom town developed there as well.

The story of the discovery of gold on Bonanza Creek and the subsequent development of Dawson and the Klondike gold fields properly belongs to the history of Canada. These wild and rollicking years had a heavy impact on Alaska, however, as thousands of people, mostly Americans, found access to the Klondike through Alaskan territory. Many naive hopes for instant wealth, in fact, were shattered before the gold-seekers even stepped foot on Canadian soil. Gold in substantial amounts was first recovered from Bonanza Creek as early as 1896, but it was not until the first shipment of the precious metal from St. Michael in the summer of 1897 that the wild scramble to the North began. Before winter some two thousand had already reached the Klondike, adding to the three thousand people already in the territory. But this was only a pale foreshadowing of the rush in the spring of 1898. Although the rapid influx led to temporary shortages of provisions, by the following spring the Canadian authorities had matters well in hand (Hulley 1958, 251-52).

The major route to the Yukon gold fields was via the Lynn Canal and the Taiya Inlet, either to Skagway and over the Coast Range through White Pass, or to Dyea and over the Chilkoot Pass. The initially favored Chilkoot Pass was thirty-five miles in length and reached an altitude of 3500 feet, whereas White Pass, which became more popular in the winter and spring of 1898, was ten miles longer but involved a climb to only 2400 feet. Both passes were situated on the Alaskan border with Canada and guarded by stalwarts of the Royal Canadian Mounted Police, who insisted that every prospector carry at least one year's provisions before being allowed into Canada.

Skagway and Dyea grew up almost overnight as staging areas for this frenzied mass migration. Both towns were filled with thousands of men and women from all walks of life, from down-and-outers and prostitutes to shopkeepers and professional persons, including many doctors. Most were inexperienced and naive, at least as prospectors, and were motivated largely by dreams of princely wealth and an easy life. A few were canny individuals who knew exactly what they wanted and how to get it. Both towns moved quickly to accommodate the influx. Many wiser men saw that money was to be gained with more certainty and less hazard by selling goods and services to the miners than by going to the goldfields themselves. Some came as miners but stayed instead as doctors, pharmacists, lawyers, barkeepers, and barbers, a few of them permanently. (*See* Figure 17.) Nor were all scrupulous businessmen. Money was conspicuous both among the gold-seekers going north and those few returning with a full "poke." Jefferson C. "Soapy" Smith and his gang relieved many miners of their cash or gold until he was killed by vigilantes in Skagway in July 1898 (Hulley 1958, 258).

During the winter and spring of 1897-1898, Canadian records show that nearly 28,000 gold-seekers, including 631 women (Alberts 1977), came over the White or Chilkoot passes to the Klondike. Most of these had arrived from Seattle or San Francisco in crowded, poorly ventilated accommodations on aging steamers that packed as many paying customers as possible on board. No navigational aids existed in the treacherous coastal waters and not a few of these ships went aground in the difficult channels of the Alexander Archipelago. A few heavily laden vessels sank with great loss of life (Brooks 1973, 427). The food on board was often described as terrible and contributed significantly, no doubt, to the prevalence of seasickness. The crowded ships also spawned much disease among the passengers, including typhoid fever, respiratory disease, and in one case a major epidemic of meningitis causing some twenty deaths at Dyea in the spring of 1898 (Satterfield 1973, 66).

The passes themselves had their own agony and potential for disaster. In April 1898 an avalanche of snow on Chilkoot Pass buried 142 persons, with at least 43 deaths (Reinicker 1984, 23-24). What every would-be miner had to suffer on the Alaska side was the long and arduous climb over one of the passes, heavily loaded with equipment and supplies. Loads could be dragged part of the way by sled but could be brought over the summit only on the backs of the miners, or in some cases Indians employed for the task. The average outfit weighed seven tons or more, requiring repeated journeys from the beach to the base of the summit and then seemingly endless exhausting climbs, one step at a time, over the summit. Many people were ill-prepared for such physical exertion and some died from sheer exhaustion on the mountain. The cold aggravated the climb, especially near the windy summits. Accidents, including falls, were frequent. In the initial enthusiasm engendered by greed, few stopped to help someone fallen by the wayside, too weak to go on. Yet in spite of all the hazards of climate, disease, environment, and human frailty, only about one percent failed to reach the Canadian side. Later, conditions improved, with the construction of a wagon road on the White Pass and an aerial tram for freight on the Chilkoot Pass (Brooks 1973, 356-357).

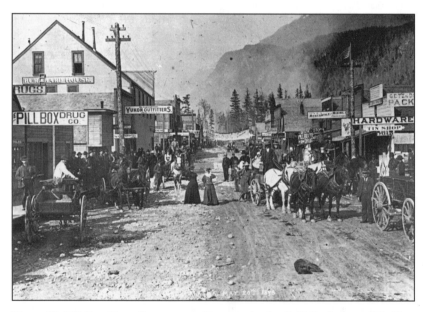

Figure 17. Pill Box Drug Company at Skagway, in the Gold Rush days. (MacKay Collection, Archives, Alaska and Polar Regions Dept., University of Alaska Fairbanks.)

Beyond the passes, however, the miners' problems were by no means over. The trail was still fraught with such hazards as stormy lakes, whitewater rapids in frail boats, and unbelievable clouds of bloodthirsty mosquitoes. From Seattle to Dawson took most prospectors at least three months (Hulley 1958, 253-54).

Not all of those on the "Trail of '98" tried to reach the Klondike via the Coast Range. Many with their heavy supplies followed the 3000-mile sea route to St. Michael and then traveled the 1800-mile journey up the Yukon by small flat-bottomed steamer. This passage took longer and was more expensive, but on the whole it was safer and probably less strenuous, especially if the traveler had a strong stomach and a willingness to stoke fires, chop wood, and perform many other essential jobs required on the way. The main problem with this route was that many miners never made it to Dawson and were dropped off on the Yukon hundreds of miles from their destination (Brooks 1973, 364-67).

Another route to the Klondike attempted by as many as three thousand miners was from Valdez, and up the Copper River valley. This idea was heavily advertised in the United States as the "All-American" route, although few had any clear idea of its practicality, not to mention its great hazards (Conger 1983, xiii-xiv). In fact, the route involved a difficult and often stormy sea voyage to Valdez, then a twenty-five-mile trek over the treacherous Valdez Glacier, which filled a pass through the rugged Chugach Mountains. Once safely past the crevasses and endless ridges of the seaward side, the miners descended on the Klutina Glacier, then built a raft or boat for negotiating the rapids-filled Klutina River, past Klutina Lake, and on to the swift Copper River, from which they ascended the Chitina River toward Mentasta Pass. Only a few of these hardy hopefuls ever reached the Klondike by this route; instead, many remained to prospect in the tributaries of the Copper River and in the Wrangell Mountains.

In many ways this was the most hazardous of all the routes to the gold fields. Horace Conger (1983, 194), who made the trip, mentions chest pain, stroke, smashed fingers, an accidental shooting, a broken leg, sore throats, and a hanging resulting from a miners' meeting—and all of this before he left Valdez. On the glacier, he or others suffered from frostbite, immersion foot, snowblindness, scurvy, and neuralgia of the jaw, not to mention the results of snow slides and falls into crevasses. A special problem was what came to be known as the "glacier demon," which supposedly strangled its victims or lured them into crevasses. Many of these hazards continued in the interior, plus the ever-present threat of drowning in the river rapids. There was never a shortage of doctors: at one time as many as twenty-five physicians were on the Valdez trail.

The winter of 1898-1899 was a disaster for the miners in this area. Food supplies ran short and scurvy, or "black leg," was a widespread problem in the Copper River mining camp, where a small hospital was established at Copper Center (Austin 1968, 68). The extent of the problem necessitated the relief effort organized by Captain Abercrombie, who previously had explored and surveyed much of this region. By the spring of 1899 most of the sick miners had either recovered or had been shipped back to Seattle (Abercrombie 1900a). (*See* Figure 18.) The Copper River district in any event no longer held much interest for the gold-seeker, nor did the Klondike, for that matter. Gold had been found on the beaches in Nome.

The last great Alaskan gold rush before the end of the century was on the Seward Peninsula, where a group of men, including Swedish Covenant missionaries and government employees working for the reindeer project, discovered placer gold near Cape Nome as early as December 1897. It is

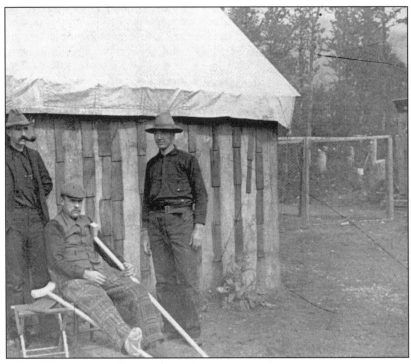

Figure 18. Scurvy hospital set up at Valdez to aid sick miners en route to the Klondike in 1899. (Abercrombie 1900a.)

interesting that two of the first men to stake claims in the rich Anvil Creek district were physicians—Dr. J. R. Gregory, a government doctor from St. Michael, and Dr. A. N. Kittelsen, employed by the reindeer project at Teller (Carlson 1946). By November 1898 news had spread widely in Alaska, and disappointed but hopeful prospectors from Kotzebue Sound, the Yukon, even as far away as Dawson, stampeded for Nome with all speed to stake their claims. By December some forty miners had marked out seven thousand acres, many of the claims proving fraudulent. Subsequent legal battles greatly raised frustrations and tempers (Brooks 1973, 375-76).

Then during the summer of 1899 a chance discovery by an old prospector distracted everyone from their legal entanglements. Gold could be found in the sands of the beach and anyone could recover it equipped with only a shovel and rocker. Nearly everyone made money, for those without a claim simply worked during the day on the beach for enough to spend on food, drink, and other less essential gratifications that night. A sea captain who arrived in 1900 found eight steamers, eight sailing vessels, and a revenue cutter in the roadstead. The beach was littered for three miles with lumber, cargo of all types, countless tents, and mounds of tailings. (*See* Figure 19.) In the town itself he noted a hospital facing the main square, a half-dozen restaurants, and by actual count fifty saloons, gambling houses, and dance halls. Most people lived in tents, although a few of the more prosperous had constructed rough board shacks (West 1965, 80-81).

In 1900 the gold rush reached its peak at Nome, although by this time the gold was getting much harder to find. In that year some 18,000 persons arrived in Nome, of whom perhaps 13,000 returned that same year in discouragement (Brooks 1973, 392). Many of those who arrived were totally unprepared for what they found in Nome and few had the means or the stamina to spend the winter in a tent in a region where wood and game were scarce.

Life in Nome in 1899-1900 had all the characteristics of the frenzied life of Dawson a few years before, but without the discipline afforded by the Royal Canadian Mounted Police. It was a cosmopolitan population, including people from many European countries as well as the United States and Canada. By the end of the summer of 1899, the more responsible element had organized a city government, including a board of health, a hospital corps, and various charitable organizations. Several doctors in the mining community practiced their profession. Drunken and disorderly conduct was punished by fine and imprisonment (Schrader and Brooks 1900, 45-46).

Considering the abominable crowding, the city remained remarkably healthy. Initially there were no public sanitary facilities but the Board of Health, frightened by the appearance of a few typhoid cases (Rininger 1985), saw to it that public latrines were erected and used by both men and women. To offset the cost, a user's fee of ten cents was extracted, with three tickets selling for a quarter (French 1901, 37). Clean water was piped in from distant streams under the supervision of the Army (McKee 1902, 34). Much of the sickness was concentrated on the beach, where few tents had floors and the subarctic winds penetrated with ease. Pneumonia was common, as was louse infestation. Some of the chronically ill were deported on southbound ships by the authorities. In July of 1900 smallpox was introduced from a ship but fortunately did not spread widely (*see* Chapter 13).

A much greater disaster in the summer of 1900 was a severe epidemic of influenza and measles which struck western Alaska causing appalling mortality, especially among the Native people. This epidemic, remembered long afterward as "The Great Sickness," led not only to deaths from the diseases themselves but also to later deaths from starvation, or from tuberculosis, pneumonia, and other chest infections (*see* Chapter 12).

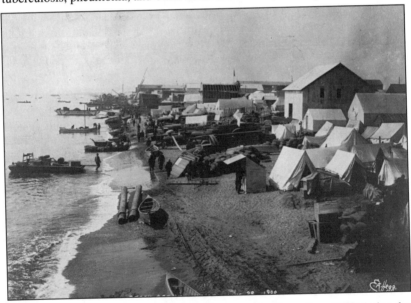

Figure 19. Sanitary conditions on the crowded beach at Nome, June 1900, during the peak of the Gold Rush. (Charles Bunnell Collection, Archives, Alaska and Polar Regions Dept., University of Alaska Fairbanks.)

10

Missions and Medicine

EARLIEST MISSIONARY EFFORTS: RUSSIAN ORTHODOX AND ROMAN CATHOLIC

The Russian Orthodox Church, which as we have seen traced its origins back to 1794 in Alaska, was only peripherally involved in the provision of medical care. Priests were taught to perform vaccinations at an early period and sometimes were entrusted with the use of a small medical kit when a *feldsher* or surgeon's apprentice was not assigned to the post (Netsvetov 1984, 82, 146, 151). As part of their normal clerical functions they comforted the sick, consoled the survivors, and even helped bury the dead during epidemics such as the one at Kodiak in 1819 (Chapter 11) or the great smallpox epidemic of 1835-1840 (Chapter 13). Sometimes hostility was directed at the priests for supposedly causing disease by their "incantations" (Oswalt 1960, 114). Despite these involvements in health, however, the Russian Orthodox Church did not sponsor medical missionaries or operate any health facilities in Alaska. The individual priests remained active in local health affairs, however, even after the sale of Alaska (e.g., University of Alaska 1936-1938, 2:48-67).

Besides the pastor of the small Lutheran church at New Archangel serving the Finns and Germans working for the Russian-American Company, the only non-Orthodox clergymen in Alaska before the American purchase were some Roman Catholic Oblate missionaries who came into Fort Yukon from Canada in 1862 via the Yukon River. A permanent station was established by the Jesuits at Nulato in 1877 by Bishop C. J. Seghers, who was assassinated there by a deranged lay assistant eleven years later (Llorente 1969, 6-7).

Three sisters of the Order of St. Ann arrived at the burgeoning mining town of Juneau in September 1886. Before long they had raised enough money to establish a small hospital on the corner of Lyon and Harris Streets, where Dr. Hugh S. Wyman served as the first physician (Balcom 1970, 50). In 1888 a larger two-story building was erected adjacent to the first at a total cost of $2300, with the interesting provision that those who had contributed to the building fund were given free care. An even larger hospital building was put up in 1897 (Hill 1977, 44), the same year the sisters also built a facility across the water at the huge Treadwell mine in Douglas. This latter hospital was operated by the Order of St. Ann under contract with the mine (Down 1966, 121).

In 1888 Father Pascal Tosi, in collaboration with the Sisters of St. Ann, established an important mission at Holy Cross seventy miles up the Yukon River from the old Orthodox center at Ikogmiut. The mission soon included a boarding school and even a farm (Renner 1979). Holy Cross and the surrounding villages suffered terribly during the epidemic of influenza and measles that struck western Alaska in 1900. Virtually every Native and most Whites in the mission community became ill and many died, including nineteen children. The sisters and priests carried on to the best of their abilities, caring for their charges, in the words of a visiting naval officer, "with a tenderness and devotion which no words can adequately describe" (Calasanctius 1947, 222; *see also* Chapter 12).

PRESBYTERIAN MISSIONS

The first Protestant mission to the Alaska Natives began in Wrangell, where Mrs. A. R. McFarland and the Rev. Sheldon Jackson arrived in August 1877. The following year the Rev. S. Hall Young took charge of the mission and Jackson moved to Sitka (Jackson 1903b, 9). Young was fascinated by medicine, although his only training in the field was a surgery book a physician uncle had given him (Loree 1935, 265). He clearly recognized that all missionaries in Alaska needed training in medicine, surgery, and dentistry and was convinced that thereby many lives would be saved. When navy ships or revenue cutters stopped at Wrangell, Young would insist that the surgeon make rounds with him to visit the sick in the neighboring Indian villages (Young 1927, 109). Dr. Robert White (1880, 36) of the Revenue Cutter *Rush* was one such surgeon, and upon his departure he left a small supply of medicines with written directions for their use, since the missionary seemed to be "the most capable person in the place for the duty."

That same year a Baptist missionary described by Jackson (1880, 228-29) as "Rev. W. H. R. Corlies, M.D." arrived at Wrangell. According to Young, however, Corleis [sic] had had only one year at Jefferson Medical College in Philadelphia, but since that gave him medical seniority over Young, he took over most of the medical duties of the mission. His training must have made him less squeamish than Young, for he treated "many loathsome cases of venereal diseases"—a class of illnesses Young would not touch (Young 1927, 108). Corlies opened a school at Wrangell and soon afterward a student residence located in the old military hospital building (Jackson 1886, 82). During his two years at Wrangell he seemed to show several lapses of judgment, the most serious one taking place in January 1880 when about fifty Angoon Indians were visiting for trade and set up a still for making "hootch," a kind of distilled homebrew. Corlies sent a Stikine Indian to destroy the still and a general melee resulted, which had to be broken up by the guns of the U.S.S. *Jamestown.* As Captain Beardslee remarked of the missionary, "Unfortunately, his zeal is not tempered with discretion and familiarity with Indian affairs" (De Laguna 1960, 152-53). The missionary and his wife then established a summer school for the Taku Tlingit, near Juneau, in 1880, and took up their residence there from 1882 until 1884 (Jackson 1903b, 24). From 1892 another missionary physician served the Wrangell mission. Dr. Clarence Thwing had left medicine for the ministry, but it is unlikely that he could have avoided providing at least some medical care during his tenure (Jackson 1903b, 10-11).

The Presbyterians were also active in Sitka at this time. In 1880 A. E. Austin, a missionary teacher, persuaded Commander Glass to let the mission use the now abandoned building once serving as the Russian hospital to house the newly established Presbyterian Boys' Boarding School, later known as the Sitka Industrial Training School. Glass agreed to detail some of his men, including a ship's carpenter, to assist in the rehabilitation of the decaying structure, using funds from the mission for the purchase of materials (U.S. House of Representatives 1882, 30). Twenty-five students and the teachers moved in and the school flourished until the building burned to the ground in late January 1882, the fire having apparently originated in a defective flue over the school room. The missionaries would have lost everything but for the brave assistance of the miners of Sitka (Blee [1986], 28-29). A few years later the Board of Home Missions erected a new building, which was operated under contract to the government. By 1886 there were plans for a curriculum which would include physiology, "laws of health," simple remedies, the proper care of accidents, and nursing the sick (Jackson 1886, 85). In 1887 a man from New York donated one thousand dollars for a girls' hospital ward, and the following year another benefactor donated enough to complete the boys' hospital section and pay the expenses of a medical missionary. Dr. R. A. Henning of Washington, D.C., was hired for the post and arrived the following May (*North Star* 1973, 24). He was replaced the next year by Dr. William F. Arnold, who in turn was followed by Dr. Clarence Thwing before he went on to Wrangell. Mrs. Josie Overend served as hospital matron (Jackson 1891, 757).

By 1891 the hospital had two twelve-bed wards. The death rate was not high but the wards were usually full, with the principal diagnoses being respiratory infections, rheumatism, consumption, and epidemic diseases. Many of the children had scrofula, sore eyes, "syphilitic taints," or consumption (Jackson 1893b, 931). The following year it was decided to combine the two establishments and a second floor was added to the boys' hospital to accommodate the girls. The expanded facility was opened on November 22, 1894, under the direction of Dr. B. K. Wilbur, assisted by a nurse named Esther Gibson. That year an appeal went out for a fracture bed, a set of trial lenses for eye refractions, and a set of ophthalmic instruments. Initially, the financial situation of the school had not permitted all patients to be accepted "without distinction," but the new hospital was thrown open to Natives from all parts of Alaska. In 1897 the hospital recorded 206 admissions, 2594 hospital days, and an average length of stay of 12.5 days. Six patients died—three from tuberculosis and three from "capillary bronchitis" (an old term for pneumonia). In addition, the doctor treated 1,119 outpatients and performed 38 operations (Jackson 1896a, 1466; Jackson 1898a, 1617-18).

At the close of the century Jackson (1901b, 1754) reported that in the previous year the hospital had had 179 inpatients and 1751 outpatients. The total financial outlay had been $2574.34, which included the salaries of one doctor and two nurses. He concluded, with paternal pride: "The Sitka Hospital is widely known, and many natives come from long distances to receive treatment herein. Much good is accomplished by the religious instruction which is imparted along with the help given to the body."

Sheldon Jackson (1903b, 26-27), the indefatigable one, also was responsible for establishing a Presbyterian mission and school at the northernmost point of Alaska, Point Barrow, in 1890. This community was a difficult challenge for the church because of the long history of tension between the Eskimos and Whites. The first missionary teacher, Leander Stevenson, arrived in 1890 and three years later was joined for a year by Dr. T. E. Beaupré (Jackson 1896a, 1451). Stevenson himself was replaced in 1896 by a young physician just out of school, Dr. H. Richmond Marsh, who remained through the end of the century (Jackson 1897a, 1446). (*See* Figure 20.) When Dr. Call of the Overland Relief Expedition arrived in Barrow in

1898, he found that Dr. Marsh had been regularly rendering medical assistance to the whalers, apparently with some success, for thus far no deaths had occurred. The missionary freely made his drugs and supplies available to his new colleague. The two apparently cooperated amicably, even performing an autopsy together, although Call reported in a cryptic remark that "our schools differed materially." Dr. Marsh, for example, would not treat an Eskimo who had previously consulted a shaman (*in* [Jarvis] 1899, 117-20).

EPISCOPAL MISSIONS

Rev. John W. Chapman arrived in the Athapaskan village of Anvik, on the lower Yukon, in 1887. Though not himself a physician, he recognized immediately the need for one, particularly because of the prevalence of serious lung disease among the people. In the summer of 1894 he was successful in bringing Dr. Mary V. Glenton to the village as a medical missionary. She plunged enthusiastically into caring for the sick and teaching

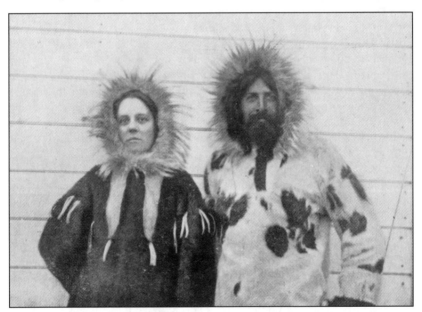

Figure 20. Dr. and Mrs. H. Richmond Marsh, Presbyterian missionaries at Barrow in the 1890s. (Call *in* Jackson 1889.)

sanitation and hygiene at the school. The following year she had plans to establish a small hospital for children and maternity cases and to train two Indian women as assistants (Chapman and Sabine 1895, 378). A hospital was reported to be still in existence in 1900 (Stuck 1920, 96). Dr. Glenton spent two years on the Yukon, dividing her time between Anvik and the St. James Mission, near the confluence of the Yukon and Tanana rivers. Although she left Alaska for reasons of health in 1896 (Jackson 1897a, 1445), she later became a long-term medical missionary to China.

The St. James Mission at Fort Adams included a boarding home, school, and small hospital, all under the supervision of Rev. Jules L. Prévost. In 1895-1896, when Dr. Glenton was still in the area, hospital statistics showed thirty-one inpatients, of whom four—all infants—died, and 347 outpatients. At that time there were plans for a larger hospital, materials for which were already on site (Sheakley 1896, 1278).

On July 21, 1890, a carpenter and several sailors from the *Bear* went ashore to help construct a school at Point Hope. Like many other schools in Alaska, this one was operated for the government under contract with a mission, in this case the Episcopal Church. The teacher who had come north was Dr. John B. Driggs of Wilmington, Delaware (Jackson 1893a, 1278), the first physician resident in northern Alaska.

Dr. Driggs encountered bitter hostility at first, the legacy of many years of strained relationships between the Eskimos and visiting whaling ships and their nearby shore stations. Initially they would not even permit the doctor to land, but after Captain Healy repeatedly assured them that this was a different sort of White man, they let him come, but with an ominous warning that if he turned out to be of the wrong sort, he would not be found the following summer (Jenkins 1943, 145). That he was indeed of the right sort was demonstrated by the fact that he survived not only that winter but remained at Point Hope for eighteen years, often as the only White man in the village. During that period he left the village three times and then only when a replacement could be found (Stuck 1920, 34-35). He worked primarily as a teacher because, as he confessed, "Should I attend to that line of my work [medicine] properly, I should have little time for anything else" (Driggs 1894, 562-63). He also refused to engage in trade, as so many missionaries were doing.

The government withdrew its support for the school in 1895 but life went on. Another missionary joined him and in the following year the school had eighty students (Sheakley 1896, 202). Plans to move into a larger school and new quarters had to be postponed that year because of a summer influenza epidemic (Driggs 1897, 608).

Influenza struck Point Hope in much greater force in 1900, as part of the vast epidemic that engulfed western and northern Alaska that year. The *Bear,* now under the command of Captain Tuttle, again rendered assistance to the beleaguered doctor. Also on board was Bishop Peter T. Rowe, who for years had tried to make the journey to Point Hope to offer his support and encouragement. He found Dr. Driggs well, having himself recovered from the disease, but the Eskimos were dying everywhere, and many were close to starvation (Jenkins 1943, 147-48).

In the later 1890s the Episcopal Church undertook to establish missions along the central Yukon to serve not only the Indian population but also the many miners and prospectors who were lured by the smell of gold. In 1893 rich gold deposits were found in the Birch Creek district and before long a large mining town known as Circle City grew up along the river. Bishop Rowe on a visit in 1896 immediately saw the need for a hospital and took steps to secure land for this purpose from the miners. Initially they promised to donate the land as soon as work began (Rowe 1897a, 19), but later it seems that the bishop had to pay eight hundred dollars for it. As an act of faith, Rowe started work on a log structure and ordered equipment, supplies, and drugs from San Francisco (Rowe 1897b, 364-65).

The hospital opened in 1897, staffed by Sister Elizabeth Deane, who had graduated from a church training school (Jenkins 1943, 91). Several months later Dr. James L. Watt arrived with his wife and child to take over the medical duties. In 1898 the bishop described the building, now called Grace Hospital, as "large, roomy and well lighted by three good sized windows. We have seven beds now and room for two more. Deaconness Deane has her room at one end, and medicines are nicely arranged on shelves at the rear" (Jenkins 1943, 92-93). The hospital was equipped for surgery, but was short on basic surgical instruments and supplies. Dr. Watt reported in 1898 that forty-two patients had been admitted, thirty-one of them Caucasians, all of whom survived, whereas of the eleven Indians treated, three died. Among the outpatients, 147 were Indian and only 20 were White, for a total of 487 visits. Only half of the total number of patients made any payment (Jenkins 1943, 92). Dr. Watt remained in the region several years, treating Natives and miners and sometimes making medical trips to the surrounding area (Jackson 1900a, 1397-98). By 1900, when he left, most inhabitants of Circle City had flocked to Nome.

Further down the Yukon River at Rampart a small hospital facility was in existence as early as 1898, built by the miners with the understanding that the church would purchase it in the spring of 1899 for five hundred dollars and thereafter operate it as a mission facility (Jackson 1900a, 1399). When Army 1st Lt. Edwin Bell visited in 1899 on a government relief expedition, however, he found that the hospital had had to close because of financial difficulties. In view of the obvious needs, Lieutenant Bell hired a building for use as a hospital for the destitute (Richardson 1900, 753). The hospital had no physician, but a lay missionary named E. J. Knapp provided constant care to the sick. The Episcopal Church later did take over the hospital, for in the education report for 1900-1901 (Jackson 1903a, 1476) a facility is mentioned there under the auspices of the church. The building had been constructed by the citizens at a cost of three thousand dollars on lots belonging to the mission. By then Rev. Jules Prévost, formerly of St. James Mission at Fort Adams, had arrived to oversee the work (Stuck 1920, 96; Jackson 1901a, 1760).

The Episcopal Church was also active in medical affairs in southeastern Alaska around the turn of the century. The principal site was Skagway, which, as the starting-point for the White Pass Trail to the Klondike, became the temporary or permanent stop for thousands of wild-eyed and lusty gold-seekers. Bishop Rowe arrived in Skagway in April 1898 and immediately recognized the need for a mission. Shortly after he had come, a committee of the townspeople visited him to ask him to establish a hospital to care for the many victims of sickness, violence, hunger, and cold who were becoming a burden on the town. Dr. I. H. Moore had already set up a makeshift hospital and this was hastily and gratefully turned over to the church (Satterfield 1973, 66). He then set about raising funds from the miners and local businessmen and before long was able to erect a sizeable log structure. A local nurse, Miss Anna Dickey, was persuaded to take on the post of superintendent. The committee was so delighted with the prompt results that it insisted the new facility be named Bishop Rowe Hospital. The hospital building consisted of a ward on the upper floor with the kitchen and utility rooms below. In 1899 a New York woman contributed funds for an operating room, bathroom, two rooms for private patients, and a variety of other improvements. Medical care was provided by volunteer physicians from the community (Jackson 1901a, 1760). In the year 1898-1899 there were 121 admissions and 19 deaths (Jackson 1900a, 1396-97).

It is said that the infamous "Soapy" Smith offered to collect funds for the hospital around this time, but when it came time for the funds to be turned over to the bishop, lo, poor Soapy had been robbed, or so he tried to explain to the churchman. Rowe insisted on an accounting, however, and Smith finally settled up for five hundred dollars, probably a good deal less than he had collected (Jenkins 1943, 94-95).

From the very beginning the Skagway hospital was put to full use. Shortly after it opened a severe epidemic of meningitis swept Skagway, and an extra wing had to be hastily added to accommodate the overflow. Another medical disaster in the early period was the great snow avalanche that killed several dozen men in the spring of 1898. In addition, the hospital staff was kept busy on a continuing basis with the inevitable medical mishaps associated with taverns, brothels, and too much ready cash.

Another hospital that could trace its origins to the tireless bishop was the one in Ketchikan, founded about 1897 with the help of Rev. Thomas Jenkins. This facility, initially under the medical direction of Dr. A. J. Campbell, later became known as the Arthur Yates Memorial Hospital (Jenkins 1943, 100-101; Jackson 1899, 1764).

Before leaving the Episcopal missions brief mention should be made of the work, beginning in 1857, of Rev. William Duncan on behalf of the Tsimshian Indians of British Columbia. His work prospered mightily for many years in Canada, but after an ecclesiastical quarrel he received permission in 1887 to move his flock to Annette Island, Alaska, where he founded the town of New Metlakatla. Among those who made the move was Robert Tomlinson, who had had some medical training and had been ministering to the sick in the Nass River District for twenty years (Loree 1935, 265). Dr. James Bluett-Duncan also accompanied Reverend Duncan to Alaska and remained for more than five years. Then from 1899 to 1901 Dr. Ernest R. Pike and his wife spent an extended honeymoon at Metlakatla (Arctander 1909, 302, 328).

OTHER PROTESTANT MISSIONS

The first missionaries of the Moravian Church, or Unitas Fratrum, arrived on the Lower Kuskokwim River in 1884, where the next year they founded the town of Bethel at the site of a trading post. One of the earliest missionaries was Rev. John Kilbuck, who was a Delaware Indian. He and his wife established a church and a school but found the Eskimos strongly resistant to cultural change. Kilbuck at an early period recognized the need for medical assistance, not only because of the poor health of the people around the mission, but also because he saw Western medicine as one of the best and quickest ways to break the hold of the shamans over the minds of the people—an essential task from the perspective of the missionaries. He and others tried to dispense simple remedies themselves, but the needed medical work was clearly beyond their skills (Henkelman and Vitt 1985, 142). As his wife's diary shows, famine, injury, and disease were almost overwhelming (*North Star* 1887-1892, 31). Among the epidemics of the early period were pneumonia in 1889 and whooping cough and chickenpox early in 1896 (Schwalbe 1951, 72).

In the summer of 1893 the first nurse missionary arrived on the Kuskokwim, Miss Philippine King, who remained at Bethel for three years before transferring to the Moravian station at Carmel, near Dillingham. There she provided health care until ill health forced her departure in 1902 (Henkelman and Vitt 1985, 65, 133, 137-38).

Edith Kilbuck's brother, as it happened, had just finished his medical training at Hahnemann Medical College in Philadelphia. Dr. Joseph Herman Romig, no doubt influenced by his sister, took some special training in surgery and finally reached Bethel in late July 1896. He remained in Alaska, though not always as a missionary, for most of his professional life. It was during his years at Bethel, however, that he became known, with ample justice, as the "Dog-Team Doctor" (E. Anderson 1942). He set up his work in a small log building divided into two rooms, one of these containing two crude beds and the other serving as an office and dispensary, including a makeshift operating table (Romig 1962, 86). In his first year he treated 470 cases, with 72 different diagnoses. One of his first patients was a local village leader who was badly injured by a harpoon. Romig's surgical skill in this case and others enhanced his reputation among the Eskimos. He operated under all kinds of conditions, in missions, igloos, *kashims,* and even steambaths. His toughest case, however, came in late 1898 when his brother-in-law developed a rapidly spreading infection of his arm secondary to a fishhook injury of his hand. With Mrs. Kilbuck giving the anesthetic, Dr. Romig amputated the arm just below the shoulder. The Eskimos who watched never forgot how the missionary died and then came alive again (Schwalbe 1951, 83).

Once they saw his skills, the Eskimos, not to mention Indians, came from far and near to seek care. Romig himself regularly made extended journeys by dog team up and down the Kuskokwim and occasionally to the lower Yukon. He often treated other missionaries and traders and their families, and, despite serious doctrinal differences, maintained close and friendly relations with the Catholic and Orthodox missionaries in the area (Romig 1962, 86).

The health of the Eskimos deteriorated rapidly during the last years of the century. Epidemics swept through the population repeatedly, notably the disastrous epidemic of 1900 known as the "Great Sickness" (*see* Chapter 12). This plague was attributed by the Eskimos to the census-takers, including Kilbuck, who had gone through the villages earlier that year. Dr. Romig himself had assisted with the census and this, plus the fact that his remedies were no more effective than those of the shamans in the face of the epidemic, discredited him somewhat for a period of time (Oswalt 1963, 100).

Despite these setbacks, Dr. Romig was one of the most successful of the early medical missionaries in Alaska. One old Eskimo named Bad Heart, after seeing what the doctor could do for the sick and injured, was quoted as saying: "Now we understand that the Savior, Jesus, not only preached, but healed as well" (Schwalbe 1951, 72).

The Swedish Mission Covenant, now known as the Evangelical Covenant Church, first established a mission in Unalakleet in 1887, under the leadership of Axel E. Karlson. He found alcohol abuse to be one of the principal health problems in the early years (Matson et al. 1941, 193), perhaps a legacy of the town's history as a trading post. The earliest Covenant outpost mission was established at Golovin in 1893, by Rev. A. Anderson and Rev. N. D. Hultberg. Associated with this station for many years was an Eskimo helper named Dora, who received some nursing training (Jackson 1897a, 1449, 1451). In 1899 Dr. Julius Quist of Worcester, Massachusetts, replaced Rev. Karlson at Unalakleet at an annual salary of five hundred dollars. Among the medical items he ordered that year for Unalakleet were syrup of quills [sic, probably syrup of squills], cascara, prune juice, and two proprietary drugs with multiple ingredients known as "Hoffman's Drops" and "Kansas Tonic." Dr. Quist left in 1901 and was replaced by Dr. C. O. Lind, who had spent the previous year at Golovin (Almquist 1962, 72).

The first Protestant mission in the Aleutians was begun in 1886 by the Methodists at Unga, near present-day Sand Point, but the deaths of two missionaries soon after thwarted the church's efforts there. In 1890 a school and orphanage, known as the Jessie Lee Home, were opened in Unalaska. Five years later a young woman named Agnes Louise Soule arrived as missionary. On her first return home, in 1898, she married Albert Newhall, who was just finishing his medical studies. Their honeymoon was a voyage to Unalaska, where they spent many years together (Middleton 1958, 34). Dr. Newhall became something of an institution himself at Unalaska, providing medical care there for over two decades, often assisted by some Aleut practitioners.

Finally, in 1893 the Baptist Women's Home Mission Society opened a large orphanage on Wood Island, just opposite the community of Kodiak. The facility, which included a school, was established to take care of the many children whose parents had died of tuberculosis and other diseases not only on Kodiak Island but in the eastern Aleutians. The mission report for 1895 mentioned a hospital, where seven men with severe frostbite were recuperating after their ship was wrecked on the southern coast of Kodiak Island. Around the turn of the century one of the government teachers was C. F. Mills, M.D. (Jackson 1903a, 42-43; Jackson 1896a, 1468-69; Jackson 1896b, 26).

When gold was discovered at Anvil Creek near Nome in the spring of 1899, gold-seekers, adventurers, and speculators poured into the town, creating within a few months a sprawling, violent, crowded sinkhole of humanity. By the fall tents were set up along a twenty-mile stretch of beach. Sanitation was of course primitive, to say the least, and before long typhoid and other water-borne diseases were spreading. In 1899 there were some fifty saloons available to quench the prodigious thirst of the miners (Hunt 1974, 113). A city government, including a board of health, was established that year and one of its first priorities, not surprisingly, was a hospital.

In October 1899 a temporary hospital was established in the library building, to care for the overflow from the military hospital. An army surgeon, James Miller, was very helpful during this period but was soon to be transferred out. The city council met and appointed a health officer, a hospital manager, and a hospital assistant. Rev. S. Hall Young offered to raise funds and to organize the ladies of the city (*Nome News* 1899 [Oct. 9], 14).

Rev. L. L. Wirt, a Congregationalist minister, had arrived several months before and immediately had been sent out with four thousand dollars collected by the miners to purchase supplies and lumber for the hospital. He and his family returned in mid-October with the materials, but the lighterage barge was driven ashore in a heavy storm and a great deal was lost in the pounding surf. Some 50,000 feet of lumber were salvaged, however, and work began on a new hospital. The temporary facility became known as the "Hospice of St. Bernard," a name taken over in late November by the new hospital (*Nome News* 1899 [Oct. 21, Nov. 18]). The facility almost immediately fell on hard times, however, as promised support from the city and other sources did not materialize (*Nome News* 1900, Jan. 20). Rev. Wirt headed south by dogteam to seek relief for the beleaguered city, where scurvy had also broken out due to shortage of fresh provisions (Wirt 1937, 44). (*See* Map 2.)

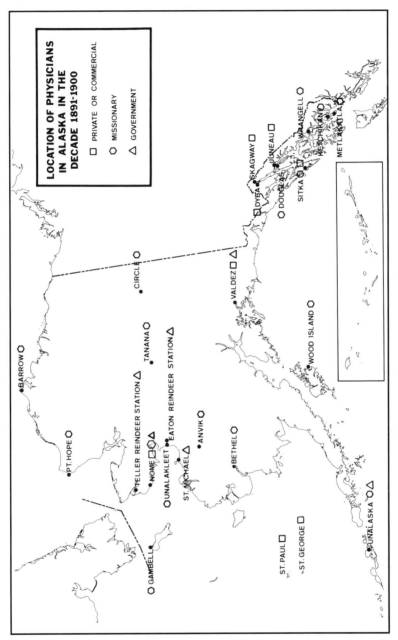

Map 2. Location of physicians in Alaska in the decade 1891-1900.

THE IMPACT OF MISSIONARIES ON HEALTH

The American missionaries who came into Alaska during the last two decades of the nineteenth century undoubtedly hastened cultural change among the Native peoples. Some of these effects were undeniably positive, since they helped the Natives to cope with the more destructive agents of cultural pressure, such as the whalers, some traders, and the miners, who were already forcing their ways, intentionally or not, on the people they encountered. Not that the missionaries were an unmitigated blessing by any means: of all the outsiders they were the ones most committed by their nature to bringing the Natives over to their own beliefs and destroying certain elements of their culture.

The most obvious impact of the missionaries on health was in the conscious and unrelenting war on shamanism. The missionaries viewed the struggle as a spiritual, not a medical one, but an important effect was that Christianity and shamanistic healing could not comfortably coexist. Sometimes a major epidemic demonstrated the helplessness of the shaman. Perhaps even more important for the decline of shamanistic healing was the growing conviction among many Natives that Western medicine in fact was more effective than their own in dealing with medical and especially surgical problems.

The missionaries had other important effects on health. For the most part they were the first schoolteachers. Although their approach was slanted by their convictions, they taught, besides the Bible and catechism, principles of hygiene, nutrition, and other subjects bearing on health. "Cleanliness is next to godliness" was a popular slogan of that era. Missionary education also laid considerable emphasis on "morality" and "virtue," which in practical terms meant opposition to polygamy and promiscuity. Such efforts may in fact have helped reduce the spread of venereal disease. Alcohol was also bitterly opposed by the missionaries, who fought relentlessly not only against its manufacture and use by their parishioners, but also against the whiskey traders who brought it into the villages.

In times of sickness and death the missionaries tried to be a help and comfort in any way they could. Even those who were not physicians and nurses usually had access to some medical supplies or drugs that might ease pain or otherwise relieve distress. During the epidemics the missionaries worked to the point of exhaustion to treat the victims, comfort the dying and their families, and bury the dead. Although it is doubtful that they thereby changed the course of the epidemic, such selfless behavior on their part often made a deep impression on the Natives.

Missionaries have become increasingly controversial in the twentieth century because of their sometimes heavy-handed paternalism. Yet in many ways the missionaries were the best friends the Natives had in a time when attitudes of some toward them ranged from indifference to their welfare to conscious exploitation. The missionaries tried to increase the quality of life of the Natives as they saw it. While many forces were destructive to health, the missionaries were a generally positive influence.

Finally, the activities of missionaries in the health field also effectively increased the acceptance of their spiritual message. This is demonstrated by Veniaminov's experience during the smallpox epidemic of 1835-1837 at Sitka. It was only after the Tlingit saw the effectiveness of vaccination and the ineffectiveness of their own shamans that they in any numbers were willing to accept Christianity (Kashevaroff 1927, 145-46; *see also* Chapter 13). The situation was particularly well expressed by a Yupik convert at the Moravian mission in Bethel in August 1895 (Henkelman and Vitt 1985, 147):

> When these teachers first came, they did not command our attention by what they preached, but when they gave us medicine, and said that this or that ailment would be cured, we looked on to see if what they said was true. And because their medicines proved to be just what they said they were, we learned to believe that what they preached was equally true. . . . So I give you counsel that whenever missionaries set out to work among the heathen, they take the Word of God in one hand and medicine in the other.

*   *   *

The principal theme in Part II of this book has not been disease, but rather the development of Western health services. The story began with the physicians and surgeons on the ships of many nationalities that came to Alaska first to explore and trade, and later to supply the new settlements. These individuals usually doubled as naturalists or scientists and spent relatively little time providing medical care. In this latter capacity, of course, their principal responsibility was to the officers and crew of their ships, but on occasion they also treated the people of the settlements, and rarely even the Natives.

The first Russian settlements such as Unalaska or Kodiak had no trained medical assistance, except when a visiting ship was in port. Essential care for illness and injury at other times was rendered by a priest, the trader, or other experienced person. Even at Sitka itself in the early years the situation was no better. The sick and disabled largely had to shift for themselves.

Around 1820 the Russian-American Company assigned a physician to the capital and established small hospitals there and at Kodiak for the benefit of company employees. It is unlikely in those early years that Aleut or Koniag hunters, or even Creoles, received much help at these facilities. Certainly the Tlingit, who were unalterably hostile to the intruders, received no care unless it in some way also clearly benefitted the Russians.

Once the medical service was established, progress was rapid. From the earliest period the doctor was assigned the task of training assistants, including conscientious Creoles, who could help not only around the hospital but also, after appropriate experience, work independently at the smaller posts. *Feldshers* also came from Russia, either as assistants under the supervision of the physician at Sitka, or to provide independent care at the larger company posts such as St. Paul's Harbor (Kodiak), Unalaska, and St. Michael. Even the smallest posts and the company ships were provided with a medical kit and written instructions for its use. All these activities were supervised by the doctor, or doctors, at Sitka, who usually traveled in the summer to visit the larger posts and provide consultation, training, and restocking of drugs and supplies. In the latter years of the company this system reached most employees, including Creoles, and probably increasingly the Natives living near the posts. For the most part, however, the Natives had no access to Western medicine and continued to rely on their shamans, herbalists, surgeons, midwives, and relatives.

With the transfer of Alaska to the United States in 1867 the Russian health care system, so painstakingly developed, was rapidly dismantled. The physicians and most *feldshers* were repatriated and the trained Creole medical assistants were no longer allowed to practice openly. The U.S. Army took over the administration of the hospitals and other medical facilities and restricted services primarily to their own personnel, although they gave some grudging care to former Russian-American Company employees and to the Natives.

Private physicians opened shop in Sitka soon after the purchase, but of course limited their practice largely to those who could pay. Additional physicians came to Alaska during the Gold Rush and set up offices in Juneau, Skagway, Dyea, Circle City, Rampart, and Nome, although it seemed that some had come more for prospecting and profit than for medical practice. A few stayed on after the gold fever had subsided.

Beginning in the late 1870s the surgeons of the Navy and Revenue Marine Service ships were the first to provide consistent but admittedly sporadic services to the Alaska Natives in the more distant coastal areas of the territory. But the ships came rarely and briefly, and the demands on the doctors' time were great. The mid-1890s saw the beginnings, at last, of regular physician services in the remoter areas of Alaska, when the first medical missionaries took up residence and established small hospitals in some of the larger Native communities such as Bethel, Unalaska, Point Hope, and Barrow.

But doctors and hospitals did not necessarily mean better health either for the settlers or the Natives. By the close of the nineteenth century, Western physicians, for all their understanding of pathology, had little more to offer by way of treatment than the shamans and herbalists did. A few basic drugs—morphine, digitalis, and mercury were the most important—were definitely helpful, in contrast to the numerous ready-made proprietary remedies and to most of the laboriously compounded prescriptions of the physicians. Only a few preventive measures, notably smallpox vaccination, were of significant value. Western obstetrical and surgical techniques, particularly when performed antiseptically, were undoubtedly safer and more effective than what Native practitioners were able to accomplish. Both Western and Native medicine, however, continued to be nearly helpless in the face of the great plagues to be described in Part III.

PART III
Special Health Problems in Early Alaskan History

This final section of the book comprises eight chapters that briefly describe in a chronological fashion certain health problems that have had an unusual impact on the history of Alaska. These problems collectively were the most important causes of morbidity and mortality in eighteenth- and nineteenth-century Alaska. Each involved the interaction between Europeans and Americans on the one hand and the Alaska Natives on the other.

Chapters 11 to 13 are devoted to the epidemic diseases that swept through the Native population again and again, causing great loss of life and social and economic disruption. Most of these epidemics were caused by viruses—notably smallpox, measles, and influenza—which were highly contagious and spread rapidly through a population that had no prior immunity and hence no natural defenses. Two of these epidemics, smallpox in 1835-1840 and influenza and measles in 1900, caused such devastation that they must rank among the most significant single events in the recorded history of the peoples they affected. Other epidemics, though less destructive than these, caused many deaths and economic hardship for smaller, often isolated groups.

The diseases discussed in Chapters 11 and 12 are presented geographically; that is, the epidemics of the Pacific rim are described first, followed by those of western and northern Alaska. To a certain extent this classification also conforms to chronology, since the more southerly areas were explored first and hence subjected to new microorganisms at an earlier time. Smallpox is treated by itself in Chapter 13 because of its importance and because it affected such a huge geographical area.

Chapters 14 and 15 also deal with infectious diseases, namely syphilis, gonorrhea, and tuberculosis. These were more insidious, though no less pernicious in their long-term effects, than the acute epidemic diseases. They also were apparently introduced from outside, but instead of causing acute illness with a rapidly fatal outcome, they often smouldered for months and sometimes years in their victims, before ending in chronic disability or death. These diseases were spread by more prolonged or intimate contact than the former group and were in fact serious and often intractable health problems at the same time among the Europeans and Americans.

Chapters 16 and 17 consider the introduction and spread of a different sort of pathogenic agent—not microorganisms, but rather substances causing physical harm as well as psychological or chemical dependency. Tobacco and alcohol were introduced into Alaska at a very early period, and led to much ill-health in the eighteenth and nineteenth centuries among both the Natives and the Euro-Americans.

Finally, Chapter 18 briefly summarizes the adverse effects on health resulting from direct and sometimes violent confrontations between the original occupants of the land and those who came later. Personal cruelty toward the Natives, including virtual enslavement of the Aleuts and Koniag by the Russians, acts of individual and collective violence between the races, and hunger resulting directly or indirectly from these interactions are all briefly discussed.

11
Epidemics I:
Southern Alaska

GENERAL CONSIDERATIONS

As medico-historical events, epidemics have always held pre-eminence because of their intrinsic interest and dramatic course. Many epidemics in early Alaskan history have been described, a few with profound and lasting social and economic consequences on families, communities, and even entire cultural groups. The smallpox epidemic of 1835-1840 (*see* Chapter 13) and the influenza-measles epidemic of 1900 (*see* Chapter 12) are both examples of historical events in Alaska that caused death, social disintegration, abandonment of traditional homes, and despair on a scale unparalleled by anything but a major war. Never would the survivors of such overwhelming personal and collective tragedy be quite the same again. Even smaller outbreaks of disease, whether affecting only a single village or a limited region, could cause great hardship within families, especially when they caused the death of a parent critical to the survival of the social unit.

Epidemic diseases strike suddenly and usually without warning. They are particularly destructive in a population without previous exposure, and therefore immunity, to the infectious agent. Most of the epidemic diseases that ravaged Alaska were totally new and incomprehensible both to the Native people generally and to their shamans and other healers. None of the magical techniques of the shamans seemed to have any effect on the course of the illness, nor did any of the traditional ministrations of the herbalists or surgeons. As the victims of some diseases sickened and often died, the Russians and other Europeans seemed to be spared, a circumstance which led many Natives to believe that the White man had unleashed these terrible powers expressly for their destruction.

Although some epidemics affected the Caucasians as well as the Natives, the emphasis here will be on the ordeals of the aboriginal population. Many epidemics will be mentioned, but probably a similar or larger number have simply gone unchronicled, especially those that spread to Native villages away from the centers of trade or government. For a large number of disease outbreaks the available narrative accounts are too brief or uncritical to permit even a reasonable guess as to the diagnosis. For others there is diagnostic confusion, with different observers holding different views on the cause of the same epidemic. In still others there can be no mistake about the nature of the disease, because the clinical description, even by nonmedical observers, is so characteristic.

RESPIRATORY DISEASES

The first mention of an epidemic of respiratory disease in Alaska was by Dr. Merck (1980, 177), who observed in 1791 that many people of Unalaska had suffered chest pain, cough, and bloody sputum during the severe winter just past, when strong winds had prevailed. Sauer (1802, 272), who was on the same expedition, may have been referring to the same illness when he wrote that many of the people of Sitkanak Island (near Kodiak) had become ill following the visit of the Russians in 1790.

The first well-documented epidemic of respiratory disease in Russian America occurred in Kodiak in 1804. It was apparently brought by the Boston ship *O'Cain,* which had just returned from the California coast with a group of Koniag who had been hunting sea otter there. Clinically the disease was characterized by a headache lasting two weeks, followed by nasal congestion, a cough, blocked ears, and constriction in the chest. The victims then lost their appetite and steadily weakened. Curiously, the disease was reported to have selectively killed off many of the shamans on the island, and spared most of the others (Pierce 1978, 136).

Two years later a severe illness broke out in Unalaska, marked by a high fever and chest congestion. After supposedly causing 350 deaths there, the following year the disease spread via a Russian vessel to Atka, where at Korovin Bay Aleuts had gathered from several surrounding islands to meet the ship. The plague spread so rapidly that soon there were not enough men left to bury the dead (Black 1984, 98-99; 1980, 100). It was reported at the time that a person who drank cold water after catching the disease immediately succumbed. So many died in the epidemic that the settlement at Atka never regained its former importance (I. F. Vasilev *in* Black 1984, 156).

In 1819 another severe epidemic caused some fifty deaths at Sitka, having apparently been brought by an American ship from Java. The company ship *Finlandia* spread the disease to Kodiak in the fall, where it raged out of control for several months. Chief Manager Ianovskii, who was visiting Kodiak at the time, has left a vivid account of the epidemic. It impressed him so much that he was instrumental a few years later in having a physician assigned to the colonies for the first time (Pierce 1986, 5-6). According to Ianovskii (*in* Pierce 1978, 83-84) the disease "began with a fever and a heavy cold, a cough, shortness of breath, choking, and three days later death followed! . . . The epidemic affected everyone, even babes in arms." The death rate was so high that many corpses lay around unburied. The chief manager made every effort to comfort the sick and dying, and in the course of his stay visited a large Koniag *kashim* where more than a hundred persons were living. "Some were lying already dying," he went on, "their bodies growing cold, next to those who were still alive; others were already dead: the groans, shrieks that were heard tore at my heart. I saw mothers already dead, on whose cold breasts hungry children crawled. . . ." Ianovskii, his wife, and children themselves contracted the disease, but he nursed them back by the use of elder-tea and warm clothing. Father Herman left his post at Spruce Island during the epidemic and, according to Ianovskii, "ceaselessly, tirelessly and at great personal risk visited the sick, not sparing himself in his role as priest—counselling those suffering to be patient, pray, repent, and prepare themselves for death." Father Herman was one of very few at Kodiak who escaped the disease, and he later built an orphanage to care for the children whose parents had perished in the epidemic (Bensin n.d., 31).

The epidemic spread from the settlement at Kodiak throughout the whole island and to neighboring islands (Ianovskii *in* Pierce 1978, 66, 83). According to Khlebnikov (1973, 105), the same disease spread that winter to the isolated island of Ukamok, despite the supposed lack of contact between its population and the residents of Kodiak.

From the clinical description and its rapid course it is probable that this disease was caused by a virulent strain of influenza virus, although Rosse (1883, 17), citing Petroff, called it measles because of a reddish rash that accompanied it. In any event the disease affected nearly everyone, including some Russians, and resulted in forty-two deaths in Kodiak and six more in outlying areas (Tikhmenev 1978, 161).

In the winter of 1827-1828 another severe epidemic of respiratory disease struck Kodiak, killing 158 persons on the island (including 57 at Three Saints' Harbor), all of them Koniag and Creoles. The symptoms were coughing, hemoptysis, chest pain, headache, and dizziness (Gibson 1982-83, 62), again suggestive of influenza.

In the fall of 1830 and extending through the spring of 1831 an epidemic of cough and chest congestion appeared on the island of Unga and later spread to the greater part of the Alaska Peninsula. More than thirty deaths occurred, nearly all in young healthy men. Children, the elderly, and all women were spared (Veniaminov 1984. 258). This illness may well have been the same one that the missionary Netsvetov (1980, 55, 74) described as "a coughing sickness" attacking nearly every inhabitant in the settlements on Atka and Amlia Islands in early 1831. At the outset of the illness in early 1831, eight persons died in Atka alone in the period of a month. The disease spread to the Rat Islands by a hunting *baidara*, exacting a heavy mortality there over the course of the year. By the early months of 1832 the people of the Near Islands were also succumbing to the illness.

At Sitka during the fall of 1843 the people suffered from catarrhal attacks of the respiratory passages, due, according to Dr. Romanovskii, to the constant southeast winds coupled with cold, humidity, and snowstorms. During that winter many developed pneumonia, pleurisy, and blood-spitting (*in* Pierce 1974, 2).

Two years later another company physician described in accurate clinical terms what must have been an outbreak of pertussis, or whooping cough, among the children of Sitka. They began to become ill in December 1845, with a fever and dry cough, followed by thick, yellowish, blood-streaked mucus lasting throughout the illness. Later in the course,

respiration, at first rapid, then became frequent, short, difficult and at the end almost ceased from spasmodic coughing; pulse beats, weak even without that, quickened so much that they became impossible to count; the skin throughout the illness was dry, pale and insensitive to local irritation through Spanish fly or mustard, except that after attacks of coughing the upper part of the body was covered with local, clammy and cold sweat. Weakness increased daily, and after several weeks the disease ended with death from general exhaustion of paralysis of the lungs (Frankenhaeuser *in* Pierce 1974, 23-24).

The exact number of cases was not reported but was said to be "remarkable."

A couple of severe epidemics of respiratory disease also occurred in the colonies during the 1850s. Dr. Rosse (1883, 17), citing Tikhmenev, mentioned epidemic pneumonia in 1852 affecting the population of Sitka (especially the children), Kodiak, and the company establishment at Bristol Bay. He further reported an outbreak in Kodiak and Sitka in 1855 in which 398 cases occurred, with 60 deaths, but P. A. Tikhmenev (1978, 372) reported only one death in what apparently was the same epidemic.

"Catarrhal grippe," probably influenza, was prevalent at Sitka in 1862 and 1863 (Pierce 1986, 42). The following winter influenza carried off fifty-five victims, including the priest at Korovin Bay on Atka (Black 1984, 105). Dr. W. T. Wythe (1870-1871, 341), who visited Alaska in 1870, reported that an outbreak of "bilious pneumonia" occurred at Kodiak during a spell of unusually warm weather. Some fifty Natives became ill but there were apparently no deaths.

According to a detailed analysis of Russian Orthodox Church records from Nushagak by Don E. Dumond (1986, 30-34), the villages of the Lake Naknek region of the Alaska Peninsula suffered severe epidemics of cough and stabbing pains in 1853 and 1860, causing 163 and 116 deaths respectively. Smaller epidemics occurred in 1859 and 1863. A high mortality from respiratory diseases, largely pneumonia, also took place in 1882 (31 deaths), 1883 (23 deaths), 1887-1888 (47 deaths), and 1889 (58 deaths). Furthermore, influenza is said to have caused 56 deaths in 1890 and 23 more in 1891. With such high mortality, and presumably morbidity, from severe lung disease, it is not surprising that the number of tuberculosis deaths also increased during these decades. Similar systematic study of church records elsewhere in Alaska would undoubtedly reveal many other epidemics not described here.

A major outbreak of respiratory disease was witnessed by Dr. Rosse (1883, 16) at Unalaska in May 1881. While the *Corwin* was anchored offshore, the Native people of the village were dying in great numbers of a disease characterized by a rapid course, with marked breathlessness, cough, sputum production, chest pain, cyanosis (blueness of the lips and skin), and weakness. Since the Alaska Commercial Company physician was himself seriously ill, Dr. Rosse and the crew of the ship lent every possible assistance to those suffering. The disease spread widely to St. Paul, Unga, Kodiak, Cook Inlet, and Prince William Sound shortly after the first vessel of the season arrived in port. The epidemic struck persons of all ages, but the case fatality was especially high in the aged. Death often came only three or four days after the first symptoms had made their appearance.

The disease spread, as noted, well beyond Unalaska. Joseph D. Aronson (1940, 33) reported many deaths from influenza at Kodiak in 1881, and an Orthodox priest described a severe epidemic of pneumonia at Iliamna that summer (V. Shishkin *in* University of Alaska, 1936-1938, 2:146). Another priest reported influenza at Kenai, Ninilchik, and Seldovia that carried off nearly all the children under two years (Nikita *in* University of Alaska 1936-1938, 1:357). In fact, throughout the next few years epidemics of acute respiratory diseases seemed to plague the people of the Aleutians and Kodiak, being brought from island to island by *baidarkas* or larger vessels (H. Elliott 1886, 112-3). These diseases carried a heavy mortality, not only by themselves but also because even those who recovered were then highly susceptible to tuberculosis. Governor Swineford (1887, 54) reported that as a result of the serious recent outbreak at Belkofski, the Shumagin Islands, Bristol Bay, and Kenai, the extinction of the Natives of the Aleutians and some parts of the mainland will occur in a "comparatively short time."

In April 1888, the day-books of the Alaska Commercial Company (personal communication, Ray Hudson 1976) indicated that all the Natives at Unalaska were "suffering more or less from influenza," some of the cases complicated by pneumonia. Likewise, Aronson (1940, 33), citing Russian Orthodox parish records, states that there were many deaths from influenza in the Kodiak District in 1889. In the following year an outbreak in Kenai led to the deaths of some forty persons (Lazell 1960, 117). Four years later another epidemic struck Kodiak Island, leaving many disabled, especially at Kodiak and Karluk (J. White 1894). Epidemics of pneumonia were also reported in the Lake Iliamna region in the late 1880s, with nine deaths in 1888 and forty-one deaths the following year alone (Townsend 1965, 333).

OTHER EPIDEMIC DISEASES

Some epidemics were described in such general terms that their nature remains obscure. In June of 1799 Baranov stopped at Yakutat, where he found the people in the throes of a severe outbreak of disease. The many victims had felt nausea, dryness of the mouth, severe constriction of the chest, and shortness of breath for a period of twenty-four hours and then had expired. He first attributed the illness to the ingestion of "sweet grass," but noted that others who had not eaten it also became ill (Baranov *in* Tikhmenev 1979, 110-11). A similar epidemic, he had learned, was raging around Kenai, where there had also been many deaths (Khlebnikov 1973, 26). Kodiak and its surrounding islands were affected that year as well (Litke 1987, 72).

Later in 1799 the ship *Phoenix* sank with all hands, including Archimandrite Ioasaf, the newly appointed bishop of Kodiak, on the voyage from Okhotsk to Kodiak. An epidemic of unknown type (possibly influenza) was raging at Okhotsk and on Kamchatka that year and company officials speculated that the crew of the ship may have been so weakened by the disease that the ship foundered (Pierce 1976, 171; Gedeon *in* Pierce 1978, 174).

In the fall of 1802 the Russian galiot *Aleksandr Nevskii* arrived in Atka with a deadly cargo. Some fifteen of her crew had succumbed en route to a contagious fever that they had caught in Okhotsk. Before going on to Kodiak the ship wintered at Atka, where the epidemic spread to the local people, causing many deaths and serious food shortages (Davydov 1977, 105).

In 1805 Baranov reported on an epidemic that had occurred the previous summer in a hunting crew near Icy Strait. Although the nature of the sickness is not clear, several died and others had to be returned home very ill (*in* Tikhmenev 1979, 141).

Many other such epidemics must have decimated the population of the Aleutians and Kodiak Island during the late eighteenth and early nineteenth century. Khlebnikov (1973, 104) alone refers to a "contagious rotting fever" that swept through the colonies in 1806, 1808, 1819, and 1824, causing many deaths. At Unalaska in 1807 and 1808 there was a severe outbreak of dysentery that ultimately spread over the whole district, causing many deaths among men and young women, but strangely enough sparing the elderly women. The disease seems to have begun following the wreck at Sanak Island of an American ship under the command of Joseph O'Cain. The local inhabitants were said to have eaten wet and spoiled rice from the wreck before becoming ill with bloody diarrhea (Veniaminov 1984, 257). Khlebnikov (1976, 5) mentioned an epidemic of diarrhea that occurred on Kodiak Island in 1810, resulting in more than one hundred cases and two deaths.

Apparently the first experience of the Alaska Natives with measles occurred on board Kotzebue's vessel *Riurik* while in the far-away Indian Ocean in 1817. At that time two young Aleuts who were being taken to Russia developed a darkish violet-colored rash associated with headache, sore gums, and pain in the neck. Both recovered after three or four days (Eschscholtz 1821, 2:343).

Dr. Blaschke (1842, 44, 64, 69), the company physician at New Archangel, described several types of epidemic disease he saw there in the 1830s. "Gastric fever," probably typhoid, was particularly common during the winter months. What he called "acute hydrocephalus" (probably meningitis) assumed epidemic proportions one winter. Diphtheria and whooping cough also were reported not infrequently among the children of the settlement.

During the early 1840s epidemics of several types were described at New Archangel in the medical reports of Doctors Romanovskii and Frankenhaeuser. An outbreak of "membranous tonsilitis" (which could be streptococcal sore throat or even diphtheria) occurred among the children in 1841, causing twelve deaths (Frankenhaeuser *in* Pierce 1974, 25). Dr. Romanovskii described a cycle of epidemics in 1843-1844, beginning with children's diarrhea in the summer, respiratory and gastrointestinal diseases in the fall, and followed by pneumonia and pleurisy in the winter months (*in* Pierce 1974, 2). Likewise, his colleague (Frankenhaeuser *in* Pierce 1974, 28) reported for the 1847-1848 period an epidemic of "blepharoblenorrhoea" of the children, "gastric fever," and tonsilitis. Two cases of "intermittent fever," no doubt malaria, were observed in persons returning to Sitka after a round-the-world voyage.

Dr. Romanovskii has left a vivid account of an epidemic of mumps that raged in southeastern Alaska between December 1843 and February 1844. The disease was first introduced as early as October in the southern Indian communities and spread northwestward from there. Nearly every Indian, Aleut, and Creole was stricken, but no Europeans, an observation that led him to the bizarre conclusion that the condition was not infectious. Mumps appeared in all its usual and unusual manifestations, including orchitis (manifested by pain and swelling of the testicle) and aseptic meningitis (causing severe headache, nausea, and vomiting). The doctor described in great detail his theories on the causation and treatment of the disease, most of which seem quaint and even far-fetched today. Only one case, with suppuration of the parotid gland, was serious, and there were no deaths attributable to the disease (*in* Pierce 1974, 3-9).

Early in 1848 measles made its appearance in the Stikine River district and rapidly spread to Sitka, where the epidemic lasted until mid-summer. Virtually all Natives and the children of the Russians became sick. Curiously, the Tlingit tolerated the illness well, but the case fatality rate among the Aleuts and Creoles was about ten percent, leading to fifty-seven deaths (Pierce 1986, 30). The epidemic then spread to Unalaska, Unga, and the Alaska Peninsula, where hundreds died, supposedly because of their refusal to accept medical help (Tikhmenev 1979, 371-2).

According to Clarence L. Andrews (1916, 293), typhoid fever carried off thirteen victims in Sitka in 1853. What is more likely, however, is that these deaths were the same as those reported for 1855 by Tikhmenev (1979, 372) among 341 cases of "typhus." The illness was said to resemble yellow fever and to have been brought to the capital by the crew of a round-the-world ship. Typhus is an acute febrile illness, often with a rash, that is spread usually by the bite of the human body louse. If the disease was really typhus (others also called it typhoid: Rosse 1883, 17; Krause 1956, 103), it is not surprising that it spread so widely among a population known to be heavily infested with body lice. According to Tikhmenev (1978, 372) severe epidemics of grippe (influenza) and scarlet fever also appeared at Sitka that same year, although with virtually no mortality.

In 1860 a widespread epidemic of measles struck the Russian colonies, affecting both adults and children and causing eighty-one deaths. The following year epidemic typhus broke out on Afognak Island but was promptly suppressed (Rosse 1883, 17). Other epidemics of the period included an outbreak of scarlet fever in 1865 and another of mumps in 1868, both on Kodiak Island (Aronson 1940, 33). In the latter year measles struck the Chugach Eskimos of Prince William Sound, spreading to the Eyak and Ahtna Indians around the mouth of the Copper River (De Laguna 1956, 3).

A severe form of measles struck Prince William Sound (Abercrombie 1900b, 399) and Kodiak Island during the winter of 1874-1875, causing many deaths. Gen. O. O. Howard (1900, 51), who was traveling in the region around that time, stated that some 515 Kodiak Natives and Creoles died in the epidemic, but these figures may well be inflated, for Rosse (1883, 18) quotes the *Alaska Herald* of August 3, 1875 as reporting a total of only 130 deaths in the region through July 1875, including 40 on Kodiak Island itself. In any event the severity of the epidemic apparently discouraged the plans of the Icelandic Society of Milwaukee, members of which were investigating the possibility of settling on Kodiak Island (Bancroft 1886, 681n; H. Elliott 1886, 113).

Measles continued to plague the people of southern Alaska in the latter part of the nineteenth century. A severe outbreak of so-called "black measles" ravaged southeastern Alaska in September 1882, causing many deaths among the Indians and "Russians" (perhaps Creoles with Russian names) at Sitka and the surrounding communities. At the mission schools in Sitka and Fort Wrangell, however, the mortality was light among the children, probably due to the careful nursing care they received (Wright 1883, 196). It may have been during this same epidemic that the captain of the U.S.S. *Adams* found two shamans torturing several hapless women and children who had been accused of causing the outbreak through sorcery (Scidmore 1885, 42).

Typhoid fever was another recurrent problem during this period, although it was not highly contagious, like measles, and therefore the outbreaks were usually limited in scope. Typhoid was described as prevalent among the Indians of the Kenai Peninsula in 1881 (University of Alaska 1936-1938, 2:63). Around the same time Abercrombie (1900b, 399) reported it as very destructive in some of the Chugach villages of Prince William Sound.

An epidemic occurred near Harris in the fall of 1881. The missionary there noted that the disease was "much like smallpox, though not fatal." Several deaths did occur despite devoted care, however, including one young woman and three children (Willard 1884, 119-20). From the clinical description and low mortality, this disease could have been a mild form of smallpox known as variola minor, or it could have been chickenpox.

At the end of the century a couple of other epidemics were recorded among the Natives people of Kodiak Island. Thirty-six were said to have died at Karluk in an unspecified epidemic in 1898 (C. Elliott 1900). In the spring of the same year twenty-four had perished at Kodiak from an epidemic said to be "similar to cholera" (University of Alaska 1936-1938, 2:88).

12

Epidemics II: Western and Northern Alaska

RESPIRATORY DISEASE

Perhaps the first recorded epidemic of respiratory disease in the more northerly parts of Alaska was the outbreak of "catarrhal fever" that occurred at Fort Kolmakov on the Kuskokwim in 1844 (Zagoskin 1967, 241, 255). Four "workers," probably Creoles, developed the illness and died.

During the following decade there were outbreaks of an influenza-like illness at several points along the western and northern coast, usually after a visit of a ship. One such encounter led to much respiratory disease and coughing around Port Clarence in the early 1850s (D. Ray 1975, 178). Likewise, it was almost certainly the arrival of a British ship of the Franklin search that brought influenza to Point Barrow in the early winter of 1851-1852, causing forty deaths (J. Simpson 1855, 920).

During his long sojourn on the lower Yukon, Father Netsvetov (1984, 84) had occasion to describe many epidemics. The first of these was in March 1848 at a winter camp near Ikogmiut, where some victims were said to be too sick to stand. Early that June a serious outbreak of a coughing disease occurred at St. Michael. This illness affected nearly everyone, young and old, and spread widely to the Native villages. By mid-July many individuals throughout the area were still sick. The nature of this disease remains speculative, although pertussis (whooping cough) must be seriously considered. One clue is Netsvetov's (1984, 99) description of those affected. "My co-servitors," he wrote, "are restless, cough and have lost their voices, but worst of all is my Vasia [his nephew] . . . at times his breath seems to stop, he chokes coughing, and there is nothing to help." As late as September some were still suffering from the sickness.

A mild epidemic of headache, sore throat, and cough occurred at Ikogmiut in March 1849 (Netsvetov 1984, 132). That July the Indians of the upper

Kuskokwim were also suffering from an epidemic. In February 1850 another severe outbreak of disease occurred at Ikogmiut. This was characterized by the sudden onset of headache, chest pains, and weakness of the limbs, a clinical picture that is suggestive of influenza. Other epidemics occurred at Fort Kolmakov and Ikogmiut the following winter. Nearly every spring respiratory illnesses arrived in epidemic force in the riverine communities (Netsvetov 1984, 190-91, 228, 240).

In July 1851 a severe epidemic of respiratory disease, this one with a rash, occurred at St. Michael. It is significant that the illness, affecting Russians, Creoles, and Natives alike, broke out about five days after the arrival of a ship. It soon spread to all surrounding villages, then made its way up the Yukon at least to Ikogmiut and probably farther. This disease was widespread throughout the summer and fall months on the Yukon and in September was brought to the Kuskokwim. The epidemic finally burned itself out during the winter months (Netsvetov 1984, 263-80). The following summer Natives were reluctant to hire out at St. Michael for fear of another epidemic. The redoubt was spared that summer, although an outbreak of cough, stabbing chest pain, and nasal congestion struck Ikogmiut in December (Netsvetov 1984, 304, 330).

Entries in Netsvetov's diary are missing for several years (1984, 393-96). Then in the summer of 1859 he described another severe outbreak of respiratory disease that spread up and down the Yukon, reaching as far as Nulato. In November it appeared on the Kuskokwim, where many died, especially children.

Father Illarion, Netsvetov's successor at Ikogmiut, himself became ill during an epidemic of respiratory disease lasting from August to November 1862. Still another epidemic ravaged the people of this area during the winter of 1867-1868, causing harm especially during periods of thaw (University of Alaska 1936-1938, 2:121-22). Beginning in October 1867, Dall (1870, 162, 193) reported an outbreak of pleurisy and bronchitis at Nulato causing many deaths. One old shaman tried to stir up trouble locally by blaming the illness on the sorceries of the Russians.

The 1870s seem to have been relatively free of epidemics of respiratory disease, but more outbreaks are recorded along the Yukon in the early 1880s. In 1882 a Tanana Indian reported to the governor that his people were dying of an epidemic (Brooks 1899, 493). In the fall of the same year, Jacobsen (1977, 106-8, 139) observed among the Ingalik a severe epidemic of respiratory illness characterized by a heavy cough and loss of voice. Two months later he encountered what he thought was the same disease among the people of Eratlewik, on the north shore of Norton Sound. The following year Jacobsen (1977, 175) learned that almost all the Natives of a village on Nelson Island had died the previous winter from an epidemic. Likewise Lieutenant Schwatka (1885, 99), traveling through the Ingalik villages of the Yukon in 1883, noted that many had died of pneumonia in the winter. Whooping cough was said to be prevalent among the children.

On the northwest coast near Cape Thompson the young Charles Brower (1960, 37) around 1885 came upon a deserted village. The Eskimos accompanying him attributed its abandonment to widespread death from starvation following an influenza-like illness a few years previously. Not long afterward, probably around 1890, a flu and fever epidemic wiped out more than a hundred Nunamiut during a trading feast on the upper Noatak (Gubser 1965, 53).

It was possibly the same epidemic that decimated the population of Wales in the late fall of 1890. This large village, by virtue of its location on the eastern shore of Bering Strait, was a natural stopping place for many trading vessels and other ships passing northward into the Arctic Ocean. On October 2, the people of the village started to become ill with severe respiratory symptoms, and by eight weeks some twenty-six persons, or five percent of the population, had succumbed. The missionary teacher attributed the mortality to a sudden wet and cold spell that caught the Eskimos unprepared. The shamans blamed the presence of the Whites and specifically some of the slates the teacher had sent home with the pupils (Thornton 1931, 25-26, 54; D. Ray 1975, 216; Jackson 1894b, 6-7). Another serious outbreak of respiratory disease occurred at Wales in October 1894, resulting in four deaths (D. Ray 1975, 244).

Another severe epidemic occurred in the summer of 1894 at Point Hope, a community that was constantly exposed to new pathogenic microorganisms by the crews of visiting whaling ships. Dr. John Driggs, the missionary schoolteacher, described the outbreak as "capillary bronchitis," an old term for bronchopneumonia. The epidemic began in July and ultimately struck three-quarters of the population, with one-sixth perishing before the disease burned itself out in August. So many people were sick and dying that bodies were left in the streets as a prey to the dogs (Jackson 1896a, 1467). Dr. Driggs (1894, 563-64) described several heart-rending incidents he encountered, including one in which he found five dead or dying individuals outside in the rain lying under a tent cloth, where they had been dragged to avoid having them die in the house. Driggs worked himself to exhaustion during the ordeal. At a critical juncture when his drugs and supplies were giving out, Captain Healy of the R.M.S. *Bear* arrived and made a timely gift of medicine. Again in the late summer of 1896 an epidemic, probably influenza, struck Point Hope (Driggs 1897, 608).

In southwestern Alaska the Moravian missionaries chronicled several epidemics in the late 1880s and the 1890s. In 1888 an outbreak called "pneumonia" raged on the Yukon and later spread to the Kuskokwim, causing twenty-two deaths around Bethel. Epidemic disease recurred at Togiak in Bristol Bay between 1888 and 1890, causing many deaths and frightening others away from the village (Fienup-Riordan n.d., 129, 150). In the fall of 1890 influenza brought a high mortality to the Kuskokwim, and interfered somewhat with food-gathering for the winter (Henkelman and Vitt 1985, 140). The summer of 1895 saw whooping cough at Bethel, claiming dozens of lives among the children (Schwalbe 1951, 72). This was followed by a relatively minor but still distressing siege of "La Grippe" (Fienup-Riordan n.d., 311).

A major influenza epidemic occurred in the fall of 1896, affecting many villages and compromising the winter food supply. In December of the following year influenza struck again and caused an estimated forty to fifty deaths near Bethel (Henkelman and Vitt 1985, 148-49). That same month the disease appeared at Tununak, probably brought by the crew of the *Bear,* which had returned north to relieve the stranded whalers at Barrow. Here the symptoms included nasal and laryngeal catarrh progressing to bronchitis and pneumonia. Some of the guides for the overland expedition were sick with the disease and apparently carried the epidemic through the whole lower Yukon ([Jarvis] 1899, 115). That same winter fourteen deaths occurred at Unalakleet due to the "grip" (D. Ray 1975, 244).

The St. Lawrence Islanders, often the first to be visited by ships sailing north, had severe outbreaks of respiratory disease nearly every spring during the 1890s (Doty 1900, 193). A particularly severe outbreak of influenza complicated by pneumonia occurred in May and June of 1898, resulting in several deaths (Lerrigo 1901, 101-2). In the fall of 1897 influenza carried off eleven persons on King Island. In 1898 Dr. Call treated some twenty-six cases of "flu" and another severe case of bronchitis at Barrow, the first victims as early as May. In his report he noted that influenza first attacked the Natives soon after the snow disappeared and again just before freeze-up. This was the pattern all the way from Attu to the Mackenzie River. Usually, he went on, the disease ran a mild course, although at Wales that spring nineteen men had died of it (*in* [Jarvis] 1899, 119, 123, 127). It was probably in 1899 that a tragedy occurred at Barrow. After a successful whaling season, the people of Barrow invited their inland cousins to a huge feast. Following a period of revelry and trading some ships appeared at the village carrying trade goods and, unfortunately, influenza. Before the Nunamiut reached their homes, as many as two hundred had perished from the disease (Gubser 1965, 8).

The mission station at Anvik on the Yukon suffered two influenza epidemics in 1899, the first during the salmon run, with the result that very little fish was put up for the winter (Chapman and Sabine 1899, 572).

Further south in Bristol Bay a foretaste of the disaster to come was beginning. Around the old Russian post at Nushagak, the Russian Orthodox church records listed 111 deaths in 1899, four times the usual number. At the nearby Moravian mission at Carmel, every child under two died (Schwalbe 1951, 72; VanStone 1967, 101).

OTHER EPIDEMIC DISEASES

A severe epidemic of unknown type swept through the Nushagak River region sometime prior to 1832, according to an administrative report by Baron Ferdinand Wrangell (VanStone 1967, 99). Five years later Thomas Simpson (1843, 153-54), the first European to reach Point Barrow from the east, was struck by the sight of an immense cemetery with the bodies laid above ground. Many of these looked so fresh that "my followers caught the alarm that the cholera or some other dire disease was raging among the Esquimaux." He and his party were unable to learn further information about the disaster, however, and speculation today would be pointless.

The earliest recorded outbreak of disease, other than smallpox, among the Athapaskans of the interior was mentioned by Zagoskin (1967, 145-46) during his sojourn at Nulato in 1842. There a sick woman was brought for care from the Koyukuk River, where people were said to be dying of an illness that was spreading widely among them. The Chandalar Kutchin and other Athapaskan groups suffered severely from a devastating scarlet fever epidemic during the 1860s, probably introduced by the Hudson's Bay Company traders that were then in the region (McKennan 1965, 21).

Many epidemics must have occurred over the next couple of decades as the Native people had increasing contacts with the whalers and other ships along the coastline. Few records of such encounters seem to have survived, however. An Orthodox priest named Theophil mentioned in passing that an epidemic occurred among the Eskimos in Bristol Bay in 1859-1860 (*in*

University of Alaska 1936-1938, 2:136). In the winter of 1861 Father Illarion (*in* University of Alaska 1936-1938, 2:111) found a great reluctance among the tundra Eskimos to accept baptism because an epidemic was then raging among the people near the mouth of the Kuskokwim. The Eskimos were firmly convinced that the priests who traveled among them were responsible for spreading the disease.

In the maritime areas an outbreak of "gastric fever," which was probably typhoid, occurred in 1862 on St. George Island (Rosse 1883, 18). A few years later a severe epidemic of measles struck the people of Point Hope. The mortality was probably increased by the practice of placing a sick or dying person outside the house to avoid having to abandon the house (Burch 1981, 15-16). One whaling captain reported that the mass starvation which occurred at St. Lawrence Island in 1879 (*see* Chapter 18) was in fact due to an outbreak of "measles or black tongue" (Rosse 1883, 21).

Reported epidemics became more frequent during the 1880s. A widespread outbreak of what was apparently diphtheria, the first mention of this disease in northern Alaska, occurred in 1882 along the Yukon River. It was reported from the territory of the Han (Osgood 1971, 32), near the Canadian border, and also far down the river in the Ingalik villages. Lieutenant Schwatka (1885, 99) wrote that the disease "completely desolated some families, and was particularly fatal among the younger members. All along the river numerous and recent graves were seen." Schwatka (1891, 292) also noted rumors of an extensive measles epidemic along the river in 1883, but found evidence only of a small outbreak with a few deaths in a single village. Other epidemics of unknown type prevailed during this period, including one that carried away half the people of Rosbouski on the Yukon in 1883 or 1884 (Wells 1975, 111) and another that ravaged the Koyukon in 1883 (A. Clark 1981, 586).

Infectious disease outbreaks were increasingly severe among the Natives in the following decade as thousands of prospectors, traders, and missionaries inundated the coasts and rivers of Alaska. In 1897 scarlet fever attacked the Kutchin (Slobodin 1981, 529), and the year after that the Ingalik suffered two localized epidemics of measles and another of mumps (VanStone 1979, 224; Chapman and Sabine 1899, 572). An epidemic of mumps also attacked the people of Eaton Station in November of 1898 (F. Gambell 1900, 71, 89).

In 1900, the year of the Gold Rush at Nome and the Great Sickness, other diseases stalked the land as well. In Nome smallpox made an appearance but mercifully failed to spread. Typhoid fever was very prevalent among the miners, a missionary at Nome estimating that one-third of the population were sick at one time. He performed eleven funerals in one week, all of them for typhoid victims (Young 1927, 393). A severe diarrheal disease, called Asiatic cholera by some, was also prevalent in parts of the lower Yukon that summer and contributed its part to the mortality caused by influenza, measles, and pneumonia (Calasanctius 1947, 222).

THE "GREAT SICKNESS" OF 1900

In the spring, summer, and fall of 1900, a disastrous epidemic of influenza, accompanied by measles, smallpox, and possibly other diseases, struck with unprecedented force the Native peoples of western Alaska. Virtually no coastal or lower riverine community from Atka to Point Hope was spared this merciless onslaught, which overall may have caused the death of a quarter to a third of the entire Native population of these regions. The epidemic seems to have been composed principally of two highly contagious diseases—influenza and measles. Each was probably introduced into Alaska at a different time and in a different manner, and each spread in its own way, sometimes overlapping the other and sometimes attacking a region by itself. An excellent detailed study of these epidemics has recently been published by Robert Wolfe (1982), and the present discussion is much indebted to his work. (*See* Map 3.)

The influenza virus probably came north with the thousands of hopeful gold-seekers who crowded aboard the scores of ships bound for Nome in the late spring of 1900. The earliest reports came in June from the Pribilofs, St. Michael, and Nome, each of which were frequent ports of call for northbound ships. From these entry points the disease spread northward as far as Point Hope, to the interior along the Yukon and Kuskokwim rivers, and to the Bristol Bay region.

The first outbreak of influenza can be precisely dated on St. Paul Island, where sickness appeared just five days after the arrival of the supply steamer on June 11. Nearly all Aleuts were affected, with the first of seven deaths occurring on June 19. The annual seal drive was delayed because of the widespread illness among the workers, who were still coughing incessantly by the early days of July. On August 28 measles appeared on the island, possibly brought by a boat from Unalaska, where the disease had been present eight days previously. The local doctor began vaccinating the people against smallpox with the first signs of rash, but soon the true nature of the

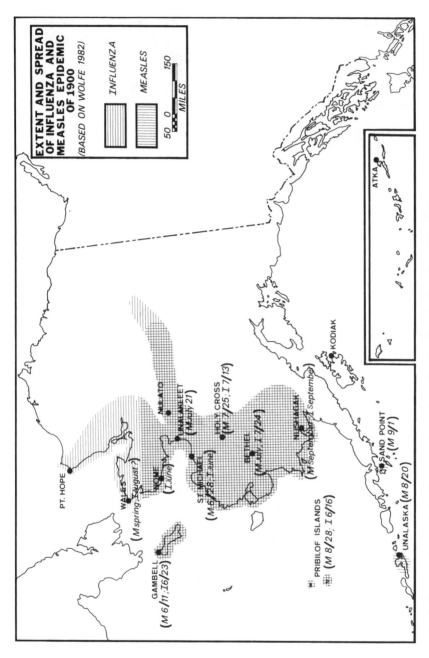

Map 3. Extent and spread of influenza and measles epidemic of 1900. (Based on Wolfe 1982.)

illness became apparent. By the early days of September the disease was widespread, ultimately attacking nearly one hundred percent of the Aleut population. Deaths began on September 5 and continued until the last of twenty fatalities occurred on October 12. Entries from the company logbooks on the island showed that measles was the more severe of the two diseases and that most of those who died were over forty and often afflicted with other illnesses (Wolfe 1982, 100-103).

On St. Lawrence Island measles struck before influenza. According to a physician-teacher on the island, measles broke out at Gambell on June 11, having been brought from Cape Chaplino on the Siberian coast by the indigenous peoples of the region, who in turn may have become ill from a passing whaler or from the people of the interior of Siberia (Lerrigo 1901, 104). The attack rate was nearly one hundred percent, suggesting that the population had never previously been exposed to the virus. About half of those affected had respiratory complications and a few had encephalitis, but the mortality was limited to two babies. Many people were left in a weakened condition, however, and fell prey to the epidemic of influenza that struck a couple of weeks later, probably brought by ships arriving June 21 and 22 (Wolfe 1982, 105). The influenza virus found a fertile field in the raw, irritated respiratory passages of the Natives and within a short time virtually every individual was sick, many with complications such as pneumonia, bronchitis, and enterocolitis. In one day Dr. Lerrigo (1901, 104) visited every house in the village and prescribed for over one hundred patients, fifteen of whom had severe pneumonia. Deaths continued to occur from pneumonia, but also from enterocolitis, until by August 1 some forty-four persons had succumbed. Over the following year Lerrigo counted another twenty who had died of tuberculosis in the village in the aftermath of the flu. In December and January another milder wave of influenza swept Gambell, affecting at least thirty and causing one death (Wolfe 1982, 106).

Measles and influenza converged on the Alaskan mainland in the early part of the summer, at a time when most families of Eskimos and Indians were scattered to their fish camps along the rivers. Influenza seems to have struck the Native people around St. Michael shortly after the beginning of summer and soon spread to many of the villages of Norton Sound and the lower Yukon. The case fatality rate was high, with many succumbing to pneumonia complicating their initial illness. Measles was first recognized in the area around July 1 and also rapidly spread to the surrounding region, although proving fatal only to a few infants (J. White 1902, 259).

Both epidemics raged in the St. Michael area into August. The U.S. Army contingent stationed there assumed the responsibility of bringing assistance to the needy, burying the dead, and providing whatever medical assistance was possible. By August 12, thirty deaths had been recorded in St. Michael (J. White 1902, 260). Conditions were particularly grim in the nearby Eskimo village of Stebbins, which an army sanitary officer visited in early August. By this time the population had already been suffering from influenza for three to four weeks. Of the forty to fifty Natives in the village, ninety percent were sick and helpless, quite unable to procure food for themselves. Eight had died in the previous week and their bodies had remained unburied until the soldiers performed this task (Brady 1900, 49-51).

From the St. Michael area the diseases rapidly spread throughout the Norton Sound region, to Nome, and to the southern approaches to Bering Strait. By early July the epidemic had reached Nome, Wales (Jackson 1901b, 34-36), and Teller, and from these larger communities spread to Golovin, Cheniko, (McKee 1902, 58-59), Port Clarence, Behring City, Sinrock, Grantley Harbor, and north of the strait (French 1901, 60). The missionary at Teller described the Eskimos as panic-stricken by the dual epidemics that had overwhelmed them. Many of the reindeer herders around the station died, leaving a number of orphans to be cared for by the mission (Brevig 1901, 140-42). A prominent Eskimo murdered the shaman at Teller in order to try to appease the evil spirit causing such devastation, but this act of desperation had no perceptible effect. The murderer himself died of tuberculosis a few weeks later (French 1901, 60). A similar incident occurred in Port Clarence not far away, where ten out of twelve Eskimos ultimately perished in the epidemic. There a dying Native seized a rifle and shot the shaman, who was himself at the brink of death (French 1901, 60l; Jackson 1901b, 10).

At Nome itself the epidemic caused little harm, but in the surrounding area the Eskimos fell ill in large numbers. Lieutenant Jarvis of the Revenue Marine Service established a temporary hospital for the sick near the new army barracks outside of town (Brady 1900, 32). This facility, located at the mouth of the Nome River, caused some problem when word got out that the dead were being temporarily kept in a morgue. The deadhouse became a source of terror to the Eskimo patients, some of whom fled down to the beach until they collapsed from exhaustion trying to escape the dreadful vicinity (French 1901, 60-1).

The Revenue Marine Cutter *Bear* cruised these northern waters throughout the summer, making several trips across the straits to Siberia, where both measles and influenza were also found in epidemic proportions (Jackson 1901b, 10). The surgeon on board, Dr. R. N. Hawley, rendered medical assistance in the villages to the extent of his abilities. Captain Tuttle of the *Bear* saw to it that food, clothing, and medical supplies were distributed, under the direction of Lieutenant Jarvis, in all the affected coastal villages. Such supplies were left with missionaries, teachers, and government officials and were responsible for saving many from starvation the following winter (Jackson 1901b, 10-11).

It is at least possible that the *Bear,* despite its mission of mercy, may have been responsible for spreading the epidemic. The vessel called at King Island on July 1, at which time there was no sickness among the people (Jackson 1901b, 34). Six weeks later, however, when the *Bear* returned from the north, many King Islanders had died and the remainder were too ill to meet the ship (Jenkins 1943, 147).

At Wales measles struck with unusual severity. Brought in the early spring by a Siberian boat, the disease persisted for several months, causing nearly universal sickness and a number of deaths among the elderly and infants (Jackson 1901a, 1755; Wolfe 1982, 96). Even as early as July 1, five Natives had died and all five of the missionary's children had been sick (Jackson 1901b, 34). It is likely that influenza also struck Wales later in the summer, for when Captain Tuttle was returning southward in September he noted that many would be destitute there (*in* Jackson 1901b, 152).

Point Hope seems to have been the northernmost limit of the epidemic. When Bishop Rowe was finally able to visit Dr. Driggs at his mission there in early August, he found the doctor well but having recently recovered from the flu. Many of the Eskimos were dying, however, and the food supplies were only sufficient for a week (Jenkins 1943, 147-48).

Very soon after measles and influenza appeared at St. Michael in June 1900, they spread to the lower Yukon, with disastrous consequences for the Eskimos in their fish camps along the river. The weather that summer was unusually hot and dry on the Yukon, a circumstance the Natives believed was associated with the epidemic (J. White 1902, 262). Once disease struck a camp nearly every individual became sick, with no one remaining to fish, cook, mend clothing, gather firewood, or even bury the dead. Most of the people became totally demoralized and lay in their tents awaiting death with resignation. The few with strength remaining fled the camp, leaving the dead and dying to their fate. The Orthodox priest at Ikogmiut (Russian Mission) wrote to the U.S. Special Treasury Agent at St. Michael around mid-July that three hundred deaths had occurred in his district and that conditions were "growing worse daily." He pointed out that the epidemic had struck just as the Natives should have been fishing to put up their winter food supply. The priest predicted that an auxiliary food supply would be essential for the coming winter and closed with this appeal: "If you could but see the miserable huts that these people occupy in winter, the conditions under which they have lived in good health, and then picture them as they are now—weak, sick, starving and poorly sheltered—you would, I am sure, hasten your Government in this errand of mercy" (J. Korchinsky *in* Brady 1900, 51).

Around mid-August the Revenue Marine Steamer *Nunivak,* under Lieutenant Cantwell, left St. Michael and ascended the Yukon, carrying on board Dr. James T. White and loaded with extra supplies of food and medicine. (*See* Figure 21.) Already in the delta itself, usually well populated with summer fish camps, they noticed that the landscape was strangely deserted. At Kwikpak Crossing they found a camp with eleven people, mostly children. Six persons had recently died there and four of the survivors were suffering from pulmonary congestion and were too sick to fish. At Andreafski, an old trading post near the present site of St. Mary's, only about twenty-five people remained. Nearly all of them were suffering from influenza or measles, the latter disease having only recently arrived. Six deaths had already occurred; another took place after the boat's arrival (J. White 1902, 260-62).

A short distance upriver was the village of Pitka's Point, with a usual population of sixty-five but now swollen with an encampment of many Eskimos who had fled from the sickness in other villages. When the *Nunivak* arrived, twelve persons had already died and all the others were sick, most of them with respiratory complications of influenza. A little further upriver they stopped at a village of five houses and twenty people, most of them sick or dying. White (1902, 263) described one house of five or six persons: "The place was dark, damp, and dismal, the fireplace was cold, and an odor of rotting fish permeated everything. The inmates were lying about on their beds, some covered, some uncovered. In one corner was a girl of about fourteen years, entirely nude, whose body was covered with the red rash of measles. Food and medicines were left for these poor people, and we hurried on."

Proceeding up the great river, the *Nunivak* visited nearly every inhabited village, treating the sick, burying the dead, and leaving behind what

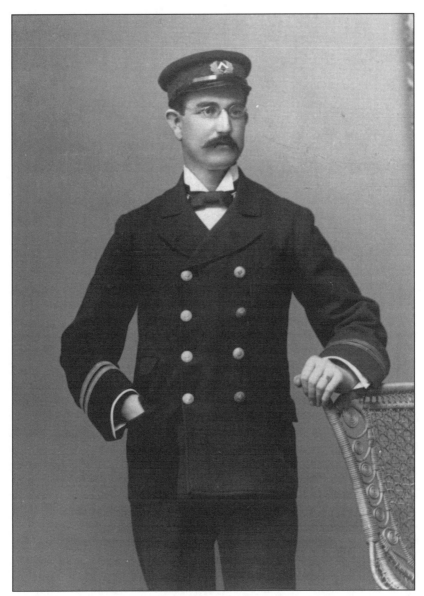

Figure 21. Dr. James T. White of the U.S. Revenue Marine Service, who reported on the "Great Sickness" of 1900. (James T. White Collection, Archives, Alaska and Polar Regions Dept., University of Alaska Fairbanks.)

provisions they could spare. At Russian Mission (formerly Ikogmiut) measles had arrived before influenza and had caused relatively little harm. When the boat arrived, however, influenza was raging through the settlement. Over the previous month twenty-four deaths had occurred, mostly in older adults, and during their brief stay three more persons succumbed. At the little village of Dog Fish, however, conditions were even worse. Of an original population of thirty or forty, only eight persons remained, the remainder having died or fled. The survivors were all sick and demoralized. Food left for them was treated with indifference, although all houses visited were without edible food or even fuel for cooking. Nearby there were salmon on the drying racks, but they were rotting for lack of care. Five persons had died recently and their corpses had remained unburied until the crew of a passing steamer had performed this melancholy office. Dogs had uncovered the shallow graves, and here and there the *Nunivak*'s crew found them gnawing on human remains (J. White 1902, 265-66). "Everywhere," wrote Lieutenant Cantwell (1902, 69), "was there the unmistakable evidence of terrible suffering, absolute neglect, and grim despair."

The villages around Holy Cross Mission were hit unusually hard, and several eloquent accounts of their misery have survived. The disease was introduced around mid-July, probably by the passengers of a river steamer, and spread rapidly not only in the settlement itself but especially in the Eskimo and Indian villages nearby. At a mission fishing camp the ten boys and four girls all survived, thanks to the devoted ministrations of a priest. At the mission itself the staff took special precautions to protect from harm the many children in the boarding school. The mission doctor personally attended the twenty boys in one dormitory, where only one died. In contrast, however, nine of the thirty-six girls in the other dormitory died during the epidemic and two more later succumbed to tuberculosis. The doctor attributed this poor outcome to the remedies used by the sisters, including coal oil, flour and water, carbolic acid, and whiskey (Wolfe 1982, 113). One special victim in Holy Cross was the mother superior of the school, who died during the epidemic as a result of "exposure and overwork" (Cantwell 1902, 69).

The total number of deaths at Holy Cross remains unclear. One witness reported that eight out of sixty-nine Indians living adjacent to the mission died (*in* Wolfe 1982, 112). Dr. White (1902, 266) stated that twelve deaths had occurred by August 22, the date of the *Nunivak*'s arrival. His commanding officer, on the other hand, mentioned fifty-seven deaths at Holy Cross, but likely he was referring to the surrounding area as well (Cantwell 1902, 69). A later historian put the total at sixty-five (VanStone 1979, 224).

The villages and fish camps near Holy Cross bore the brunt of the disease and suffered a high mortality. The mission staff had neither the strength nor the resources to provide assistance to these villages except for a periodic visit by the priests and the older boys to bury the dead.*

At one such camp the priests found fifteen unburied corpses (J. White 1902, 266). In one of two fish camps within a mile of the mission, everyone but a single man died; in the other all perished except a woman and two children (Wolfe 1982, 112). The Natives were either too sick to bury the dead or they refused to touch the bodies for fear of contagion (Balcom 1970, 59). The task of gravedigging became so burdensome that mass graves were necessary. Sometimes a large canvas tent was simply lowered over a group of corpses (Savage 1942, 92). A vivid image of what conditions must have been like in these camps was captured by an eyewitness:

> You enter a tent and you see a man and his wife and three or four children and some infants lying on a mat, all half naked, coughing up bile with blood, moaning, vomiting, passing blood with stools and urine, with purulent eruptions from the eyes and nose, covered with oily and dirty rags, all helpless, and wet and damp day and night (A. Parodi *in* Wolfe 1982, 95).

Further upriver, the territory of the Ingalik was also devastated by the epidemic. Some twenty-six died around the village of Shageluk (VanStone 1979, 224). When the *Nunivak* arrived at Anvik, nearly all the children from the Episcopal school there were suffering from both measles (which had arrived first) and influenza, including thirteen who were being treated in the small hospital (J. White 1902, 266). Some debate exists about the total number of deaths at this village. Dr. White reported only five, whereas Lieutenant Cantwell on the same vessel recorded thirty-seven, with more expected (Cantwell 1902, 70). In recent times VanStone (1979, 224) put the total at twenty. A few miles further upriver at Grayling, White found ten out of thirty-two individuals sick, only five of whom had complications of influenza. Six had died, however, before the arrival of the boat (J. White 1902, 267). At one Ingalik village a visitor found the only living creature to be a dog. "Here and there," he reported, "bodies wrapped in skins, mats, and

---

*In 1965 in Holy Cross the author interviewed an elderly man named Jimmie Walker, who had assisted in this task as a lad of seventeen.

old garments were lying about. Our search discovered eight. . . . The whole village reeked with the filth of every kind and the ground was strewn with all kinds of tools, cooking utensils, fishing tackle, and numberless other things, left behind by the panic-stricken people" (A. Sipary *in* Wolfe 1982, 113).

At Nulato, Dr. James White (1902, 268) found twenty persons ill out of the fifty at the Catholic mission, most of whom had dysentery and pulmonary problems. Measles had swept through in early July and many had become sick a second time when influenza struck. A total of twenty-seven deaths had occurred by the end of August, and another 220 persons were ill in the surrounding area.

The last village on the Yukon affected by the epidemic that summer was Big Bend, thirty-one miles northeast of Ruby, where fifty of the population of sixty-five were sick, sixteen of them with measles and the remainder with respiratory problems (J. White 1902, 269). Further upriver there were scattered cases of both influenza and measles but not in epidemic proportions, except perhaps around Dall River (near present-day Stevens Village), where the *Nunivak* tied up for the winter. (*See* Figure 22.)

Measles and influenza also spread from the Yukon to the Kuskokwim, probably via the traditional portage between the two great rivers from Russian Mission to Kalskag. John Kilbuck, who was helping with the U.S. Census that year, noted its appearance July 25 in the upper river villages (Fienup-Riordan 1988, 438). Dr. Romig, the Moravian missionary physician at Bethel, was also assisting with the census and wrote that somewhere above Tuluksak his boat met another that had just come across the portage and was filled with men with fever, pains, and cough. These influenza victims reported that other villages were suffering from a similar illness. At the Moravian mission at Ogavik (just below Kalskag), Romig found that influenza was already widespread. Before long he and his family were also ill. After ten days at Ogavik, his party set off for Bethel. All along the river he found the villagers sick or dying. Prostrate individuals lay at the water's edge and in the tents hungry infants were found trying to suckle their dead mothers' breasts.

At Bethel and the villages of the tundra the same desperate conditions prevailed. At Quinhagak the shaman blamed the trader for importing the disease with his goods and accused Dr. Romig of sending the wrong medicine, for which he threatened to burn the mission buildings. It was estimated that nearly half the Eskimos of the region perished. Fifty-seven died at Bethel and some 212 were counted dead between Ogavik and Bethel (Schwalbe 1951, 84-85). Below Bethel the mortality was also frightful

(Fienup-Riordan 1988, 443). In one village only 20 survived from a population of 121. As a result of the epidemic several villages along the Kuskokwim and on Nelson Island were permanently abandoned (Wolfe 1982, 114).

As on the Yukon the Eskimos were unable or unwilling to bury the dead, and this task fell largely to Dr. Romig and the other missionaries. The weather, quite unlike that on the Yukon, was an incessant and exasperating downpour (E. Anderson 1942, 196-8). Pneumonia was the immediate cause of death in many cases. Dr. Romig graphically described the situation along the lower Kuskokwim (*in* Henkelman and Vitt 1985, 153):

> The misery of the people seemed to be complete. They were cold, they were hungry and thirsty and weak, with no one to wait on them. The dead often remained for days in the same tent with the living, and in many cases they were never removed. Those that recovered left the tent to fall on the dead as the only covering for the remains of relatives and friends. Children cried for food, and no one was able to give it to them. At one place some passing strangers heard the crying of children, and upon examination found only some children left with both parents dead in the tent. Thus the situation continues from the source to the mouth of the river.

The shamans meanwhile tried desperately to deal with these unseen powers of sickness. They ordered bodies to be thrown in the river or from the tops of the *kashim*, but without effect. It was not lost on the Eskimos that the Whites usually recovered after only a mild illness, whereas they themselves were desperately ill and dying. Hostile feelings developed against the missionaries that took several years to dispel. Dr. Romig himself, who had worked miracles of medicine in the eyes of the Eskimos, never fully recovered his reputation (E. Anderson 1942, 198-200; Oswalt 1963, 100).

From the Kuskowkim, or perhaps from ships supplying the canneries, the epidemic swept into Bristol Bay, causing heavy mortality at Carmel, the Moravian mission there (Schwalbe 1951, 60). Many deaths also occurred along the Nushagak River drainage and in the Tikchik Lakes region. In some of the villages one-third to one-half of the population perished. The village of Manasuk was abandoned, as was Tikchik itself, as a result of the epidemic. In the latter village, excavations revealed bodies stretched out full length on sleeping benches inside the homes (VanStone 1971, 34, 119).

The "Great Sickness" of 1900 was probably the most calamitous event in the history of the Alaska Native people since the smallpox epidemic of 1835-

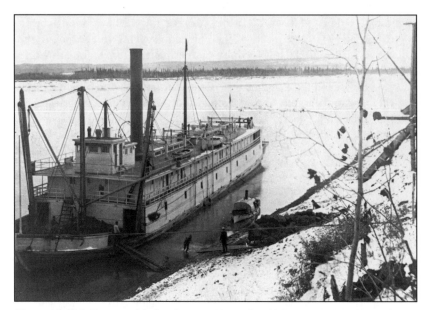

Figure 22. U.S. Revenue Marine Steamer *Nunivak*, which ascended the Yukon in the summer of 1900, at the time of the "Great Sickness." (James T. White Collection, Archives, Alaska and Polar Regions Dept., University of Alaska Fairbanks.)

1840. In the earlier epidemic, however, the disease spread more slowly, and even in more localized areas was abroad for as much as a year. In 1900, however, influenza and measles struck with lightning force and within days whole villages were sick or dying. No one knows the full extent of deaths the epidemic brought, but official estimates, perhaps conservative, ran as high as two thousand (Brady 1901, 28). In some areas the mortality surely ranged between twenty-five and fifty percent. So great was the toll and the impact on the people in some areas that for many years later events were reckoned from that date (Schwalbe 1951, 84).

13

Epidemics III: Smallpox

EARLY ENCOUNTERS

More than any other disease, smallpox struck terror into the hearts and minds of the Alaska Natives in the eighteenth and nineteenth centuries. It was an overwhelming force against which they could find no defense either in their religion or in their tradition. The plague swept through villages like a tundra fire, leaving in its trail dead, dying, and the permanently disabled. Those who escaped a rapid death were condemned to days of high fever, headache, and aching bones, with their faces and extremities swollen with countless pustules. The young were not infrequently left blind or developmentally retarded, and all survivors had to face life with permanent disfiguring scars and haunting memories.

Smallpox had long been known—and probably no less feared—in Europe, where it periodically snuffed out the lives or scarred the faces of countless persons from all walks of life, including many of the royal houses (Hopkins 1983).

The Russian official Kyrill T. Khlebnikov (1976, 29) reported on a meeting with a Tlingit headman called Saigakakh, who remembered as a small child what was perhaps the first smallpox epidemic in Alaska. Spreading northward from the Stikine about 1770, the disease swept through his village leaving only one or two survivors in each family. The old man attributed the pestilence to the crow [Raven?] as a punishment for his people's continual internecine wars.

In August 1787 Portlock (1789, 271-76), while trading with the Tlingit along the western coast of Chicagof Island, noted an elderly man and a girl of about fourteen to be "very much marked with the small-pox." With the aid of an interpreter the captain was able to learn that the disease had carried away no fewer than ten of the man's own children, each of whom was commemorated by a tattoo on his arm. Since none of the marks represented a child younger than ten or twelve, Portlock deduced that the epidemic had occurred about 1775, probably brought by Spanish explorers. Juan Pérez and Bodega y Quadra, in fact, were in Alaskan waters around that time. Portlock speculated how the vessel carrying the disease must have passed near Cape Edgecumbe, since many Indians from that area were pockmarked, he later learned, but none from the westward.

Portlock felt comfortable (and just a bit righteous) in assigning the blame to the Spanish, "a nation designed by Providence to be a scourge to every tribe of Indians they come near." We should not be overly hasty in blaming the Spanish, however, since the records of their voyages make no mention of smallpox either among the crew or among the Indians, despite the fact that Bodega y Quadra spent the greater part of a month in the waters around present-day Craig. In fact, according to Rosse (1883, 25), Bodega's pilot Mourelle observed what he thought were smallpox scars among the Indians of Bucareli Bay in 1775, thus suggesting an introduction of the disease prior to that date. Further north, when the surgeon of Marchand's expedition in 1791 questioned the Tlingit about their scarred faces, he received the reply that they had suffered from a disease which had made their face swell with virulent pustules leading to severe itching. They observed that the Frenchmen themselves bore similar scars and thus must have been acquainted with the disease (Fleurieu 1801, 2:221).

In 1795 Potap Zaikov sailed from Kodiak to Yakutat Bay to trade. According to Bancroft (1886, 350), growing hostility between the Koniag hunters and the local Tlingit was cut short by the appearance of smallpox in two Koniag, whereupon the Indians fled in panic. If true, the source of this outbreak is something of a mystery, for about a decade earlier Shelikhov (1981, 55) had remarked that smallpox had never occurred on Kodiak Island, nor had there been a report since that time. Zaikov's ship was manned only by Koniag hunters and a few Russians who had presumably been stationed in the colonies for some time. In 1818, however, the French explorer Camille de Roquefeuil (1981, 85) noted a considerable decrease in the population of Kodiak, which, he said, "is particularly ascribed to the small pox."

As early as 1768 Catherine the Great had led the way in the effort to prevent smallpox by her warm espousal of variolation for herself and her family. At the time Edward Jenner's much safer and more effective method of vaccination became available in 1798, it was again the royal family that took the initiative; in 1804 the Empress Dowager had the new vaccine imported from Prussia. Vaccination became compulsory in Russia in 1812, and by 1814 some two million Russians had received it (Hopkins 1983, 65-70, 81-82, 86).

Well aware of the devastation that could be caused by smallpox in a population with no prior exposure to it, the directors of the Russian-American Company were quick to seize on Jenner's new vaccine. As early as 1808 they sent a supply to their distant colonies, with instructions for its administration to all Russians and to as many Natives as possible. Dr. Mordgorst, surgeon on the *Neva*, was charged with demonstrating the technique of vaccination and teaching the method to capable company employees (Tikhmenev 1978, 161-62). A priest en route to Kodiak in 1815 (University of Alaska 1936-1938, 4:169) was told:

> The Board of Directors considers it its duty to request you to learn how to vaccinate from the local medical officers, in order to be useful to the people in the Colonies. . . . You will have enough time for this study while you wait at Yakutsk for your sailing in the spring. The operation is not difficult or incomprehensible.

A serious problem with the vaccination program was the availability and stability of the vaccine itself, which had to be shipped halfway around the world by sea, or overland through the endless expanses of Siberia. Moreover, it was chronically in short supply and no doubt expensive. Methods for administration were not standardized, nor was the potency of the vaccine reliable. Dr. Eschscholtz (1821, 2:339-42) of Kotzebue's ship *Riurik* described a severe reaction in several Aleuts whom he had had vaccinated with a single needle prick in Manila in 1817. Other attempted vaccinations probably did not "take" at all. Not only the Russian employees, but understandably also the Creoles and Natives were reluctant to submit to the needle.

Despite these difficulties, however, the company directors were persuaded that vaccination was worthwhile. In a letter to Chief Manager Baranov in 1817 (University of Alaska 1936-1938, 4:142), they suggested that promising young Creole boys be sent to the capital for training as pharmacists, physicians, and bookkeepers, but only after vaccination, since one such talented Tlingit had already died of smallpox while in Russia. In fact Count Rezanov had suggested as early as 1805 that such apprentices be vaccinated in Irkutsk before going on to Moscow or St. Petersburg (Tikhmenev 1978, 92).

In response to the orders of the company, about two hundred Russians, Creoles, and Aleut hunters in Sitka had been vaccinated by 1822, thanks to the arrival of a large vaccine shipment from Okhotsk. A special mass of thanksgiving was celebrated on March 12, 1823, to mark this event. The next priority for vaccination was the people of the outlying districts, but this goal could not even be attempted until October 1828, when a new shipment of vaccine permitted the Creole *feldsher* Aleksandr Repin at Kodiak to send his assistant Galakhtion to the outlying areas of Kodiak Island. Native vaccinators were used whenever possible to increase acceptance of the procedure on the part of the reluctant and often suspicious villagers. By April 1829 nearly three hundred additional Tlingit and Koniag had been vaccinated (Sarafian 1977b, 47-48).

THE GREAT SMALLPOX EPIDEMIC OF 1835-1840

The smallpox epidemic that swept through Alaska from 1835 to 1840 ranks as one of the most significant events in the history of the Native people. From Prince of Wales Island to Norton Sound the disease devastated the population, leaving in its wake as many as one-third dead and many of the remainder scarred, blind, or otherwise disabled. Beyond the physical harm, however, smallpox left demoralizing losses of a different kind: the destruction of family groups, communities, religious faith, and in some areas even a way of life. The Alaska Natives were never the same after this catastrophe. (*See* Map 4.)

Smallpox first appeared in Sitka in late November or early December 1835. How it was introduced remains an enigma. Some feel that it had spread from the British dominions to the south and east, or from the mainland Tlingit, but the most likely hypothesis is that it was brought to the capital by a trading ship (Gibson 1982-1983, 67; Arndt 1985, 2-3). According to the eyewitness account of Father Veniaminov (1972, 47), the disease first appeared in a Creole boy living at the fort, and next spread to the Creoles and hunters, initially killing some 14 out of 160 affected, principally the elderly. Over the next four months a total of one hundred unvaccinated Creoles and Aleut hunters died of the disease, despite the best available medical care in the colonies (Sarafian 1977b, 48). No Russians and only one Finn contracted the disease, presumably because of prior immunity, but in the adjacent Tlingit village, where the disease had appeared in January 1836, about three hundred persons died in a two-month period, sometimes as many as eight to twelve a day. Veniaminov (1972, 47) attributed the high mortality among the Indians to their practice of throwing themselves into the sea or eating ice and snow to cool their burning fever. By April 1836 the disease had largely disappeared in Sitka, leaving a total of four hundred Tlingit dead in the region (Tikhmenev 1978, 198).

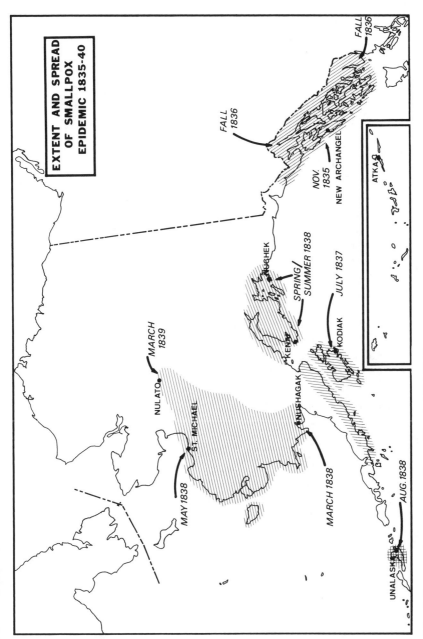

Map 4. Extent and spread of smallpox epidemic 1835-1840.

During these early months of the epidemic Dr. Eduard Blaschke, who had arrived just before the outbreak, was working long hours with his staff to treat the afflicted and comfort the dying, while at the same time vaccinating appproximately two hundred Aleuts, Creoles, and Russians who were still susceptible (Sarafian 1977b, 48). The Tlingit, however, who were suffering the brunt of the disease, at first refused to be vaccinated, preferring instead the traditional ministrations of their own shamans. The latter tried in vain to deflect the disease from their own people to the Russians, even, it was rumored, by contaminating the fish and meat they sold to them with fresh scabs from smallpox victims. When the Russians failed to become ill, however, many Tlingit lost confidence in their shamans, and soon some three hundred were clamoring to be vaccinated by the very enemies they had previously scorned. Three months previously, according to Father Veniaminov (1972, 47-48), a Tlingit forced to submit to the needle probably would have torn the very flesh from his vaccinated arm. Once they saw its effectiveness, however, they began to accept other things Russian, including the Orthodox faith.

The epidemic soon spread to other Tlingit villages, where there was no more immunity and no less resistance to vaccination. Some of the first to be hit were Kutznahoo, near present-day Angoon, and other villages in the straits. By April, when the disease had largely run its course in the area around Sitka, it was just reaching the Stikine River, but it apparently caused few deaths there (Tikhmenev 1978, 198). In the summer and fall of 1836, however, smallpox broke out with renewed intensity over a wide area of southeastern Alaska from the Lynn Canal to Tongass (Arndt 1985, 3). In the village of Tongass itself 250 died in a population of 900 (Bancroft 1886, 560), and in other Indian communities some households were left with no survivors (Tikhmenev 1978, 198). The Haida and Tsimshian villages, the latter in British North America, were especially hard hit (Gibson 1982-1983, 69). Sometimes when the disease struck a home, those who were not sick fled to other villages, carrying the virus to new potential victims (Belcher and Simpskinson 1979, 22). The disease continued to take its toll in the Panhandle throughout the winter and spring of 1837 and had finally fizzled out by August. Sporadic cases continued to appear in Sitka, however, as new susceptibles arrived from outlying districts (Arndt 1985, 3).

Ivan Kupreianov, chief manager of the Russian-American Company at this time, clearly recognized the need to extend control measures promptly to other parts of the colonies. In March 1836 he issued regulations requiring the captains of all company vessels to vaccinate their crew members, air out all items taken on board, isolate all cases of smallpox, lie at anchor for at least two days in a port of arrival, and prohibit mingling of their crews with people on shore. In May he had Dr. Blaschke write down instructions for the prevention of smallpox and send them to all colonial medical personnel (Sarafian 1977b, 48). He also sent vaccine to Kodiak five times between October 1835 and the spring of 1837, but apparently only the last batch retained its potency (Arndt 1985, 7).

Despite these precautions, however, smallpox broke out in Kodiak on July 8, 1837. Fearing the worst, Kupreianov dispatched a Dr. Volynskii and two *feldshers*, Kalugin and Zykov, to vaccinate the Koniag living in the villages on the northern and southern sides of the island. By the time the team arrived in October, however, some 265 Koniag had already died, and despite their best efforts, another 473 died before the epidemic burned itself out there in January 1838 (Sarafian 1977b, 48). The Koniag, like the Tlingit, resisted vaccination and consequently they suffered a heavy mortality from the disease (Veniaminov 1984, 321). Dr. Volynskii reported seeing smallpox victims lying naked on beds of straw and covered with sores (Gibson 1982-1983, 73). Many ran away and hid from the vaccinators, or relied in vain on their own shamans. Some of the vaccine used may also have been of poor quality and thus ineffective (Veniaminov 1972, 48; Sarafian 1977b, 48).

Dr. Volynskii then sent his assistant Kalugin to the Alaska Peninsula, but before he could arrive, Kastylev, the company foreman there, had already succeeded in vaccinating some 243 persons, using lymph from recently vaccinated Aleuts (Arndt 1985, 8). Only twenty-seven, all of whom had refused vaccination, succumbed to the disease in the entire area (Gibson 1982-1983, 70; Tikhmenev 1978, 199).

Dr. Blaschke himself sailed to Unalaska on the company ship *Polyfem* to try to prevent a similar disaster. Arriving in early June 1838, he immediately set about vaccinating the Aleuts, compliance being assured by a "most peremptory order" of the commander of the district (Bancroft 1886, 561). Even without this pressure, however, the Aleuts were prepared to accept and even assist with vaccination because they were persuaded of its benefits (Veniaminov 1984, 321). Having vaccinated the people of Captain's Harbor, Blaschke departed at the end of June for the eastern part of the district, leaving *Feldsher* Repin to vaccinate the residents as well as visitors in the villages around the Russian settlement. The doctor successfully completed his task in the eastern region, but on his return to Captain's Harbor on August 9 he found that Repin not only had just begun to vaccinate, but he had also failed to enforce a proper quarantine as instructed. Despite belated vaccination efforts by Blaschke, smallpox rapidly spread to the western part of the district. By the time the disease had run its course, Blaschke had vaccinated a total of 1086 persons in a three-month period. Fifty-four of these (five percent) had died, some of whom may not have had a successful "take" from the vaccine. An additional ninety unvaccinated persons succumbed to the disease in the Unalaska District (Arndt 1985, 11-12).

In the Atka District, the vaccination order was received via the brig *Okhotsk* as early as May 1838, but vaccination could not begin until a new supply of vaccine had arrived from Kamchatka. By August of that year it had still not been received, and in fact it is uncertain whether it arrived at all until several years later. Meanwhile, all was in readiness. The Orthodox priest Netsvetov, himself a Creole, was specifically requested by the chief manager to assist in persuading the Aleuts to accept vaccination, as was the Aleut chief Nikolai Dediukhin. Despite these preparations, or perhaps because of them, the disease seems to have spared the islands of the district (Netsvetov 1980, 163-64, 176, 250, 258; Sarafian 1977b, 48).

In the spring and summer of 1838 smallpox ravaged the Natives around company posts in Cook Inlet and Prince William Sound (Arndt 1985, 4; Osgood 1937, 19; De Laguna 1956, 256; De Laguna and McClellan 1981, 643). The trader Malakhov was entrusted with the vaccination program in Cook Inlet, but had little success because a large percentage refused to be immunized. *Feldsher* Kalugin had similar results on the Kenai Peninsula and Prince William Sound. A few villages were entirely wiped out, such as Chichenof, where the survivors fled leaving the sick to die and the dead to rot (Bancroft 1886, 561-62n; Aronson 1940, 29).

Afanasii Klimovskii, who was about to leave Kodiak for an extended overland journey to St. Michael, was assigned the task of vaccinating as many persons as possible while en route. Accompanied by a Yakut with considerable vaccinating experience in Siberia, Klimovskii reached Fort Aleksandovsk at Nushagak on March 3, 1838. Following a week of intensive effort in that area, the two set off northward, arriving at Ikogmiut on April 17 and at St. Michael on May 14. Their efforts were only a little too late. Smallpox broke out at Nushagak on March 12, the virus having probably been introduced just before their arrival. The disease seems to have preceded the vaccinators all the way to St. Michael, where the first fatal case appeared on the day of their arrival (Arndt 1985, 10).

Despite Klimovskii's earnest endeavors to limit the disease in southwestern Alaska, smallpox exacted a heavy toll. At Nushagak eighteen workers and six children died. In the region around Bristol Bay and the Kuskokwim and Holitna rivers some 552 were said to have perished, with only 351 survivors, but these figures are almost certainly incomplete (Arndt 1985, 10). The vaccinators probably did not receive a friendly welcome in many places and might have even encountered open hostility. During the course of the epidemic about a dozen Yupik from the Kuskokwim portaged across the Yukon to Ikogmiut, where they killed several company employees and seized the furs stored there. This act of violence seemed to result at least partly from the belief that the Russians had deliberately introduced the deadly plague among them (Oswalt 1980, 12).

Lieutenant Zagoskin (1967, 204, 281), who traversed this region on foot and by boat from 1842 to 1844, found that at Paimiut (below present-day Holy Cross) one-sixth of the total population had been carried off by the disease, and that at Pastolik on the Yukon delta the population had diminished by fifty percent in the five years since the epidemic. Petroff (1882, 40), during his journeys through the region for the 1880 census, estimated the mortality from the epidemic to have approached fifty percent, based on the evidence of Native tradition and the many abandoned villages "converted into cemeteries by the burial of the dead in their own dwellings." If the mortality indeed reached this level, it probably included not only those who died from the disease itself but the many who starved or succumbed to other diseases in their weakened state.

After smallpox reached the fort at St. Michael in May 1838, it continued to spread through the nearby villages during the summer and fall, carrying off as many as fifty percent of the Natives (Arndt 1985, 4-5, 10). Although vaccination had been offered to the people of the post and nearby villages, it probably arrived too late to be of much help. The nearest Eskimo village, once populous, was reduced to a population of nineteen. In fact, the whole southern coast of Norton Sound was rather heavily populated when the Russians built their post in 1833, but a mere nine years later only 283 persons remained in eight scattered settlements, most of the rest having died in the smallpox epidemic. Zagoskin (1967, 100) expressed the Russian perspective of the matter when he remarked, "The affliction sent them by Providence was great, but the blessing that resulted was likewise, as all those who are left are Christians." Along the coast from St. Michael to Unalakleet Zagoskin (1967, 92-93) found ruins of four summer camps which had been abandoned since the disease swept through in 1838. At a fifth camp only one elderly Eskimo and his grandchildren were living, the sole survivors of the epidemic.

A large Eskimo village had formerly been situated on the south bank of the Unalakleet River, across from a small Russian trading post. By the time of Zagoskin's visit in 1842 the thirteen survivors had moved across the river to two small winter huts a quarter of a mile from the company post. This settlement later grew to the present day town of Unalakleet (D. Ray 1975, 125-26).

Just how far north smallpox spread remains uncertain. Dorothy Jean Ray (1964, 64), the premier authority on the area, says that it stopped at Unalakleet, while another recent writer claims it reached Golovin (Koutsky 1981, 2:59).

The Ingalik of the middle Yukon River were perhaps the hardest hit of all the Natives of this region. When the trader P. V. Malakhov established his trading post at Nulato in March 1839, the smallpox epidemic was in full swing there. By spring dead bodies were being gnawed by the starving dogs in the villages. When Zagoskin (1967, 188) visited the post in 1843 the Native population consisted of two men, five women (three of whom were pock-marked), and seven children. A similar situation was evident in other villages nearby, some of which were abandoned and others populated by a few scarred survivors. As he traveled downriver from Nulato, Zagoskin (1967, 193) noted that the disease had struck villages with different intensity. In several instances he found the current population to be less than half of what it had been at the time of Glazunov's visit to the area in 1835. Overall there is reason to believe that the Ingalik may have lost fully two-thirds of their people to smallpox and its aftermath (VanStone 1979, 60).

AFTER THE GREAT EPIDEMIC

Once the epidemic had exhausted the supply of susceptible individuals within its reach, it sputtered and died, probably in early 1840. The surviving Natives of southern and western Alaska found their world in ruins. Between one-quarter and two-thirds of their people had died outright and many others bore ugly scars both on their skin and in their minds. Many of those who escaped death were left an easy prey to secondary infections of the skin or the respiratory tract, particularly tuberculosis.

Starvation was a grave threat to many families, since the loss of hunters precluded the storage of food for the winter. Numerous hunters and fishermen who survived the epidemic missed the seasonal salmon runs or the favorable ice conditions for the taking of seals or walruses. Families were broken up everywhere, with widowers, widows, and children having to find shelter and food with other relatives or friends, most of whom were already having difficulty in providing for their own families.

Discouragement and despair were everywhere. During the epidemic people had found themselves helpless against the overpowering forces that assailed them. The chants of their shamans echoed hollowly and their traditional remedies were wholly without effect. Ominously, it was only the Natives and not the hated Russians who were getting sick. Those who ultimately accepted vaccination were faced with having to admit the inadequacy of their own culture to deal with this scourge.

The Koniag, who suffered heavy losses in the epidemic, probably experienced the greatest change of all. Faced with having to provide food and shelter for countless families devastated by the disease, Russian-American Company officials, led by Chief Manager Etholin, consolidated sixty-five Koniag settlements on Kodiak Island into a mere seven. At these new sites the Russians built frame houses, storehouses, and community buildings. Those unable to provide for themselves were given new clothing and other amenities. The reluctant Koniag were then introduced to farming and sheep and cattle raising as a means of lessening their traditional reliance on the sea (Tikhmenev 1978, 200). Although Russian motives for such changes were probably based on humanitarian considerations, as well as a desire to streamline administration, the Koniag by and large bitterly resented these poorly disguised efforts to make over their lives (Bancroft 1886, 561-62; Okun 1979, 202; Tikhmenev 1978, 200, 347).

The Tlingit, Chugach, Yupik, Tanaina, and Ingalik also were forced to make difficult adjustments in the aftermath of the epidemic. Many lost confidence in their own shamans and religious beliefs and became more susceptible than before to the efforts of the missionaries. For numerous families a strong tradition of self-reliance and independence had to be replaced by dependency on relatives, strangers, or worst of all, the Russian trading post. Their elders, carriers of cultural wisdom and experience, had perished with their memories, leaving a younger generation unsure of themselves and their ability to survive. Village sites and hunting grounds which had been occupied for centuries had to be summarily abandoned for unfamiliar ones where fish and game were uncertain.

Some inkling of the numbers who perished in the great epidemic may be gleaned from the population figures published by Tikhmenev (1978, 447) in 1863. According to him, the total number of person in Russian America declined from 10,989 on January 1, 1836, to 7574 on January 1, 1840, a decrease of 3415, or thirty-one percent. These figures of course do not include the many Natives who died uncounted in villages remote from the Russian posts. The Aleut and Koniag population alone declined by forty-three percent during the period of the epidemic (Sarafian 1977b, 49).

The Russian-American Company was determined that such a tragedy would not repeat itself. To this end the vaccination program which had begun in earnest during the epidemic was continued thereafter. In addition to the four thousand immunizations carried out during the period 1836 to 1840, some 1200 more were carried out in Sitka alone during the administration of Chief Manager Etholin from 1840 to 1845 (Tikhmenev 1978, 371). Dr. Romanovskii, the chief medical officer at the capital, also supervised an extensive vaccination program on Kodiak Island, the Alaska Peninsula, and around company posts in the Aleutians, the Kenai Peninsula, Bristol Bay, the Pribilof Islands, and St. Michael. By 1845 he felt that the colonies were "definitely" protected from the further threat of smallpox (*in* Pierce 1974, 18-19). His colleague Dr. Frankenhaeuser (*in* Pierce 1974, 26, 28, 32) also noted the continuing vaccination program in the outlying areas, using fresh vaccine shipped from Sitka. Since many adults were already immune from having survived an attack of the disease, the emphasis of the program was rightly shifting to children.

Once memories of the great epidemic faded, the vaccination effort lost some of its impetus, until Johan Furuhjelm (chief manager from 1859 to 1863) revitalized it during an inspection tour of the colonies. Using vaccine obtained from California, a doctor accompanying the chief manager immunized people throughout Russian America and apparently taught others the technique (Tikhmenev 1978, 371). As in the earliest years of the company, not every employee willingly accepted this added responsibility. Most *feldshers* seemed to consider vaccination part of their regular work (Netsvetov 1980, 250, 258), but in smaller posts the job was assigned to traders and priests, some of whom kept poor records (Golovin 1979, 63), and others complained of the tiring extra burden (University of Alaska 1936-1938, 2:57). In a few areas, such as the lower Yukon, the vaccinators still met some resistance from the Natives (University of Alaska 1936-1938, 1:379).

Despite these renewed efforts to protect the population, the disease itself broke out again in 1862 in southeastern Alaska. Once more it spread northward from Canada, where at Fort Simpson, British Columbia, some five hundred deaths occurred (Arctander 1909, 155-56). The epidemic affected many of the Tlingit and Haida villages but largely spared Sitka, where the level of immunity was still high (Tikhmenev 1978, 371).

SMALLPOX IN THE AMERICAN PERIOD

Although the American government apparently made no effort to maintain immunization levels in Alaska, smallpox seems to have been largely absent during the latter part of the nineteenth century. It may have been present around Haines in 1881, as suggested by a missionary account (Wright 1883, 231), but the diagnosis is at least questionable. Likewise, Lieutenant Cantwell (1889, 81) saw what he thought were typical smallpox scars in a Kobuk River Eskimo and speculated that the disease was sporadically introduced from the Koyukon Indians. There is, however, no corroborating evidence that it was ever prevalent in this area.

The only time smallpox seriously threatened under American rule was in the summer of 1900, at the height of the Nome Gold Rush. According to Dr. James White (1902, 257-59), two vessels from Seattle, the *Oregon* and the *Ohio,* were found in June to have smallpox on board while lying at anchor off Nome. Passengers had already gone ashore from the *Oregon,* but the second ship was immediately quarantined by the authorities, with the three of her passengers showing clinical signs of the disease being put ashore at Egg Island, a small rocky islet about ten miles off St. Michael. There under the supervision of a physician the victims were cared for in a cluster of tents erected for the purpose.

One of the other ships quarantined at Egg Island, the *Santa Ana* from Seattle, had also had a case of smallpox on board while at sea. A fellow passenger described the boredom of the 450 persons on the ship, who passed their time in quarantine by holding a mock presidential election (William Jennings Bryan won), and a kangaroo court. The fruit the ship carried as cargo soon began to rot and so the passengers took up a collection and bought large quantities as a gift for the sick on the island. Fortunately, no other cases of smallpox occurred on the ship (Mallory 1986, 218-19).

Smallpox broke out in Nome within a week of the arrival of the *Oregon.* The situation was especially dangerous not only because of the crowded, unsanitary conditions in Nome itself, but also because many disappointed miners were leaving Nome for St. Michael and the Yukon River. There the disease was in danger of causing devastation among the Native villages, which were already under siege from the epidemic of influenza and measles.

In late June Gen. George Randall, commander of the Department of Alaska, arrived in Nome and was asked by the Chamber of Commerce to declare martial law, in order to prevent anarchy if a serious disease outbreak of smallpox should occur. On July 2, 1900, he issued an order forbidding all vessels from Nome from landing at St. Michael until they had spent two weeks in quarantine at Egg Island. This period was later shortened to eight days, "just long enough," according to Dr. White (1902, 257-58) of the Revenue Steamer *Nunivak,* "to cause considerable inconvenience to commerce and insufficient to prevent the landing of smallpox."

Quick control of the epidemic led to a lifting of the quarantine on July 24, but not before some twenty-one ships had been quarantined at Egg Island. No cases of smallpox appeared on the vessels, yet hygienic measures were strictly enforced, including the fumigation of all mail by perforating the letters and blowing sulfur dioxide gas through them (J. White 1902, 258-59).

At Nome itself the general's orders forced several needed improvements in sanitation. A total of eighteen cases of smallpox occurred in the city but prompt isolation in a pesthouse one-and-a-half miles from town was effective in containing the disease, thus preventing a potentially serious epidemic (Cole 1984, 71). The scare, however, was sufficient to make the sprawling settlement more health-conscious and to lead to the cheerful acceptance of vaccination by many of the miners (McKee 1902, 34).

Another smallpox outbreak occurred late that year, beginning in Ketchikan. An Indian from there was on his way to Sitka by steamer to get married when he broke out with the telltale rash and was quarantined with his contacts on a small island. Nevertheless, the disease spread to the village of Saxman, where nearly everyone became sick and a few died (Jackson 1903a, 1459). Later that winter a group of Indians traveling to Hoonah for a feast broke out with smallpox. The disease spread rapidly through the susceptible population, resulting in some fifteen deaths, including two students. The disease also appeared in Sitka, where it caused a few deaths among the elderly and debilitated, and at Killisnoo, Juneau, and Douglas (Brady 1901, 50). In the latter two communties nine persons with the disease were held for a two-week period in a makeshift pesthouse (Leonhardt 1901, 1616). During this time physicians of the Marine Hospital Service were urgently vaccinating the Natives of the villages and canneries of southeastern Alaska in order to prevent further spread. Governor Brady lent his full support, with even his ten-year-old son contributing his part by showing off his vaccination scar to the Indians (Hinckley 1979, 41). Fortunately for all, the epidemic was soon brought under control and did not spread to the many unvaccinated individuals in other parts of Alaska.

14

Sexually Transmitted Diseases: The Gift of Venus

THE ALEUTIANS AND KODIAK

Ethnohistorians seem to agree that syphilis and gonorrhea were not present among the Native people of Alaska prior to the first European contact (Oswalt 1967, 75; VanStone 1958, 9; Laughlin 1980, 101). The few available studies of early human remains confirm this view. The earliest written record of such diseases in Alaska seems to be from the diarists of the third Cook Expedition. In October 1778, while the ships were visiting Unalaska, the captain himself (Cook 1967, 3(1):468) wrote: "The Russians told us they never had any connections with the Indian [Aleut] women, because they were not Christians; our people were not so scrupulous, and some were taken in, for the Venereal distemper is not unknown to these people." On the same occasion Surgeon David Samwell (*in* Cook 1967, 3(2):1144) also noted that several of the ship's company had contracted venereal disease from the Aleuts. Samwell indeed was one of those who were "taken in" (to use the captain's phrase) by the charms of the local women, some of whom slept on board despite Cook's specific prohibition (1967, 3(1):265) against such behavior in January, while the ships were in Hawaiian waters. It is interesting to note that this rule was being strictly enforced when the ships had passed near Unalaska in June of that year, though Samwell even then (*in* Cook 1967, 3(2):1121) felt compelled to boast that he was able to procure sexual favors by presents of tobacco.

It seems clear that venereal diseases were already present in the Aleutians by the time of Cook's sojourn there. Cook's own second in command, Capt. Charles Clerke (*in* Cook 1967, 3(2):1337), was well aware that only the Russians had been there before the English when he wrote that the Natives were afflicted with "that heavy Curse attending every set of People, who are unfortunate enough to get by any means European connections." The Russians had probably arrived in this region in the 1750s, most of them unencumbered by the pious restriction about relations with non-Christians.

It is more than likely that Cook's men themselves carried not only syphilis but also gonorrhea. The word "syphilis" is never used by any of the Cook diarists with respect to the Aleuts, but rather polite circumlocutions such as "the curse," and "venereal distemper." Moreover, in the eighteenth century syphilis itself was not always clearly distinguished from gonorrhea. In what is the most detailed discussion available on this subject, Sir James Watt (1979, 153) indicated that gonorrhea was very prevalent among the crews of Cook's third voyage, having been spread in both directions between the sailors and the Society Islanders. Both syphilis and gonorrhea, and perhaps other sexually transmitted diseases, were left by the crew on the newly discovered Sandwich (or Hawaiian) Islands in January 1778, and also apparently bestowed on the Indians of Nootka Sound after Cook's visit there. At Samganoodha, however, gonorrhea seems to have been already present and presumably of Russian origin.

In 1790 Dr. Merck (1980, 176) described the Aleuts of Unalaska as suffering from "wounds of the venereal kind," which they had only known, according to him, since the arrival of the Russians. A generation later Father Veniaminov (1984, 258) wrote that syphilis appeared in the Aleutians as "the gift of the Russians," and reached its peak there about 1798, when sometimes entire families, young and old alike, were affected. By 1825 the disease had declined markedly and appeared seldom thereafter except after the visit of ships. Dr. Eschscholtz (1821, 2:335) was unable to find syphilis at Unalaska in 1817, "considering the numerous ships of various nations that have resorted hither since 1742." And Golovin (1979, 63), writing in the early 1860s, reported that syphilis, although once widespread, was now almost nonexistent in the Aleutians.

With the arrival of the Americans, however, came a resurgence of the disease. Dr. Robert White (1880, 39-40) found a "marked prevalence of venereal diseases in all forms" among the people of Unga Island, a situation he attributed to the many Caucasians who were fishing there. He found many manifestations of syphilis, including the congenital form in children, that would have done credit, he said, to a venereal disease clinic in Paris or Vienna. The situation was much the same in Unalaska, where many whalers refitted each summer on their way northward. In other islands the prevalence of syphilis seemed to parallel the amount of contact the people had with the "outside."

About a decade later Dr. James White (1890), noted a marked prevalence of syphilis at Belkofski, where "the whole village with very few exceptions is diseased, men, women, and children." On a subsequent visit to the village, White (1894) found more syphilis than anywhere else on the Aleutian Chain.

A more skeptical voice was that of Dr. Samuel Call (*in* [Jarvis] 1899, 124), who spent five years with the Alaska Commercial Company at Unalaska, during which time he claimed to have visited every Native village from Attu to St. Michael once or twice a year. In all this area he saw only two chancres (the earliest manifestation of syphilis), both in non-Natives, but was not so sure about the nature of the large, deep, destructive, and foul-smelling ulcers that he conceded may have been the result of "hereditary syphilis."

The earliest mention of sexually transmitted disease on Kodiak Island was by Shelikhov (1981, 55), who founded the first permanent Russian settlement there in 1784. He noted that the Koniag were free from communicable diseases "with the exception of venereal disease, which has been observed." A few years later Dr. Merck (1980, 107) remarked that syphilis, or *ytungunakhtak,* had been present among the Koniag "from long ago."

While two ships of the Billings expedition were wintering in Unalaska in 1791-1792, a party of Russians and Koniag arrived from Shelikhov's settlement in search of brandy, tobacco, and syphilitic remedies. The latter were given them by surgeons Michael Robeck and Peter Allegretti, together with instructions on their proper use (Bancroft 1886, 294-95). Whether these remedies (probably mercury) were intended for the Russians or the Natives is unclear.

Father Ioasaf (*in* Black 1977, 84) remarked in the early 1800s that the Koniag were afflicted with venereal disease, due to their unsanitary ways, and that they treated it by a special diet. The Koniag, in fact, employed several complex and seemingly effective traditional remedies for treating the disease. This suggests that they had known it for several generations, perhaps as far back as 1763-1764, when Glotov first wintered on the island. Around the same time Lisianskii observed that syphilis was among the commonest disorders affecting these people (Lisiansky 1814, 201), although Davydov (1977, 178) thought that the Russians overdiagnosed it, seeing it in every cold or other minor indisposition.

In the 1830s Chief Manager Wrangell sent a Dr. Meier to Kodiak Island to examine the people of the district for signs of syphilis and remove those who were infected to the hospital at St. Paul's Harbor (Sarafian 1971, 196). Again in 1840 the chief manager at Sitka received word that syphilis was rapidly increasing in the outlying posts, and this time sent Dr. Romanovskii to initiate control measures. After sending infected individuals to Kodiak from the company post at Nuchek, he allegedly examined all inhabitants of the island and dispatched the syphilitics to the hospital for mandatory treatment. Presumably as a result of these measures syphilis disappeared from Kodiak for a number of years, its reintroduction being prevented by the required inspection of all ships' crews embarking for the island (*in* Pierce 1974, 16-18).

In the later years of Russian administration syphilis remained rare in Kodiak except when occasionally introduced accidentally by the crew of a visiting ship (Golovin 1979, 63). In the American period, however, the disease once again spread widely, probably due to the influx of cannery workers. An Orthodox priest lamented in 1898: "The cannery at Kodiak, depriving the Aleuts of everything, of their souls and bodies, does not give anything in return except whiskey, lewdness and syphilis" (T. Shalamov *in* University of Alaska 1936-1938, 2:87).

SOUTHEASTERN ALASKA

Early records of syphilis in southeastern Alaska are scarce. The disease was apparently rare among the Tlingit around 1800 (Tikhmenev 1978, 83), but by the time that V. M. Golovnin made his tour of the colonies in 1818, it had become common in New Archangel. According to Golovnin's view of the matter, the Russians were acquiring it from the Tlingit, who were getting it from the Indians of the outlying villages. These latter, in turn, were said to be infected by the crews of foreign ships, mostly American, who were carrying on illegal trade in Russian waters (Bancroft 1886, 712n). The traders probably got the disease from their contact with the indigenous peoples of the South Sea Islands, where the disease was then rampant (Romanovskii *in* Pierce 1974, 10).

Although foreign trading vessels undoubtedly played a part in the introduction and spread of syphilis, the blame cannot be laid so easily and conveniently at their door only. The Russians had established their first post in the region in 1799, bringing with them Koniag and Aleut hunters, who as we have seen were heavily infected at this time. The Russians themselves were also a source of the disease; Capt. Adam von Krusenstern (1813, 2:108), for example, observed in 1804 that many of the employees of the

Russian-American Company about to embark from Kamchatka for the colonies were infected with syphilis.

Indeed, by the 1830s syphilis was prevalent among company employees in Sitka, but it was apparently a mild form of the disease, at least among the longer-term residents of the capital. Most cases were successfully treated by diet alone, without the need for mercury. The disease was spread mainly through sexual relations between the Russian men and certain Tlingit women from the nearby village. Zagoskin (1967, 68) remarked in 1842 that since Baranov was himself a bachelor, he had been "obliged to permit his subordinates free reign with Indian and Aleut women." By 1840 there were strict rules against such liaisons with the Tlingit, but they continued as before, especially between the Russians and a group of Indian women who lived in the woods surrounding the fort (Romanovskii *in* Pierce 1974, 10). Most of the latter were infected with syphilis, a disease they treated with indifference, probably considering it a necessary inconvenience in their line of work (Golovin 1979, 64).

The authorities tried various means of coping with the problem, finally lighting on a policy of forced treatment of the infected women. Chief Manager Etholin issued the necessary orders in 1842, apparently after consultation with Tlingit leaders and elders. The infected women were rounded up by the soldiers and brought to the fort, where they were confined and treated in a special section of the hospital until they were considered no longer a threat to others. In 1845 alone some seventy women were brought in, of whom thirty-three were found to be syphilitic. After a course of mercury treatments, they were allowed to return to their homes (Romanovskii *in* Pierce 1974, 11).

Although these draconian measures were helpful, they did not completely solve the problem. Dr. Romanovskii (*in* Pierce 1974, 11-14) clearly saw the reasons:

1. The Tlingit were a proud and independent people who did not readily submit to authority;

2. They constantly engaged in trade with other tribes, thus leading to spread of the disease to other villages and later reintroduction to Sitka;

3. Infected Tlingit slaves were often sold by their masters to other villages;

4. The women, whether slave or free, resisted treatment and often hid out in inaccessible places;

5. Tlingit leaders resented enforced treatment of the women, some of whom were their slaves or concubines, and often insisted on their release before treatment was completed; and

6. The Tlingit in any event attributed the disease to sorcery and therefore preferred to resort to their own shamans for help instead of to the Russians.

Despite all these impediments, however, Romanovskii noted that gradually the Indians were becoming more willing to cooperate, probably because they began to appreciate better not only the greater effectiveness of the Russian methods of treatment, but also the advantages of maintaining good relations with the company.

Dr. Frankenhaeuser (*in* Pierce 1974, 20-21) a few years later complained that syphilis would probably never be eradicated at Sitka, as it had been at Kodiak, because the Tlingit were never going to cooperate fully. Yet the program did demonstrate some results, the number of syphilitic men at the fort falling from sixty-two in 1841 to only twenty-four just two years later.

By 1840, when syphilis was reaching its peak in southeastern Alaska, gonorrhea was also prevalent (Blaschke 1842, 67, 73). Dr. Romanovskii (*in* Pierce 1974, 15) noted that urethral discharge among the men and cervical discharge among the women were common problems at New Archangel, although he considered these signs to be a manifestation of syphilis. It is also at least possible that the epidemic of profuse eye discharge among Sitka children in 1848 was ophthalmia neonatorum, a form of gonorrhea acquired from the mother during delivery (Frankenhaeuser *in* Pierce 1974, 28).

Control measures against venereal disease must have lapsed somewhat over the next decade or so, for by the time Chief Manager Furuhjelm arrived in the colonies in 1859, syphilis was again a serious problem at Sitka. Wasting no time, he ordered the destruction of all the huts near the fort being used in illicit relations, then had a special building constructed near Lake Lebiazhe, with a sentry posted on top. Infected women from the area were again rounded up and brought to the hospital for forcible treatment. The women continued to resist these measures, however, and usually managed to escape to the village within a few days. To show that he meant business, however, Furuhjelm then announced that any woman who ran away from the hospital would have half her hair shaved, a punishment the Tlingit found particularly humiliating. This threat was enough to ensure cooperation on the part of most (Golovin 1979, 64).

It goes without saying that syphilis was not confined to the Tlingit women, but was also widespread among the company employees at the fort. In addition some Tlingit men and some of the women of the fort no doubt were infected also, but probably did not contribute much to the spread of the disease. Company officers and others with money to spend sometimes tried to purchase uninfected Tlingit slaves, but this arrangement was beyond the means of most employees, who resorted rather to casual liaisons with the women of the forest and thus became infected. A few of these workers actually seemed to encourage the disease so that they could lie at ease in the hospital for a few weeks while undergoing treatment. The chief manager took a dim view of this practice, requiring a periodic examination of all employees and docking the pay of anyone undergoing hospital treatment for syphilis. These measures were successful in greatly diminishing the incidence of syphilis by the end of the Russian period (Golovin 1979, 64).

The abrupt arrival of American soldiers in 1867 to garrison the town largely neutralized these efforts, and syphilis once more became a serious problem. The army authorities were quick to blame the resurgence of syphilis on the plethora of street prostitutes, some as young as twelve or thirteen. The inspector general piously (or naively) wrote: "No one having knowledge of these wretched people could believe that they were corrupted by the troops. . . . [T]he presence of the soldiers only afforded opportunity and incentive for the practice of vice" (U.S. Army, Alaska 1962, 20). Another slant on the matter came from the medical director for the Army Department of Alaska, who wrote to the Indian agent: "A greater mistake could not have been committed than stationing troops in their midst. They mutually debauch each other and sink into that degree of degradation in which it is impossible to reach each other through moral or religious influences." Another army doctor wrote that syphilis was one of the commonest diseases among the Indians, "aggravated and diffused by unrestrained intercourse with the troops, and affects both sexes equally" (Tonner *in* Colyer 1869, 1023-24). Nor were the Indians the sole victims. Stories were told of how drunken soldiers would take possession of a Russian family's house at night and beat or frighten the women into having sexual relations (Bancroft 1886, 606-7).

Indeed, the extensive abuse of alcohol on both sides no doubt played a major part in the spread of venereal disease. Special Treasury Agent William Gouverneur Morris (1879, 62) had a flair for rhetoric in his fulminations against the "debauchery and degradation of the native women by a licentious soldiery." But beyond the troops a new element—the miners—were arriving, "who seem to have emulated the sons of Mars in the prosecution, performance, and mad riot of the quintescence [sic] of vicious enjoyment."

The disease also seemed to be prevalent in all its forms beyond Sitka, in the areas most frequented by Whites (Wythe 1870-71, 341). It was common wherever soldiers were garrisoned or where numbers of miners were to be found (R. White 1880, 33; Young 1927, 96).

After the advent of civil government in 1884, the governor sent Dr. Zena Pitcher to Sitka to report on health conditions there. She found that the Natives were suffering generally under a heavy burden of disease but especially of syphilis and gonorrhea and their many complications (Swineford 1886, 29). A report from the next governor a few years later described "hereditary diseases" (a common euphemism of the period for syphilis and sometimes tuberculosis) to be "frightfully prevalent" (Knapp 1889, 21-22).

In the 1890s, however, the sexually transmitted diseases seem to have declined in importance, probably because Sitka was becoming less of a frontier town once the soldiers and miners had left. Missionaries were increasingly active in the capital during these years and had established a small hospital as an adjunct to their school. In 1892 Dr. Clarence Thwing, a Presbyterian missionary, was able to write that venereal diseases had not been "prominently frequent" during his two-year stay (*in* Knapp 1892, 57).

WESTERN AND NORTHERN ALASKA

Ivan Vasilev, during his explorations of the western end of Bristol Bay in 1829 and 1830, found the people there already infected with syphilis (Zagoskin 1967, 110). The Russians had first explored this area in 1818 and 1819, when the post at Nushagak (Aleksandrov Redoubt) was established. This rapid spread of the disease among the coastal Natives led Zagoskin to make a plea that all Russians selected to serve in such distant areas be first adjudged healthy.

The Yupik Eskimos of the Yukon-Kuskokwim Delta were still free of the disease by 1844 (Zagoskin 1967, 110). Indeed, it appears as if syphilis never gained a serious foothold in this region (Oswalt 1963, 94). None of Hrdlička's (1931, 132) skull specimens and only one of Richard Holcomb's (1940, 182) (from Paimute on the Yukon) showed the telltale lesions of syphilis.

In Norton Sound, however, the situation was less clear. Khromchenko (1973, 71) visited Stuart Island, near present-day St. Michael, in 1822. There he wrote, with some assurance: "For the first time in all my years on the northwest coast of America, I observed a pernicious venereal disease which had spread to such a degree that many of those suffering from it were greatly disfigured. The face and body of such persons were covered with deep sores." The women, he thought, were more often infected because more women than men had part of their nose eaten away. Whether these people truly had syphilis (the destruction of the nose is suggestive that they did) can not be settled on the available evidence. Certainly ships of several flags, including Russian, British, and perhaps American, had already visited these waters prior to Khromchenko. Other outside possibilities include a spread northward from Bristol Bay (D. Ray 1975, 178-79), or even introduction from the people of Siberia, whom the Eskimos of the Seward Peninsula frequently visited for the purpose of trade. Syphilis was definitely known from eastern Siberia in the eighteenth and early nineteenth centuries (Holcomb 1940, 179; Krasheninnikov 1764, 217-19).

When Zagoskin (1967, 110) visited St. Michael in 1842, he attributed the syphilis he found among the Eskimos to the arrival of the Russians in 1833. A quarter of a century later American troops were garrisoned there to "protect" the new Alaska Commercial Company interests and keep the peace. In the latter third of the century the post became increasingly important as the staging area for Yukon River traffic, especially after the rush for gold began in Alaska in the 1890s. Even before the thousands of miners poured into St. Michael, however, a navy surgeon had described syphilis as so common that the Natives had come to consider it a "necessary, or at least unavoidable evil" (Knapp 1890, 24). At the peak of the Klondike Gold Rush Dr. Edmonds (1966, 30) found scarcely any group at St. Michael without active signs of congenital or acquired syphilis.

Gonorrhea also seemed to be prevalent around Norton Sound at a relatively early date. Zagoskin (1967, 110) on his visit to the region in 1842 found that the Eskimos already had their own methods of treatment for the disease, suggesting that they had known its effects for some time.

The disease may not have reached St. Lawrence Island until as late as 1885 (Foote 1964, 19). In 1899 a missionary teacher mentioned it as among the more prevalent diseases (Doty 1900, 194). A physician serving as teacher the following year observed that syphilis was much less common on the island than on the mainland, although sometimes he did see secondary and tertiary cases, not to mention signs of congenital syphilis among the children (Lerrigo 1901, 103-4). The disease was also late in reaching the Natives of the interior. By 1884, for example, syphilis was still uncommon along the Kobuk River (Cantwell 1889, 83).

The crews of Yankee whaling ships were responsible for the introduction of syphilis into some of the Eskimo communities along the northwestern and northern coasts of Alaska. The first of these vessels passed north of the Bering Strait in 1848 and they began overwintering in the 1880s. The men were a coarse lot who were not above kidnapping Eskimo women for a period of enforced companionship on shipboard (Oswalt 1979, 293). Sexual favors were also sometimes a profitable trade item between the Eskimos and whalemen, especially in exchange for alcohol (Bockstoce 1986, 194). Even the usually disciplined crews of the British Royal Navy could succumb to the temptations of a long voyage. A Moravian missionary on board M'Clure's ship off northern Alaska in 1850 confided to his diary that "the men—and this includes high ranking officers—behave themselves so shamelessly that here one will soon have an Anglo-Eskimo colony" (Miertsching 1967, 37).

Syphilis was noted to be a problem in this area by the medical officer on the 1881 cruise of the Revenue Marine Steamer *Corwin* (Rosse 1883, 27). A few years later, at Barrow, Murdoch (1892, 39) found gonorrhea common in both sexes but syphilis apparently absent "in spite of the promiscuous intercourse of the women with the whale men." Another, in contrast, reported that half the population of Barrow was "tainted" by secondary or tertiary syphilis (Bockstoce 1986, 194). A doctor visiting Barrow a short time later found venereal disease so widespread that he spent his time largely in treating cases of syphilitic origin (U.S. Dept. of Interior 1893, 141-43). He went on to predict that this disease would, if unchecked, depopulate the coast, since nearly every infant born in Barrow showed "marked indications of the curse." Dr. Call, however, who spent five months at Barrow in 1898, treated only nine cases of hereditary syphilis in Eskimos and saw no primary syphilis either among the whalers, many of whom were stranded there, or among the Native people (*in* [Jarvis] 1899, 127). The disease in any event was not confined to Barrow, but probably was also prevalent in other villages, such as Point Hope, where the people had frequent and prolonged contact with the whalemen (VanStone 1962b, 24).

CLINICAL MANIFESTATIONS AND TRADITIONAL THERAPY

Syphilis used to be known in medical circles as the "great imitator" because of its protean clinical manifestations. The disease normally has three stages of development. The primary stage, or chancre, takes the form of a painless indolent ulcer, usually in the genital region, which comes on about three weeks after infection and may last for about three weeks before spontaneously resolving. The secondary stage consists of several types of eruption on the skin or mucous membranes, which again disappear spontaneously after a few weeks. The first two stages are confusing enough, but the third stage can be exasperating. Here the disease can have destructive effects in nearly any part of the body, including the skin, mucous membranes, bones, liver, spleen, heart and aorta, meninges, and brain. Tertiary syphilis progresses slowly but inexorably for many years and ultimately can cause insanity, crippling, or death. One of the most tragic forms of the disease is congenital syphilis, an infection of a newborn baby acquired from the mother during the latter part of pregnancy. An infected infant is often afflicted with blindness, hearing loss, heart disease, deformity of the nose and teeth, and various skin lesions.

A disease with such diverse manifestations could confuse experienced physicians, much less an untrained observer. As a consequence, syphilis was probably overdiagnosed in Alaska, as several early doctors suggested (Call *in* [Jarvis] 1899, 124; Lerrigo 1901, 102-3; Eschscholtz 1821, 2:335). On the other hand, many of the "stigmata" of syphilis were so typical (and so widespread in Europe at this time) that a non-medical observer could accurately diagnose the disease.

Syphilis in its primary stage was infrequently mentioned, not surprisingly since the lesion is usually transient and found on the genitals. Dr. Romanovskii (*in* Pierce 1974, 15) noted that the primary ulcers of syphilis (the "chancre") had a mild course among the Natives. A Russian physician working at Sitka in the 1850s treated 139 cases of syphilis among the Tlingit, of whom 70 had a primary chancre (Govorlivyi n.d., 12). Dr. Robert White (1880, 39) saw only a single chancre, at Atka, during his extended voyage on the *Rush* in 1879. Perhaps no doctor of the period had greater clinical experience among the Natives than Dr. Call (*in* [Jarvis] 1899, 124), who in a five-year period saw no chancres in Natives and only two in Caucasians.

Only a few reports of secondary syphilis are available from the nineteenth century, again because the manifestations are brief and usually unassociated with symptoms. Dr. Romanovskii (*in* Pierce 1974, 15) found buboes, or enlarged lymph nodes in the groin, to be rare and mild in the syphilitic cases he treated. Dr. Govorlivyi (n.d., 12) reported a number of the manifestations of secondary syphilis among his Tlingit patients, including rash, swollen glands, and the so-called condylomata lata, or growths around the anus and genitals. In 1879 Dr. White (1880, 39) observed several florid cases of secondary syphilis at Unga. On St. Lawrence Island Dr. Lerrigo (1901, 103) reported many cases of secondary syphilis characterized by skin rashes and enlarged lymph nodes.

The situation is less clear for tertiary syphilis, since the varied manifestations of this stage can be easily confused with other diseases.

Romanovskii (*in* Pierce 1974, 15) noted that syphilitic insanity (general paresis) did not occur among the Natives. Govorlivyi (n.d., 15) knew of many persons with chronic syphilitic skin ulcers who sought relief in the warm sulfur springs south of Sitka. Also in southeastern Alaska Robert White (1880, 53-54) described "rupia" (an old term meaning a rash beginning with blisters and progressing to scabs), and "phagedenic" (or rapidly spreading) ulcers of the genital region as manifestations of advanced syphilis. In the Aleutians he (1880, 39) observed extensive skin ulcers in women and children "which had reached a condition horribly repugnant to civilized senses." On St. Lawrence Island Lerrigo (1901, 103) felt syphilis was overdiagnosed but conceded that the worst cases of skin ulcer were probably syphilitic in origin.

Chronic inflammation of the bone and periosteum is also a well-known form of tertiary syphilis. Govorlivyi (n.d., 12) found frequent cases of syphilitic periosteitis among the Tlingit. Tertiary infection of the bone has been found in archeological remains from Kodiak, the Aleutians, and the lower Yukon (Holcomb 1940; Laughlin 1980, 101; Hrdlička 1940). Tertiary syphilis of the joints was mentioned by a few observers in Alaska. At Unalaska Dr. Eschscholtz (1821, 2:335) found many arthritic complaints among the Russian foxhunters being attributed to syphilis, but he personally doubted such a cause.

Congenital (or what was in the nineteenth century called "hereditary") syphilis also could have many manifestations, one of the most characteristic being a sunken or "saddle" nose. Lisianskii described a Koniag with destruction of the nasal cartilage that may have been syphilitic (Lisiansky 1814, 202). At Unalaska Dr. Eschscholtz (1821, 335) examined a man with a sunken nose who claimed to have treated himself successfully with fumigations of cinnabar (mercury ore). And we have already seen that Khromchenko (1973, 71) in 1822 saw several Eskimos women "without noses" at Stuart Island. Without giving clinical details, Dr. Robert White (1880, 40) mentioned several cases of syphilis in children in the Aleutians, two of which he considered to be congenital. By the turn of the century, congenital syphilis was reported from St. Michael (Edmonds 1966, 29-30), western Alaska (Call *in* [Jarvis] 1899, 124), and in southeastern Alaska (Jones 1914, 223). Dr. Lerrigo (1901, 103-4) gave a textbook description of congenital syphilis in a child on St. Lawrence Island who had stomatitis, peg-like (known as "Hutchinson's") teeth, and generalized swollen glands.

Infertility can be the result of several types of sexually transmitted diseases, including syphilis and gonorrhea. Venereal disease, according to

Veniaminov (1984, 187-88, 247), was a major cause of infertility among the Aleuts until about 1825. When the epidemic was at its peak only about ten percent of women of childbearing age gave birth. At Sitka the wives of Aleut and Koniag hunters were said to be infertile due to the prevalence of venereal disease among them (Khlebnikov 1976, 104). Even at the end of the nineteenth century many young Native women were unable to have children because of their high rate of infection with venereal diseases (Young 1927, 159).

Dr. Romanovskii (*in* Pierce 1974, 15-16) was of the opinion that syphilis among the Natives was less severe than among the Europeans, and that Natives were less likely to suffer late complications. He rejected the idea that these differences were due to the Tlingits' frequent use of mercury-containing cinnabar as a body paint, and attributed them rather to the simple way of life of the Indians. Later Dr. Govorlivyi (n.d., 13-14) had similar notions about racial differences in susceptibility. At Sitka he found that Creole men and Europeans were a highly susceptible group who often suffered complications, whereas the Tlingit acquired the disease easily but displayed few serious manifestations. In a third group he placed Creole women, who for some reason, despite frequent exposure to the organism, only rarely became infected.

The high prevalence of syphilis and gonorrhea in certain parts of Alaska, dating from the earliest years of contact, led to the development of many indigenous methods for treating their manifestations. The Aleuts were said to treat "venereal wounds" in the same way they treated other wounds. One such treatment was boiled *Angelica* roots, either taken internally or applied externally. Another method was to drink an extract of the roots and leaves of sorrel (Merck 1980, 176). On Kodiak Island the Natives developed several treatment methods, reflecting the serious problem they had with these disorders. It is said that some Native herbalists even specialized in the treatment of venereal disease. One practitioner's technique was to wash the patient's lesions twice daily with the extract of a certain root similar to sarsaparilla, then give the same root to eat. Her cures were reported to be quite successful, even in patients with advanced disease (Davydov 1977, 177). Around the same time, Father Gedeon (*in* Pierce 1978, 130) described two plants, not identifiable today, which were used for the treatment of venereal diseases. One was the extract of a powdered root drunk twice daily, whereas the other was a grass that grew on the northern side of the island. The grass was boiled in a sealed dish and the extract given to the sufferer to drink, followed by a certain root to chew. The resulting saliva was said to be bitter and astringent.

It might be mentioned here that the only effective European treatment for syphilis at this time was the use of mercury in various forms. Among the Russians at Kodiak the standard therapy was to have the patient sit in a hot room and breathe cinnabar smoke, after which he was rubbed down with mercuric chloride and quicksilver and then given a solution of mercuric chloride to drink. As Davydov (1977, 177-78) remarks, with unconscious irony, "Is it not surprising that the most persistent condition cannot stand such a mercurial storm?"

In southeastern Alaska syphilis was often treated by the shaman, since it was thought to be a manifestation of sorcery. Dr. Romanovskii (*in* Pierce 1974, 17) tried hard to learn about Indian methods of cure but could only come up with the use of the warm sulfur springs. Occasionally the Tlingit tried to remove a syphilitic ulcer by simply cutting it from the skin with a knife, or by applying a cauterizing substance (Govorlivyi n.d., 16). Much later an old man from Sitka showed John R. Swanton ([1908], 447) a "syphilis medicine" to be taken only after the patient had drunk some of his own urine.

Little information is available on this subject from other parts of Alaska. Some Athapaskans were said to use a decoction of boiled alder buds for syphilis (Carroll 1972, 50). The Eskimos probably used shamanistic methods for the most part, although Zagoskin (1967, 110) found those around Norton Sound to be taking dried, ground beaver penis as a specific remedy for gonorrhea.

Sexually transmitted diseases were thus an important cause of illness, if not death, in eighteenth- and nineteenth-century Alaska. Almost certainly introduced by the Europeans, these diseases were at their worst when a "frontier" mentality ruled, such as in the times of the *promyshlenniki* in the Aleutians and Kodiak, the early days at Sitka under Baranov, the first years of U.S. rule in Alaska, the heyday of the whalers on the north coast, and finally during the breathless excitement of the Gold Rush. Promiscuity and alcohol, as in all times and places, contributed to the spread of these diseases. The record shows that, as people began to live a more ordered existence under local government, and as basic public health measures were introduced, the sexually transmitted diseases declined to a manageable though never fully acceptable level.

15

Tuberculosis: The Scourge of Alaska

BACKGROUND

No subject in the history of medicine in Alaska seems to hold a greater interest than tuberculosis. When many of the great plagues of the eighteenth and nineteenth century, such as smallpox, syphilis, and typhoid, were a thing of the past, tuberculosis was still a deadly scourge and within the memory of most older Natives now living. In fact, tuberculosis as a slow but inexorable epidemic probably did not reach its peak of destructiveness until the years immediately after World War II, following which it was finally brought under control by a concerted program effort and the development of the first effective antituberculosis drugs (Fortuine 1975a, 14-19; Fortuine 1986, 21-23).

Tracing the early history of tuberculosis in Alaska is fraught with difficulties. No one has ever seriously proposed that the disease was indigenous to Alaska, yet recent evidence strongly suggests that it was indeed found in pre-Columbian times in certain South American Indians (El-Najjar 1979). Although no conclusions may yet be drawn about the disease in the Arctic, human remains from the precontact period in Alaska have shown chronic granulomas of the lymph nodes which, although called histoplasmosis (Zimmerman and Smith 1975; Zimmerman and Aufderheide 1984) are not unlike those found in pulmonary tuberculosis.

What is particularly frustrating about searching for early evidence of the disease in Alaska is that the symptoms and signs of tuberculosis are nonspecific. For example, a person with pulmonary tuberculosis usually has a productive cough, perhaps associated with chest pain, sweating, breathlessness, and hemoptysis (blood in sputum), any of which can be associated with bronchitis, pneumonia, or even heart disease. The body wasting and progressive loss of strength of tuberculosis ("consumption") may also be caused by cancer, diabetes, or other chronic diseases. Tuberculosis of the kidney, meninges, or other internal organs has no characteristic external signs that would alert anyone but a perceptive and experienced physician to the presence of the disease. Only tuberculosis of the spine (causing a typical hunchback deformity), chronic suppurative joints, or tuberculosis of the lymph nodes of the neck ("scrofula") are specific enough to permit a clinical diagnosis of tuberculosis with reasonable certainty.

THE RUSSIAN PERIOD

The first mention of tuberculosis in an Alaska Native seems to come from the report of a voyage by the Russian trader Afanasii Ocheredin, who spent about five years on Umnak and Akutan Islands. Upon returning to Russia in 1770, he took with him two Akutan Aleuts, both of whom died of consumption in Siberia while on the way to St. Petersburg (Bancroft 1886, 154n). These unfortunate victims could have developed tuberculosis from their five-year association with the Russians or could have acquired the disease during their long overland journey through Siberia.

Tuberculosis was known to be rampant in Europe at this time, where it was no respector of age, sex, or social class. Paupers, poets, and princes were among the victims of this relentless enemy (Dubos and Dubos 1952).

Perhaps the most eminent (and certainly the best documented) victim of tuberculosis in early Alaskan history was William Anderson, the scientist and surgeon on Captain Cook's voyage to Alaska in 1778. Anderson was already ill with tuberculosis before the expedition left England in 1776, and his condition continued to deteriorate during the many months of the voyage. On August 3, 1778, the surgeon died and was buried at sea not far from the eastern end of St. Lawrence Island (Burney 1819, 233; Cook 1967, 3(1):444; 3(2):1130). Just over a year later Captain Clerke, Cook's second in command, also died of consumption while the ships were in the Bering Sea (James King in Cook 1967, 3(1):699n, 700). The latter, at least, had extensive face-to-face contact with the Natives and might have transmitted the disease. In passing, it is curious to note that in a rare navigational lapse, Cook named the eastern end of St. Lawrence Island "Anderson Island," and a month later called the western end "Clerke Island," not recognizing that it was a single island, which had been discovered and named by Bering in 1728 (Fortuine 1984a, 59-60).

Other eminent explorers had tuberculosis as well. Alexei Chirikov was said to have died of consumption after his return to St. Petersburg (Aronson

1940, 31), as did the son of Vitus Bering, who was an officer on the Billings expedition (Sarytschew 1807, 2:79). It is also possible that Kotzebue was suffering from tuberculosis when he prematurely ended his explorations in 1817 (VanStone 1960, 158), although there are other explanations for his symptoms (Chamisso 1986, 68). If the officers were sick on the major expeditions, then undoubtedly also the seamen were, who lived in damp, crowded, and poorly ventilated quarters for many months at a time. Collinson (1889, 134), for example, had to discharge a marine in 1851, after a winter in the Arctic, because of "pulmonary disease," very likely tuberculosis.

By the end of the eighteenth century most Aleuts and Koniag had had regular and sometimes intimate contact with the Russians, often for extended periods. Since many of these Native people were also subjected to repeated acute respiratory infections, malnutrition, and to great stress, it is little wonder that many of them developed pulmonary tuberculosis. In 1791 Merck (1980, 177) noted that many of the Aleuts were dying of chest diseases characterized by pain in the side, coughing, and spitting of blood. Although these symptoms could be due to influenza and pneumonia, tuberculosis is also a strong possibility. Fifteen years later Lisianskii found consumption to be one of the most common diseases of the Koniag (Lisiansky 1814, 201).

By 1824, when Father Veniaminov arrived in Unalaska, tuberculosis already seemed to be a "native" disease in the Aleutians. In describing the various ills to which the people were subject he wrote (1984, 291-92): "There were recognized two kinds of *chakhatka,** both of which were considered incurable. One of these was believed to result from the decay of the lungs. The symptoms are coughing with spitting of blood and shortness of breath [*udush'e*]." The second type of *chakhatka* was believed to be caused by a decay of the liver and was associated with colic, loss of appetite and rapid emaciation of the body. Both of these illnesses could well have represented tuberculosis, although again there are other possibilities, especially for the second type. Veniaminov (1984, 292) goes on to describe Aleut treatments for spitting blood, such as using herbs, or piercing the patient on either side of the chest below the ribs to let out the soured stagnant blood.

Most Native groups, in fact, at a fairly early stage developed methods for the treatment of hemoptysis, cough, and consumption, suggesting that

* A Russian term usually meaning consumption.

tuberculosis became widespread rather rapidly in Alaska. The Tlingit considered consumption the result of sorcery and treated it accordingly (Veniaminov 1984, 407). For hemoptysis one remedy was to dissolve slugs in water to form a slime, which then was given to the patient to drink (Swanton [1908], 448). Other Tlingit remedies for the symptoms of tuberculosis are given by Dr. Blaschke (*in* Krause 1956, 283-84). According to later authorities, the Chugach treated hemoptysis by drinking the decoction of a certain pulverized plant and by applying hot stones (Birket-Smith 1953, 117), whereas the Yupik had many treatments for hemoptysis, including drinking Labrador tea (*Ledum palustre*) or chewing the tops of the pineapple weed *Matricaria matricarioides* (Ager and Ager 1980, 37-38). The Eskimos also boiled willow leaves or bark (*Salix* spp.) to make a strong liquor that was said to be helpful in treating hemorrhage from the lung (Lantis 1959, 24). Another early remedy for hemoptysis in this area was the oily substance derived from the anal glands of beavers (Wrangell 1970, 19). Some Athapaskans also used empirical remedies, for example, chewing the root of the coltsfoot plant (*Petasites* spp.) for hemoptysis (Osgood 1937, 160).

Tuberculosis seemed to spread rapidly wherever the Russians established their bases of operation. At Atka Netsvetov (1980, 145, 183, 193) officiated at several funerals for victims of consumption during the 1830s. At Sitka Dr. Blaschke reported during the same decade that consumption and scrofula were both common among the Natives (Aronson 1940, 31). When Sir George Simpson visited Sitka in 1842 (1847, 2:190), he found pulmonary complaints and hemoptysis unusually common among the people of the coast, a judgment echoed by Dr. Romanovskii (*in* Pierce 1974, 2) around the same time. A dissenting view is that of a later company physician with a long experience in southeastern Alaska. Govorlivyi (n.d., 7-9) found that as many as sixty percent of the Tlingit suffered from chronic cough, sputum production, and hemoptysis, yet, curiously, he denied that any of them had tuberculosis.

Dr. Frankenhaeuser (*in* Pierce 1974, 29-30) wrote in detail of the devastation that tuberculosis was causing among the people in the colonies. Some ten persons out of a total of thirty-five who died in from May 1, 1847, to May 1, 1848, suffered from "consumption of the lungs;" the corresponding figures from Kodiak were five out of thirteen in 1846. The disease affected chiefly the Natives, a finding he attributed either to an inherited tendency or to their way of living. He further speculated that the prevalence of the disease was due to the adverse influence of the local climate upon the Native children, thus predisposing them to recurrent respiratory infections that weakened their lungs. Europeans, he noted, had no more consumption in the colonies than they did in their home countries, whereas the Creoles followed the pattern of disease of the full-blood Native children. Another official of the Russian-American Company noted that the Creoles were particularly susceptible to consumption and that many died at an early age from the disease, a circumstance he attributed to their "undisciplined use" of alcohol and their sexual promiscuity (Golovin 1979, 63). He might also have added that the Creoles, more than any other Natives, lived in close daily proximity to the Russians, many of whom must have had active tuberculosis.

Besides the Aleutians, Kodiak, and southeastern Alaska, tuberculosis had begun to spread to the more peripheral areas of the colonies. Wrangell in 1839 (1970, 11, 19) noted that the Kenai (Tainana) Indians had many humpbacks among them (possibly resulting from tuberculosis of the spine) and that the people of the Kuskokwim already had local remedies for hemoptysis. Lieutenant Zagoskin (1967, 110) in the early 1840s described consumption, along with eye diseases and abscesses, as the most prevalent diseases of the people of the lower Yukon. Later he (1967, 255) compared the Natives of the Kuskokwim to the Aleuts and Creoles in that they all had "weak lungs. It is the exceptional one who does not cough blood by the time he is 20." In 1857 and again in 1859 Father Netsvetov (1984, 366, 395) performed burial services on the lower Yukon for victims of consumption.

THE AMERICAN PERIOD

Throughout the latter third of the nineteenth century tuberculosis appeared to spread in ever-widening circles as more and more Native people came into regular contact with the thousands of Americans, Europeans, and Asians who swarmed into Alaska to seek their fortune. Once established in a Native family, the disease soon spread throughout the household because of the crowding and poor ventilation characteristic of most dwellings. Tuberculosis had none of the lightning-like contagiousness of measles, influenza, or smallpox, yet all the same it ran an inexorable course, like an epidemic in slow motion.

Ivan Petroff (1882, 43), who visited many parts of Alaska collecting statistical information for the census of 1880, gives this pessimistic view of the condition during the early American period:

Consumption is therefore the simple and comprehensive title for that disease which destroys the greatest number throughout Alaska. . . . The Aleut, the Indian, and the Eskimos suffer from it alike, and they all exhibit the same stolid indifference to its stealthy but fatal advancement—no extra care, no attempt to ward it off, protect, or shelter against it, not even until the supreme moment of dissolution.

After consumption, according to Petroff, the next biggest killer was scrofula, which is a type of tuberculosis of the lymph glands of the neck. This disease, he wrote, takes "the form of malignant ulcers, which eat into the vitals and destroy them. It renders whole settlements sometimes lepers in the eyes of the civilized visitor; and it is hard to find a settlement in the whole country where at least one or more of the families therein have not got the singularly prominent scars [on the neck] peculiar to the disease." Petroff believed that both major forms of tuberculosis were aggravated by the style of living of the Natives, and he was frustrated by the peoples' seeming resignation to their fate.

The Indians of southeastern Alaska, who had the most intensive contact with the new wave of immigrants, seemed the most affected of all. An important medical witness to the situation was Robert White (1880, 34-5), who stopped at several ports in 1879. At Kazan Bay and later at Fort Wrangell, several Indians were found to be suffering from an advanced stage of phthisis (an old name for consumption) and from other chronic chest infections. Tuberculosis of the neck glands, or scrofula, was also present, and was being treated by the liberal external and internal use of "hooligan" (or eulachon) oil. At Sitka he reported that most of the deaths each year were from chronic pulmonary disease. Other shipboard surgeons of the period (*in* Holcomb 1940, 187) also remarked on the extreme prevalence of pulmonary disease and scrofula in this period.

A doctor from the Marine Hospital Service visiting around the turn of the century reported that he saw many tuberculosis cases. In some he elicited a history of hemoptysis, and many others with symptoms of cough had a "very suspicious looking profuse expectoration." Many individuals were suffering from scrofula and from infections of the bones and joints. The prevalence of tuberculosis he attributed in large part to the crowded, dirty homes, where expectoration could often be seen on the floor. His solution (and one that was belatedly adopted) was the establishment of government hospitals for the care of those with tuberculosis (Fox 1902, 1615-16).

Many other visitors to southeastern Alaska were witnesses to the extent and destructiveness of tuberculosis in its various forms. The missionary S.

Hall Young (1927, 96) at Fort Wrangell reported that "nearly all the younger men and women had either running sores or scarcely healed cicatrices on their necks," presumably due to scrofula. When he visited Indian homes (1927, 107) he found one or more sick in almost every dwelling. "Consumptives rolled ghastly eyes from their filthy cots; little children, emaciated and covered with sores, wailed and shivered before our sympathetic eyes."

The missionary John Brady, later to become governor, made every effort to teach some of his charges the natural history and prevention of the disease, but they persisted in their conviction that sorcery was the root cause (Brady 1904, 1499; Hinckley 1979, 41). Another wrote that, although consumption carried away the Indians in numbers, they took no precautions to prevent its spread, relying rather on their usual shamanistic methods of treatment (Scidmore 1885, 89). At Fort Wrangell a visitor entered a home in which she found "an old man dying, a woman lying ill with a fever, and a whole brood of children, . . . all this life and sickness and death being the state of existence of a single family—a horrible picture of squalid misery and misfortune." Elsewhere she wrote that nearly all the children were "tainted with marks of scrofula" (Collis 1890, 82-3, 104). Still others echoed these findings (Knapp 1892, 57; Jackson 1893b, 931; Swineford 1886, 29).

In addition to scrofula and pulmonary hemorrhages, Livingston F. Jones (1914, 224) frequently found tuberculosis of the hip among the Tlingit. Involvement of the spine, causing the typical hunchback deformity known as Pott's disease, was also widespread and not infrequently the cause of paralysis or death. Charles Elliott (1900, 741) also saw many deformed Indians among those affected with tuberculosis, and speculated, quite possibly with justice, that the disease was being spread by Oriental cannery workers being brought to the area in large numbers.

The situation was hardly better in the Aleutians, where of course tuberculosis had been known for well over a century. Dr. Robert White (1880, 41) found the manifestations of scrofula "very common," including scars, swellings, and eruptions, all of which caused considerable disfigurement among both young and old. "Pneumonic phthisis," or what we would today call pulmonary tuberculosis, caused a large proportion of deaths on the Pribilof Islands, a sentiment echoed by Henry W. Elliott (1886, 238) a few years later. Scrofula was also said to be prevalent in the Pribilofs, having caused three deaths on St. Paul Island in 1880-1881 (Rosse 1883, 18). Scrofula, in fact, seemed to be widespread among the Aleuts generally. Both Dr. James White (1894) and Isabel Shepard (1889, 44) remarked on its frequency at Belkofski, near the western end of the Alaska Peninsula, and others noted it elsewhere (Holcomb 1940, 187; Athearn 1949, 59).

Along the north Pacific rim, tuberculosis was also taking its toll. The Chugach suffered much from "an inherited tendency to pulmonary disease" (Abercrombie 1900b, 399), which usually carried them off by the age of fifty. Likewise, a later visitor considered them an unhealthy people, with "consumptive tendencies being common among them" (Schrader 1899, 367). Frederica De Laguna (1956, 86) has excavated a late Chugach burial site containing a skeleton with tuberculosis of the spine.

On Kodiak Island Dr. Robert White (1880, 38) again found scrofula and chronic tuberculous infections of the lungs to be among the most prevalent diseases. Pulmonary tuberculosis he attributed in large measure to the recurrent colds from which the people suffered and the ease of spread of respiratory infections in the close, unventilated huts in which the people lived. According to Elliott (1886, 110-1), consumption was the illness which caused more deaths than any other, yet the Natives showed no attempts either to protect themselves from it or to prevent its progression. "Often," he wrote, "a comely young girl or man will, in turning suddenly, reveal under the jaws or on the neck and throat, a disgusting, red eruption which a scrofulous ancestry has cursed the youth with." Other testimonies of the ubiquitous disease on Kodiak Island can be cited (University of Alaska 1936-1938, 2:87; Jackson 1896a, 1468-69).

Tuberculosis also ravaged the Eskimos of western and northern Alaska during the American period, beginning with those in the closest and longest contact with Whites. Although some spread had undoubtedly occurred from such older trading centers as St. Michael, Port Clarence, Unalakleet, and Ikogmiut, the disease found a new lease on life on the one hand from crews of the many whaling ships that sailed north beginning in 1848, and on the other hand from the hordes of miners, prospectors, and camp followers who streamed into northwestern Alaska in the closing decade of the century.

Whaling crews were a tough lot who were often infected with tuberculosis (Rosse 1883, 15; Cook and Pederson 1937, 219). Their disease could only worsen, not to mention spread, in the damp, crowded fo'c's'le quarters in which they slept during voyages not infrequently lasting three or more years. Beginning in the 1880s steam whaling ships began to overwinter east of Barrow, allowing ample opportunity for the spread of the disease to the local population. Likewise, shore stations around Point Hope and Barrow itself afforded intensive contact between the Eskimos and whalemen.

Miners and others crowded into western Alaska in great numbers in the 1890s, mostly in the region around Norton Sound, St. Michael, and the Seward Peninsula. When the gold rush at Nome began in 1899, the numbers greatly increased, again comprising many individuals from the lower economic strata of society, some of them afflicted with infectious tuberculosis.

Among the earlier witnesses to tuberculosis in the Eskimos of western Alaska was army Capt. Charles Raymond (1870-71, 21, 165), who as early as 1869 found consumption prevalent among the people of the lower Yukon, a view echoed a decade later by Nelson (1899, 29). Rosse (1883, 27) reported scrofula, plus "bronchial and pulmonary troubles" among the principal diseases of the coastal Eskimo. Sheldon Jackson (1893a, 1290) listed scrofula and consumption among the causes of a high death rate among the Eskimos, and a similar view was voiced by Governor Knapp in his 1890 report (1890, 23-24). Around Nome during the gold rush days there are reports of Eskimos dying of consumption (McKee 1902, 37; French 1901, 59). On St. Lawrence Island a teacher attested to the prevalence of scrofula and lung hemorrhages among the people (Doty 1900, 193-94), while a teacher colleague, who happened to be a physician, pointed out that tuberculosis often followed other respiratory diseases such as bronchitis and pleurisy (Lerrigo 1901, 103). In Barrow Murdoch (1892, 39) observed that many cases of lung hemorrhage, some fatal, followed the many coughs and colds that were prevalent every summer and fall.

Tuberculosis seems to have come rather late to the Athapaskans of the interior, most of whom had their first intensive contacts with outsiders during the 1880s or even the 1890s. In a list of diseases of the Ingalik prepared by Dall (1870, 195), tuberculosis and scrofula are not mentioned, although he does call attention to the prevalence or pleurisy, pneumonia, and bronchitis. In 1881 the Orthodox missionary Nikita at Kenai called tuberculosis "prevalent" among the Indians who lived some distance away, but of course these people had been trading with the Russians for nearly a hundred years by this time (*in* University of Alaska 1936-1938, 2:63).

By the turn of the century the Athapaskans were not only in regular contact with traders and prospectors, but also increasingly with government officials, some of whom themselves suffered from tuberculosis, such as a young soldier at Tanana (Farnsworth 1977, 215). One observer noted specifically that pulmonary diseases were increasingly common wherever Native customs had been most modified by White influence (Mendenhall 1899, 339). Around Cook Inlet the Indians were said to be rapidly disappearing due to consumption and other pulmonary diseases, which the writer attributed to their extensive use and misuse of the Russian steambath (Learnard 1900, 666-67). In the isolated reaches of the upper Kuskokwim, however, a government surveyor found the Indians only occasionally consumptive (Herron 1901, 69).

Although there must remain some doubt about the origin of tuberculosis in Alaska, it seems likely that the disease was introduced in the eighteenth century by the Russians and other Europeans. Clearly the spread of the disease paralleled closely the number and distribution of Russians and Americans in the territory. Wherever explorers, traders, miners, settlers, and missionaries went, the incidence of the disease in all its forms began to increase among the Natives. The conditions for spread—poverty, malnutrition, crowding, and weakened resistance from repeated infections—increased with the pace of settlement. By 1900 tuberculosis was already exacting a terrible toll in Alaska. Over the following half-century, however, the disease was to increase yet further and even pose a serious threat to the survival of the Alaska Native peoples.

16

The Use of Tobacco: Smokers, Sniffers, and Chewers

INTRODUCTION AND SPREAD IN SOUTHERN ALASKA

When in 1741 Steller (1988, 72) landed for the first time on Alaskan soil, at Kayak Island east of Prince William Sound, he took away several artifacts from an abandoned Native home site, in return for which a few objects were later left in exchange. Among these were a Chinese pipe and a pound of tobacco, although he seemed certain that the Natives could not have known the proper use of either. In a rare display of humor, he noted that "if they tried [the tobacco] out wrongly, they could conclude that we wanted to do them in."

Several weeks later, while the ship was pausing in the Shumagin Islands to take on water, several Aleuts paddled out to meet the Russians. The latter offered presents, including again two Chinese pipes, which were examined carefully and placed on top of their *baidarkas*. After Lieutenant Waxell had offered some brandy (or gin), which the Aleut spat out, he tried to give other presents to smooth things over (Waxell 1962, 94). Although Steller advised against it, the sailors "tried to make up for one annoyance with a new one [and] presented him with a lighted pipe of tobacco, which he, to be sure, accepted, but, displeased, he paddled away" (Steller 1988, 99-100). Such was the introduction of tobacco to the Alaska Natives by Europeans.

Captain Chirikov (1922, 1:304), in command of Bering's other vessel, also encountered Aleuts around the same time, probably on the island of Adak. He tried to lure them close to his ship with small gifts, including Chinese tobacco and a pipe, which one of the Aleuts accepted and placed on the deck of his *baidarka*. They accepted these and other objects indifferently, as if they did not know to what use to put them (Del'Isle de la Croyère 1914, 319).

The use of tobacco spread rapidly in the Aleutians in the eighteenth century. Chuprov offered pipes and tobacco as gifts on Agattu in 1745 (Bancroft 1886, 103) and other *promyshlenniki* used tobacco as an inducement to hunt or as a reward for services (e.g., Shelikhov 1981, 128-29; Masterson and Brower 1948, 91).

By the time of Cook's voyage in 1778, the Aleuts were well acquainted with tobacco and craved it. Ellis, one of the surgeons, wrote that the people of Unalaska "perfectly understood the use of tobacco, which they asked for by that name; and when it was given them, immediately put it in their mouths; some likewise made signs of taking snuff" (Ellis 1782, 1:284). Cook himself said there were few if any who did not smoke, chew, or take snuff, "a luxury that bids fair to keep them always poor" (Cook 1967, 3(1):461). Lieutenant King noted that they preferred tobacco to "all other things" (*in* Cook 1967, 3(2):1442).

This inordinate craving for tobacco in all its forms led to the bestowal of sexual favors by some of the women. Several officers as well as sailors took shameful advantage of the situation, the most notorious being David Samwell, assistant surgeon on the *Resolution*, who candidly boasted that, although a young woman could be had for a leaf or two, "we were so much inclined to encourage this kind of traffic that we generally gave them ten times more than that they would have been satisfied with and this well timed Generosity procured us as many fine Girls during our stay here as we wanted.... " (*in* Cook 1967, 3(2):1121).

Cook's men were generous with tobacco but apparently the Russians were not, since it always seemed to be in short supply. In any event, the Russian traders rarely felt obligated to reward the Aleuts, or even trade with them, since by that time they held the local Natives in firm subjection. At the time of the Billings expedition in 1791, Lieutenant Sarychev found the Aleuts eager to trade for tobacco; in fact, once they heard it was available "they flocked to us from the remotest parts." During the winter he spent at Unalaska he distributed a large quantity of tobacco in exchange for sea otter and fox skins (Sarytschew 1807, 2:38; Sauer 1802, 275). Dr. Merck (1980, 105) at the same time noted that, despite the demand for it, tobacco was rare at Unalaska.

The Aleuts seem to have maintained their craving for tobacco well into the nineteenth century. Dr. Langsdorff (1814, 2:48) found them "passionately fond of snuff" and willing to work a whole day for a single leaf, while Archibald Campbell (1819, 44) described them as "immoderately fond" of it. In 1789 Lt. George Mortimer (1791, 59) observed that an Aleut who had been out fishing for the Russians for the greater part of a cold, bleak night was "perfectly satisfied" by the payment of a pinch of snuff. Father Veniaminov (1984, 182) said that an Aleut was prepared to give his last morsel of food or his best arrow for a leaf. In the missionary's time, more than half of some hunters' income was spent on tobacco, either for chewing or for snuff. He added that, despite their addiction, a few had given up the habit of their own free will.

Tobacco was presumably also introduced to the Koniag by the *promyshlenniki,* probably Glotov, as an article of trade, since by 1784 Shelikhov found they were already using snuff "with great gusto" (Shelikhov 1981, 78). Only a few years later Captain Meares (1790, 306) reported the Natives of Kodiak requesting snuff in trade. Dr. Merck (1980, 105) also found the Koniag eager for snuff, although women less than men. Up to that time they had not learned how to prepare snuff for themselves from crude tobacco.

By the early 1800s the Koniag were passionately fond of tobacco and were cursing the Russians for having made them so dependent on it. They used it primarily as snuff placed in the mouth; few sniffed it and no one smoked, according to Davydov (1977, 176). Around the same time Lisianskii noted that a Koniag would go twenty miles out of his way for a pinch or two of snuff. He often distributed small amounts as favors for services rendered (Lisiansky 1814, 179n).

The Russian-American Company regularly used tobacco as a treat or as an incentive for Aleut and Koniag hunters at Sitka or at the posts on the Kenai Peninsula. When the new redoubt was established at Nushagak in 1819, the trader was encouraged to use tobacco among the local Natives to show the good will of the Russians (Pierce 1984, 36, 60, 155).

In the later years of the century tobacco seemed to be holding its charm for the people of Kodiak. Holmberg (1985, 43) found it to be universally used, but still primarily as snuff rather than as a smoke. By 1874 an observer remarked that the Natives were "greatly addicted to smoking, using Circassian tobacco when it can be had, which is exceedingly strong." Many also continued to use tobacco in large quantities as snuff (Huggins 1981, 6).

The people of Cook Inlet and Prince William Sound must have been introduced to tobacco by the English, Russian, and perhaps Spanish explorers and traders who frequented this region in the 1780s and 1790s. The habit, however, did not seem to catch on at first, since when Meares offered tobacco as a trade item at Cape Douglas on the Alaska Peninsula, it was refused (Meares 1790, xi). Likewise, while Billings was at Montague Island in 1790 he could evoke no interest in tobacco (Sauer 1802, 188).

In southeastern Alaska the Indians in precontact times cultivated a tobacco-like plant which they mixed with lime and chewed. Lieutenant Whidbey of Vancouver's expedition observed the plant being grown in Chatham Straits, the only crop the Tlingit were known to cultivate (Krause 1956, 108). It was also raised among the Haida of the Queen Charlotte Islands (Drucker 1955, 9), and among the Tsimshian (Arctander 1909, 82). Captain Dixon (1789, 172) observed the use of this plant as far north as Yakutat Bay. The leaves of this "tobacco" were dried over a fire, ground up in a stone mortar and finally pressed into cakes. It was always chewed, rather than smoked or inhaled (Krause 1956, 208). In the 1780s and beyond, as intensive trade with European ships began, the native tobacco fell into disuse.

The Indians found the new European tobacco stronger and easier to obtain and soon they had learned to smoke it as well as chew it. Tobacco began to take on a ceremonial value and was often used by the Tlingit after a shamanistic ceremony (Holmberg 1985, 34), or given to the relatives and friends of a sick man (H. Elliott 1886, 50). The Russians used it in return for favors (Zagoskin 1967, 73) or for a job well done (Kotzebue 1830, 2:60). In the nineteenth century smoking became increasingly popular, with leaf tobacco mixed with pulverized bark being smoked in short, beautifully carved wooden or clay pipes (Krause 1956, 108). Smoking became so popular in Fort Wrangell, according to Dr. Robert White (1880, 34), that Indian men sometimes made their daughters or wives available to a miner for a few pounds of tobacco. After the prospecting season was over, the women returned home, only to be offered again the following year.

INTRODUCTION AND SPREAD IN NORTHERN ALASKA

Tobacco first reached northern Alaska not by European ships but over traditional trade routes with the natives of Siberia across the Bering Strait. According to Dorothy Jean Ray (1975, 101-2), it became an article of trade around the 1750s, originating in Circassia, Poland, or Sweden, and ultimately finding its way to the Chukchi traders in eastern Siberia.

Nikolai Daurkin, a Chukchi who supposedly visited the Diomedes in the period 1763-1765, reported that the first request of the Natives was for leaf tobacco. "I presented them with several leaves, in return for which they gave me a whole suit of sable and marten fur, and entertained me and my traveling companion with their best provisions" (*in* Masterson and Brower 1948, 65-66).

In 1789 a large trading market was established at Anyui on the Kolyma River, where Alaskan furs were exchanged for tobacco and other European goods, which then passed through several more Native middlemen before reaching the Seward Peninsula. Tobacco did not become an item of regular exchange in Alaska until the late 1700s and early 1800s (D. Ray 1975, 98-99, 101). Trade between Siberia and northern Alaska continued to flourish throughout the nineteenth century, with the major centers located on the north coast of Kotzebue Sound and at Port Clarence on the Seward Peninsula. From there and other points trade goods, especially tobacco, moved to the north coast and into the interior via the major river systems (Bockstoce 1986, 188).

In the vicinity of Kuskokwim Bay Captain Cook encountered Eskimos who were unfamiliar with the use of tobacco. In Norton Sound, however, he met people near Cape Denbigh who eagerly traded for knives and "had no dislike to tobacco" (Cook 1967, 3(1):403, 438), although the phrase is ambiguous on the question of prior use or knowledge. When Billings' ship visited Cape Rodney in 1791 the Eskimos were eager to trade for many European goods, but apparently not tobacco (D. Ray 1975, 49).

In 1816 Otto von Kotzebue was first greeted by the Eskimos of St. Lawrence Island with a chorus of pleas for tobacco. When he handed them a few leaves they immediately put them into their mouths. Later he saw them smoking small stone pipes, about the size of a thimble (Kotzebue 1821, 1:190). While in the vicinity of St. Lawrence Island the Russians traded freely with the Eskimos. So eager were the latter for tobacco that they would give up an elaborately decorated gut parka for a few leaves, the amount one might consume in a morning (Chamisso 1986, 16).

The Eskimos of Shishmaref Inlet also clamored for tobacco, which they seemed to enjoy chewing as well as smoking (Kotzebue 1821, 1:209). Again they freely traded their clothing for tobacco, the item they most desired (Choris *in* VanStone 1960, 147). This love of tobacco impressed the captain, who found it remarkable that it had penetrated into parts where no European had visited (Kotzebue 1821, 1:209).

When Captain Beechey landed on St. Lawrence Island in 1826 he again found tobacco to be the great object of all trade. A similar situation prevailed at a village near Cape Prince of Wales (Beechey 1831, 1:332, 339). Throughout his stay in the Arctic he and his men found the Eskimos from St. Lawrence Island to Barrow willing to trade nearly everything for their favorite commodity (Beechey 1831, 1:352, 359; 2:263). On one occasion the sailors bought four hundred pounds of caribou meat for four pounds of tobacco (Bockstoce 1977, 108). Beechey (1831, 2:304) noted that the northern Eskimos generally smoked a short pipe with a tiny bowl, although some to the south of Bering Strait chewed tobacco and the St. Lawrence Islanders took it as snuff. The tobacco was often of poor quality and extended with dried wood.

The first European to reach Barrow was Thomas Elson of the Beechey expedition in 1826. There he found tobacco well known and readily marketable (*in* Beechey 1831, 1:423). Eleven years later Thomas Simpson of the Hudson's Bay Company made his way to Barrow from the east. At Dease Inlet he encountered Eskimos who immediately clamored for tobacco, of which they were all—men, women, and children—"inordinately fond." He speculated that they had become acquainted with tobacco through indirect intercourse with the Russians, since the Eskimos around the mouth of the Mackenzie River were not familiar with it. At Barrow he found tobacco to be the "grand article in demand." A single inch of it was equivalent in trade to the most valuable articles they possessed (T. Simpson 1843, 147-56).

Over the following fifteen years a number of English ships engaged in the Franklin search stopped at Barrow and a few spent the winter there. The British sailors found it necessary to be well stocked with tobacco, not only as a trade item but also as a return for favors, an aid in negotiations, an inducement to cooperation, and even as an indemnity for an accidental death (Maguire 1857, 362-95). Capt. Robert M'Clure (1857, 73), according to his editor, "became his own Master of the Mint, by cutting tobacco sticks into pieces about three inches long, and paying with them as he thought fit." In Wainwright Inlet Captain Collinson (1889, 137) found that a man would give all his clothing and even some of his wife's garments for some tobacco.

Robert F. Spencer (1959, 462-64) has presented interesting information on the role of tobacco in traditional Barrow culture. The small pipes they used were of the Siberian or Russian type and were cleaned before use, with a caribou hair placed in the bowl to prevent tobacco flakes from entering the stem. Men's pipes were small and portable, while those of women had longer stems. Bowls might be made of ivory, metal, or clay. Tobacco was obtained from the Diomede Islands-Cape Prince of Wales area and was brought in special caribou skin sacks, each containing about forty leaves. The price of tobacco was quite high: in one instance, a man paid five caribou, five tanned fawn skins and a quantity of cured sinew for twenty leaves. Smaller quantities were kept in pouches made from walrus gut. Nearly everyone used tobacco in some form, including the children. Besides smoking, many chewed the leaves; snuff was introduced by the whalers at a somewhat later period (Spencer 1959, 462-63). The Eskimos were quite particular about the quality of the product they used. Most preferred black Russian leaf tobacco or common navy-plug, the latter first traded by the ships of the Franklin search (P. Ray 1885, 47).

Further south the Eskimos also used tobacco that they had obtained in trade from Siberia or perhaps from the Russians in the Aleutians, Kodiak, and Prince William Sound. Khromchenko (1973, 48) found the Bristol Bay Eskimos using prodigious amounts of snuff. At Stuart Island, near present-day St. Michael, he intimates (1973, 71) that the people were immoderate tobacco users. Glazunov, the first European to explore the interior of southwestern Alaska, found the Natives already passionately fond of tobacco, which they smoked and took as snuff (*in* VanStone 1959, 43).

Zagoskin (1967, 100-102) noted that the Eskimos of Norton Sound were already using tobacco when the fort at St. Michael was established in 1833; in fact, tobacco and a few metal implements were the only trade items sought. The Eskimos of this area were grateful to the Russians for having brought tobacco in greater quantities than they had been able to procure before. Zagoskin (1967, 183-84, 200) complained, however, that trade at St. Michael was being undermined by large quantities of Circassian tobacco that was being traded on the Chukchi Peninsula, after which it came over the strait to Kotzebue Sound and thence to Norton Sound. As in the more northerly areas, tobacco was expensive on the Yukon, forty pounds being traded for fifty beaver skins or 250 silver rubles. Father Netsvetov (1984, 175) mentions paying his workmen with tobacco at Ikogmiut in 1849. Because of its value it was often mixed with wood shavings or powdered fungus to stretch it and give it additional flavor (Seemann 1853, 60; Ager and Ager 1980).

Nelson (1899, 271-72) offers considerable detail on the tobacco habits of the Eskimos of the Seward Peninsula and southward. The women did not often smoke tobacco, but rather chewed it or used it as snuff, whereas the men used all three methods. For chewing, the tobacco was cut into shreds on special boards, mixed with ashes from a tree fungus (obtained from interior Indians), then rolled into pellets, or quids, which were often briefly chewed by the women to mix the ingredients more thoroughly. The women often prepared four to eight pellets daily for use by their men the following day. The latter usually did not chew the quids but rather held them in their cheek pouch. When eating or drinking, they would take out the quid, roll it into a ball and stick it behind their ear until ready to use it again (Adams 1982, 113-14). For smoking, the tobacco was cut very fine. The pipe bowls were cylindrical with a wide rim. A small tuft of fur was placed at the bottom, then a wad of tobacco stuffed in to fill the bowl. After lighting the pipe with flint and steel, the smoker took two or three deep draws and held the smoke in the lungs as long as possible. The oily tobacco extract that remained in the pipestem was cleaned out from time to time and added to the chewing quids for extra flavor and strength. For snuff the tobacco was finely shredded, thoroughly dried, and then ground into powder in a wooden mortar and pestle. The snuff was then sifted to remove the larger particles. Snuff could either be sniffed or placed inside the lip.

Captain Hooper (1881, 60) reported that the Eskimos often made their own pipes, the bowl constructed of brass, copper, or iron, and the stem of wood, up to ten inches long. The bowl held little more than a pinch of tobacco at a time. The well-appointed Eskimo carried a skin bag around his or her neck containing pipe, a cleaner, tobacco, flint and steel, and a quantity of Alaska cotton soaked in gunpowder for use as tinder. (*See* Figure 23.)

On St. Lawrence Island an observer near the end of the nineteenth century described the Eskimos as "complete slaves to tobacco" (Bruce 1894, 104-5). All of the men and most women smoked, as well as most children over six. Many of the women also chewed, always swallowing the juice. Old chewing quids were dried and smoked, to extract the last hint of flavor. Snuff was made from finely ground tobacco mixed with pulverized charcoal. Sometimes a certain shrub growing wild on the island was also smoked when tobacco was unavailable. Bruce concluded: "An Eskimo who is without tobacco is as wretched as a confirmed drunkard without his whiskey, and he will go to as great extremes to secure it as he would to procure food for himself and family." An Orthodox missionary on the Yukon echoed, "Tobacco to a savage is as valuable as bread to a Russian" (Illarion *in* University of Alaska 1936-1938, 2:99).

Most Athapaskan Indians of the interior adopted tobacco directly or indirectly from the Russians. For example, the Han Indians of the upper Yukon were in contact with Russian traders as early as the 1840s, and traveled long distances to obtain tobacco and snuff in exchange for furs (Osgood 1971, 34). Likewise, the Upper Tanana and the Ahtna groups probably received tobacco in trade from the Russians in Prince William Sound, as well as from the Kluane region (McKennan 1959, 40), while the Upper Kuskokwim Indians probably obtained it from the Tanaina living around Cook Inlet. The tribes bordering the Eskimos, such as the Ingalik, probably first received tobacco in trade from the Eskimos, for they already were using it regularly when the first Russians reached their territory in 1834 (Glazunov *in* VanStone 1959, 46, 43).

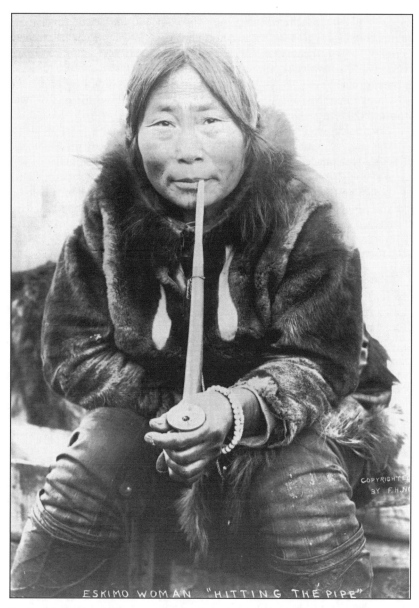

Figure 23. Eskimo woman smoking a traditional pipe. (Edith Fish Collection, Archives, Alaska and Polar Regions Dept., University of Alaska Fairbanks.)

Several of the Athapaskan groups also smoked the dried leaves of an indigenous plant, probably even before the arrival of Europeans (McKennan 1965, 30). The Tanaina chewed a mixture of fungus and cottonwood bark (*Populus balsamifera*) (Osgood 1937, 40), and similar combinations of ashes, dried fungus, or local plants were known from other groups. The Eskimos imported from the Indians the fungus they used for mixing with tobacco (Nelson 1899, 271).

Athapaskan men seemed to be very fond of smoking, at least along the Yukon, and often inhaled deeply (McKennan 1959, 41). They used the small Chinese-type pipe also favored by the Eskimos. Women and children, as well as the men, found delight in chewing (Adams 1982, 180). Zagoskin (1967, 192) also noted snuff to be used extensively among the Ingalik of the lower Yukon, another habit probably borrowed from their Eskimo neighbors.

HEALTH IMPLICATIONS OF TOBACCO USE

The Alaska Natives used tobacco in such a manner that it was certain to be harmful to health, in light of what is now known about its effects. Furthermore, the kind of tobacco available to the Natives was by its crude form and primitive methods of curing even more likely than modern tobacco products to have long-term adverse effects. An added dimension of harm could have resulted from the many questionable substances which extended the tobacco, such as lime, charcoal, wood shavings, moss, and fungi. Most Natives—men, women, and children—used tobacco whenever they could obtain it, presumably over their lifetime. The only practical limit was the plant's availability and high cost. Once it was acquired, moreover, it was used and re-used for economy's sake until the last traces of nicotine and other toxins were extracted.

What is particularly striking is the use of tobacco by children, some of whom were very young indeed. Murdoch (1892, 70) reported that at Barrow nursing children of two or three years were often pacified with a quid of tobacco. Along the Kobuk River mothers were sometimes known to take a child from the breast and put a quid of tobacco or a pipe in its mouth (Stoney 1900, 100). Another heard of a nursing Eskimo child of four years asking for a chew of tobacco and then returning to the breast (Snow 1867, 262). George Adams (1982, 180) had an Athapaskan child of five ask him for a chew of tobacco and go off with it as pleased as if it were a piece of candy. Others report Native children of four or five smoking a pipe, taking snuff, or chewing a quid (Bruce 1894, 104; Thornton 1931, 216). Dr. John Simpson

(1855, 927) observed a child of four at Barrow ask his father for a chew of tobacco and when it was not immediately forthcoming, struck him a severe blow on the face with a piece of wood.

Each of the methods of using tobacco had its harmful aspects, but it was the Native manner of smoking that was perhaps most hazardous. Although several descriptions are available, perhaps the most detailed is that of Capt. C. L. Hooper of the *Corwin* (1881, 60):

> The pipe is lighted with flint, steel and tinder, and the native commences to draw vigorously, swallowing the smoke, which he retains in his lungs as long as possible. A fit of coughing follows, which I at first thought would certainly terminate the life of the smoker in several instances. It is not an unusual occurrence for a native, who has been without tobacco for a long time, to retain the smoke in his lungs until he falls over senseless, having the appearance of a person under the influence of opium. This state lasts but a few minutes, however, when the same performance is gone through with again.

Other early accounts speak of "a momentary stupefaction" (Dall 1870, 81), "a stage similar to intoxication" (Krause 1956, 109), and "a state of unconsciousness or stupor" (Zagoskin 1967, 192). Adams (1982, 180) described how the Athapaskans along the Yukon "give two or three whifs, drawing the smoke down into their lungs, and slowly exhaling it, for a minute after exhaling the smoke, they set like on in a stupor. Their heads drop on their breasts and breathe like one with a severe attack of the Athma [sic]. The young ones when learning to smoke cough for some minutes after smoking very violently. . . ." Stoney (1900, 100) wrote that the Inupiat suffered "exhaustive attacks of coughing resulting frequently in complete prostration." Seemingly, the stronger the tobacco, the more highly it was regarded. When Glazunov (*in* VanStone 1959, 43) distributed some pipe tobacco and snuff, at the conclusion of a meeting with Indians along the Yukon, "Some were so much dazed by the smoke that they fell unconscious, while others inhaled such a quantity that they could not stop sneezing."

Early observers seemed to be of mixed views on whether smoking was harmful. According to Davydov (1977, 176) the Koniag, who certainly had no scruples about chewing tobacco or even taking snuff, refused to smoke it because they feared it would impede their breathing. Dall (1870, 81), always the scientist, felt that tobacco, especially the black Circassian variety that was so popular, had a deleterious effect on the lungs and that many habitual users died of asthma or of congestion of the lungs. He attributed these diseases to the saltpeter with which the tobacco was impregnated. At Barrow, Murdoch (1892, 39) felt that the smoking habit was responsible for aggravating several cases of lung hemorrhage that he saw. Khromchenko (1973, 71) speculated that too much smoking might account for the weak constitution he observed in the Stuart Island Eskimos.

A few early writers, although impressed with the physical effects of smoking, could not ascribe any permanent harm to the habit. A missionary at Wales felt that the Eskimos would doubtless be better off if they did not smoke, but thought the amount of outdoor exercise they took probably diminished any harm that might come from the habit (Thornton 1931, 216). A teacher on St. Lawrence Island likewise observed that "one whose nerves are all unstrung from the habitual use of tobacco is never seen and that a shattered constitution or emaciated form resulting therefrom is not to be found" (Bruce 1894, 105). His own theory was that the Eskimos' diet of fish and oil might neutralize the effect of the tobacco.

Despite these speculations on both sides of the issue, it seems likely that the excessive use of tobacco was indeed harmful to the health of the Native people. Although the most dramatic effects resulted from acute intoxication by smoke, the greater hazard to health was probably the repeated use over a long period. The Natives all inhaled deeply when smoking, and what they inhaled was from a very crude form of tobacco usually mixed with other plant products or other substances of doubtful ancestry. No type of cancer can be directly linked to smoking in the early period, but it is reasonable to suggest that bronchitis, tuberculosis, and other infections might have been encouraged by repeated damage to the airways. Breathlessness, as the early Koniag suggested, might also have been the consequence of repeated smoking, since tobacco is now known to be a major cause of emphysema. Other methods of heavy tobacco use are also likely to have been harmful. Repeated violent sneezing from the inhalation of snuff probably did no damage; on the other hand, we now know that the constant use of snuff behind the lip or of a quid of chewing tobacco in the cheek pouch may lead to cancer of the mouth.

Whatever the hazards of tobacco use, it is clear that the Alaska Natives derived much pleasure from it, and, unfortunately for their health, still do. Adelbert von Chamisso (1986, 16), the German poet and naturalist on the Kotzebue voyage, described it best:

> Whoever does not suspect the magic which dwells with [tobacco], let him watch the Eskimo fill his small stone pipe with the precious herb,

which he has thriftily mixed half and half with wood shavings, let him see him carefully light it, then eagerly with closed eyes and long, deep puffs breathe the smoke into his lungs and blow it out again into the air. Meanwhile the eyes of all are fixed on him and the one next to him is already stretching out his hand to receive the instrument so that he too may draw a puff of happiness. . . .

17

Alcohol: Alaska's Curse

It is notable that the Russians offered an alcoholic drink in friendship to the first Alaska Natives they encountered. While Bering's ship was pausing briefly in the Shumagin Islands to take on water, an elderly and eminent-looking Aleut, after some hesitation, came in his *baidarka* to the longboat where Lieutenant Waxell was waiting to greet him with gifts. According to the Russian, "I handed him a beaker of gin which he put to his lips, but spat the gin out again at once and turning to his fellows screeched most horribly" (Waxell 1962, 94). Steller, who was also aboard the longboat, adds that the Aleut drank the cup rapidly, following the example of the Russians, and after spitting it out, "act[ed] strangely about it, and did not seem at all amused by this supposed trick" (Steller 1988, 100).

Although Davydov (1977, 176) asserted that the Koniag in precontact times knew how to prepare an alcoholic beverage from fermented raspberry and bilberry juice, it seems that most Alaska Natives had no prior experience with alcohol before the arrival of Europeans. During the eighteenth century, however, all the peoples of the Pacific rim became acquainted with the joys and heartbreak of alcohol, which they either received illegally in trade, or which they learned how to prepare themselves.

The Russian *promyshlenniki* were by and large a boisterous and hard-drinking lot. By imperial edict, however, they were forbidden to traffic in alcohol or to operate a still, since distilled liquor was a strict monopoly of the crown. What the thirsty seafarers were permitted to carry on board or to manufacture was *kvass,* a kind of beer usually brewed from grain, apples, or roots, and thought to be a preventative against scurvy (Chevigny 1965, 37; Merck 1980, 87, 99). It was not long before this technology reached the

Natives—first the Aleuts and Koniag and later others (Tolstoy *in* Andreyev 1952, 28; Korobitsyn *in* Andreyev 1952, 169).

During the eighteenth century, however, alcohol abuse in Alaska was more of a problem of the Russians than of the Natives, especially after the Russians began to overwinter at Unalaska, Kodiak, and other sites. John Ledyard (1963, 94-95) of the Cook expedition visited a Russian settlement near Unalaska, taking along some rum as a gift. There he found his hosts to be "very fond of the rum, which they drank without any mixture or measure." When Captain Billings's ship was wintering near Unalaska in 1791-1792, a party of Russians came all the way from Kodiak in search of brandy, tobacco, and syphilis remedies (Bancroft 1886, 295). Likewise when Captain Meares (1790, 207) visited Kodiak in 1788 it was brandy and tobacco that were the most popular items of trade with the Russians.

Alcohol became a major problem among several of the prominent Russians in Alaska and surely must have affected the rank and file equally severely. Baranov himself once complained in a letter to Shelikhov that Gerasim Pribylov, the discoverer of the islands that bear his name, had drunk a whole flask of brandy or vodka that was being shipped to him (*in* Tikhmenev 1979, 71-72). Shelikhov himself wrote to Delarov, one of his successors at Kodiak, advising him to be temperate and not to let his men get drunk. One of his men, named Bacharov, "has been drinking ever since the day he arrived. . . . I can not sober him up" (*in* Tikhmenev 1979, 20).

Baranov himself was a particularly heavy drinker. In 1795 he felt compelled to write rather defensively to Shelikhov from Kodiak:

> It is not true that we drink vodka all the time. Nobody with the exception of myself and Izmailov makes it, or at least if the hunters make it too, it is done in such secrecy that I never hear of it. But when I make it I do so only once or twice per year: . . . It seems that the law does not prohibit the manufacture of wine from berries and roots, if it is for one's own use. Besides, it is beyond the Russian boundaries and in a new part of the world. Making wine with mercury, I have rescued from death many who were perishing from venereal diseases. . . . [N]ow that I remember it, when we were laying out and launching a ship in Chugach, I made twice a bucket of vodka out of berries and roots. The second time I added six pounds of the company's flour in your honor, and we all had drinks and I was drunk. The men drank a glass or two, and some more and became intoxicated (*in* Tikhmenev 1979, 67).

Indeed, Baranov was said to have allowed his men to drink freely, to ensure their loyalty, and to have manipulated the accounts to hide the evidence (Tikhmenev 1978, 466).

The chief manager continued to drink throughout his stay in Russian America. He suffered from pains in the arms and legs in the cold, damp climate and seemed to get some relief, or at least a measure of oblivion, from alcohol. By the time Baranov left the colonies in 1818 he was being accused in St. Petersburg of "ill management, drunkenness and dissoluteness" (University of Alaska 1936-1938, 4:178).

The widespread abuse of alcohol in the early days of the company led Rezanov to describe the colonies to the directors as a "drunken republic" (*in* Tikhmenev 1979, 172). The count saw clearly the dangers of unrestrained drinking, but also recognized that it would be unwise to forbid alcohol at the end of the workday, "because to get intoxicated is considered the greatest pleasure among unenlightened people." He warned, however, that fighting would not be tolerated and that half the men should always be sober and ready for defense (University of Alaska 1936-1938, 3:181).

In the earlier period the workers were allowed their *kvass,* a large vat of which was always fermenting, but they were permitted to drink their fill only when off duty or on Sundays and holidays. At sea sailors were in addition allowed a ration during stormy weather (Pierce 1976, 177, 180; Pierce 1984, 119). Later, after Baranov's time, the workers could purchase rum or vodka at the company store (Sarafian 1971, 109).

Workers continued to be largely recruited from eastern Siberia, especially Okhotsk, where few healthy, temperate individuals could be found (Gibson 1976, 48). One contemporary described the labor pool as "given to drink in a way that was an insult to the human race, and the police did not find itself in a position to put an end to the daily drinking and rowdyism" (*in* Okun 1979, 176). Some were said to barter their clothes for a last drink and be carried to the ship stark naked to begin their voyage to America (Andrews 1916, 29; Berkh 1979, 29). Given this background it is not surprising that the workers were willing to give their last kopeck for alcohol, which "next to articles of clothing and footwear was dearer to the workers than anything else in the world" (Baranov *in* Okun 1979, 179). The company rather cynically used this craving for alcohol as a way of keeping the workers continually indebted (Tikhmenev 1979, 169). And to insure that they gave their soul to the company store, each was required to sign a contract which read in part: "Everyone in the service of the Company is forbidden . . . to distill liquor from herbs, roots, berries, Company grain, and so forth; or to buy or barter liquor from visiting foreigners and trade in it on Company premises, to make loans or give money to each other for drinking purposes, then drink the liquor or use it in any way at all" (*in* Okun 1979, 178-79).

These restrictions applied to all company employees, which of course included most Creoles and not a few Aleut and Koniag hunters living at New Archangel. Some of these Natives were also serious alcohol abusers and resorted to many deceits, according to one official, to receive vodka and other drinks illegally (Khlebnikov 1976, 104).

With the departure of Baranov in 1818, the control on alcohol tightened. Chief Manager Hagemeister was well aware of the harm to worker productivity that drinking caused. He insisted that alcoholic beverages be permitted at Sitka and other company posts, or aboard company ships, only on special holidays. He admonished the new manager of the Kenai posts to turn people away from drunkenness by setting a good example. Above all he should not allow the local inhabitants to gather berries for the manufacture of vodka (Pierce 1984, 59, 65, 119).

The introduction of liquor to the Tlingit probably occurred in the 1790s and was said to have been first brought as an article of trade by the French ship *La Flavie*. Various New England trading ships soon took advantage of this new market, trading both firearms and alcoholic beverages for furs (Sherwood 1965a, 306; Gibson 1976, 155-56). Before long many acquired a taste for strong drink, which they freely obtained in trade from the many trading vessels that illegally plied the countless bays and inlets of the archipelago (Golovnin 1979, 127). In 1829 an American bark was trading with the Tlingit when the excessive use of alcohol led to a quarrel in which an Indian was killed and the ship's mate badly wounded. The vessel put into Sitka seeking medical help, but this was refused by Gov. Petr Chistiakov on the grounds that the Americans should suffer the consequences of their illegal trade (Andrews 1916, 29).

The Russians in general tried to keep the Tlingit from using alcoholic drinks, but were known on occasion to seal a bargain or treaty with a gift of brandy (Lisiansky 1814, 223; Kotzebue 1830, 2:61; *see also* Vancouver 1798, 2:391). After one such occasion none of the principals was left standing at the end of the banquet (Bancroft 1886, 439). Some Tlingit were reluctant to use alcoholic drinks because they knew liquor deprived them of their senses (Langsdorff 1814, 2:131). Others, however, acquired a ready taste for it. In later years Governor Furuhjelm (*in* Golovin 1983, 129) is reported to have boasted rather cynically that all Tlingit could be converted to Christianity for a blanket, a dinner, and two cups of vodka.

At outlying posts alcohol restrictions also applied, but the Natives usually found ways of obtaining it anyway, either through illegal trade or by fermenting their own. Campbell (1819, 44) found the Aleuts of Sanak Island to be "immoderately fond of spirits" at the time of his shipwreck in 1806. At Unalaska a few years later Capt. Peter Corney (1965, 136, 140) traded rum for fish and noted that all the Natives of the area were "extremely fond" of rum, often parting with their clothing and hunting gear to purchase a small quantity. Veniaminov (1984, 181-82) wrote that although some Unalaska Aleuts used no vodka at all and some saved it up for special occasions, the others without exception drank as much as they could whenever they obtained it. He described a few living in close proximity to the Russians as drunkards who would give everything they had to obtain alcohol. Veniaminov described the Aleuts, when drunk, as becoming merry and garrulous, but not disposed to quarrels or violence. In his later years in the islands the priest was pleased to note that tea was becoming so popular that it was sometimes even exchanged for a shot of vodka (Veniaminov 1984, 279).

Despite the company's attempts to monopolize the importation, manufacture, and sale of distilled beverages, it was unable to prevent effectively the brisk trade in strong drink that continued to occur from British and American vessels visiting the northern coasts. In 1824 the Russian government and the United States concluded a treaty which allowed American vessels the right to trade with the Natives in Russian America, but with the specific exclusion of spirituous liquors and all types of firearms and munitions. The United States agreed to prevent their citizens from selling such items to the Natives, but refused to permit their ships to be searched for contraband. Similar provisions were incorporated into a convention between Russia and Great Britain in the following year (Golovin 1979, 216, 8). The illegal trade continued, of course, since effective enforcement was all but impossible (Bancroft 1886, 542-43n) There was some suggestion that the Hudson's Bay Company in particular did not always make serious efforts to fulfill the terms of the agreement (Golovin 1979, 92; Gibson 1976, 200).

In 1832 the Russian-American Company began the practice of selling spirits to the Indians at Sitka, because the directors had to admit that they were powerless to prevent the smuggling of liquor by the illegal trading vessels. The Hudson's Bay Company shortly after followed suit, although both companies recognized that this step was contributing to the rapid deterioration of the Indian people (G. Simpson 1847, 2:87-88).

In 1841 Sir George Simpson, Chief Factor of the Hudson's Bay Company, visited the Russian colonies and was so disturbed by the drunkenness of the Indians that he proposed to Governor Etholin that by the end of 1843 both companies should agree to abolish the trading of liquor (G. Simpson 1847, 1:132). The two-year delay was meant to provide adequate time to fortify the trading posts against possible violence by the Indians who might be angered by their enforced abstinence. When Simpson returned to Sitka in the spring of 1842, however, an incident occurred at the Tlingit village which led the officials of the two companies to reconsider their decision. Two prominent Indians had engaged in a drunken quarrel and one had stabbed the other to death. The friends and relatives of the deceased turned out to the number of a thousand strong and a civil war was narrowly averted by the pointed threat of turning the guns of the fort on the participants. This incident, and another recent one at Stikine, where the factor John McLaughlin had been shot by drunken Indians, convinced both Simpson and Etholin that their companies should immediately discontinue selling alcohol to the Natives (G. Simpson 1847, 2:88). The agreement went into effect on May 13, 1842, and lasted throughout the remainder of the Russian period in Alaska. Although the Natives continued to obtain smuggled liquor, the ban on trade in alcohol did much to restrict the flow into their villages (Tikhmenev 1978, 354-55). No violent reaction occurred on the occasion of the ban, as some had feared, but the Sitka Tlingit "retired in sullen silence" when they learned that they had been subjected to unwilling prohibition (G. Simpson 1847, 2:88).

The ban on trade, of course, did nothing to staunch the flow of alcohol among the employees of the company. Many kinds of alcoholic drinks were available, including rum, gin, port, and sherry, most of it brought to Alaska by American ships. The use among the workmen and soldiers was limited by the officers of the company, who themselves seemed to have alcoholic drinks freely available. Workmen received one or two measures of strong drink on feast days, but often obtained more illicitly. Sailors were issued a measure of rum during stormy weather (Blaschke 1842, 55-57). One observer noted that "drunkenness, debauchery, violence, laziness and insubordination [were] very, very common, especially among soldiers and laborers" (Golovin 1979, 14). Likewise, Hjalmar Furuhjelm described the workmen at the Russian coal mine on the Kenai Peninsula as "hard-drinking good-for-nothings" whom the company had enticed to come to America (*in* Pierce 1975, 106).

Simpson (who was on a round-the-world voyage at the time) called Sitka the most drunken place he had ever visited. "On the holidays, in particular," he wrote (1847, 2:88), "of which, Sundays included, there are one hundred and sixty-five in the year, men, women, and even children, were to be seen staggering about in all directions." Governor Etholin, who was one of the more enlightened managers of the colonies and sincerely concerned about alcohol abuse, had to recognize that it was impossible to live in Sitka without rum, which served as a sort of unofficial currency (Zagoskin 1967, 69, 74; Golovin 1983, 117).

At St. Michael, far from the fashionable life at the capital, only a single barrel of rum was allowed annually, and this was usually consumed at a glorious three-day drunk at the time of the arrival of the supply ship. Lieutenant Zagoskin (1967, 91-92) who observed this annual rite in 1842, noted that if alcohol gladdens the heart, "some superintendents manage to be gladdened beyond this limit of three days, but only because they keep the means to gladness in their own possession."

The company could not bring itself to outlaw alcohol altogether for fear of losing many of its best artisans, who were not prepared to remain in far-off Alaska without the comforts of strong drink (G. Simpson 1847, 2:88). In the early 1860s the free sale of spirits at Sitka was still prohibited, in order to curb drunkenness. Rum and vodka could be purchased only from the company warehouse, and even this privilege was denied to Creoles, who sometimes employed extreme measures to obtain liquor through intermediaries. Among the "lower classes of Creoles," according to a visitor, "husbands calmly peddle their wives' favors. . . . In exchange for a bottle or two of rum, a man will give his wife's services for a day or two or a week, depending on the terms. This is done openly" (Golovin 1983, 116-17).

SOUTHERN ALASKA IN THE AMERICAN PERIOD

Even as negotiations for the transfer of Alaska to the United States were proceeding, the Treasury Department moved to control the importation of "ardent spirits" into Alaska (De Lorme 1975, 145), yet only weeks after the new flag was raised, saloons were already opening in Sitka (Bancroft 1886, 600). By the summer of 1868, when the Customs Act was extended to Alaska, public and private drunkenness was already a serious problem. In May 1869 the *Alaska Times* of Sitka carried advertisements for six saloons, a brewery, and a store that sold wines and liquors (Becky Smith 1973). An early visitor, Dr. Emil Teichmann (1963, 187), complained that almost every evening and especially on holidays the whole community became drunk and merry, and that "the noise made by the workmen, maddened by drink, resounds throughout the eerie settlement."

For lack of any form of civil government, the Army was charged with the responsibility for controlling the importation of alcohol on behalf of the customs collector. Yet the Army was itself responsible for much of the abuse in the early years. Vincent Colyer, a special Indian agent who traveled north in 1869, was outraged to see cases of champagne and port, ten barrels of ale, and five barrels of rum, whiskey, and brandy offloaded from the government quartermaster vessel at Fort Tongass. All this alcohol was consigned "for the use of the officers of the post," of whom there were merely four. Colyer was certain that the liquor was meant for trade with the Indian village only five hundred yards away.

He had a similar experience at Fort Wrangell, but by a strong protest was successful in having at least the distilled liquor brought to Sitka. Some nine hundred gallons of "coal oil" landed by the steamer were found to be pure ethanol and confiscated by the customs collector, who after a short time sold it at public auction right back to the members of the community (Colyer 1869, 979-81). From there the liquor was openly sold or bartered to everyone who could pay or offer value in return, including the soldiers and the many Indians living near the post. The medical director of the Army's Department of Alaska was particularly concerned about the adverse effects of a drunken soldiery on the Indians. "Whiskey has been sold in the streets," he wrote (*in* Colyer 1869, 1023), "by government officials, at public auctions, and examples of drunkenness are set before the Indians almost daily, so that in fact the principal teaching that they are at present receiving is that drunkenness and debauchery are held by us . . . as indications of our advanced and superior civilization." Some Indians, for their part, seemed reluctant to see the liquor traffic expanded, for they well knew the destructive effects of drunkenness (Colyer 1869, 982).

Despite earlier attempts to declare Alaska "Indian country," it was not until March 1873 that Congress acted to extend to Alaska the 1834 law prohibiting the sale of "spirituous liquors" to Indians and forbidding the operation of distilleries in the territory (Gruening 1954, 501). The attorney general upheld this provision in November 1873 and ruled that the War Department had jurisdiction over the importation of all alcohol to Alaska, not only that intended for the use of the officers and troops (Morris 1879, 57). The following June the commandant issued orders prohibiting all importation of alcohol except by special permit issued from Pacific Headquarters (U.S. Army Alaska 1962, 15). In 1875 the duties of Indian agent were bestowed upon an army officer stationed at Sitka.

Alcoholic abuses continued to mount through these years. The Indians could always find means of acquiring liquor illegally, while the soldiers continued to obtain it legally through their own supply channels. A Russian named Stepan Ushin, who kept a diary during this period, wrote in June

1874, "In our Sitka, inebriation has developed without limits. . . . [A]lmost all Sitka gets drunk daily, is unruly, fights and so on" (*in* Shalkop 1977, 104). In most of the encounters that took place the Indians were the clear losers (Gruening 1954, 502). The army command did what it could to suppress drunkenness whenever it occurred, but they enjoyed limited success, since no longer was it simply a question of importation and sale but rather of home manufacture.

Although the details are often unclear, there is general agreement that the Tlingit learned to make a distilled liquor known as "hootch" sometime during the early years of the American occupation. Various accounts attributed the formula and method to a trader named Brown (Krause 1956, 108), a discharged soldier named Sullivan, or another named Doyle. Still another account attributed the introduction of the nefarious substance to an escaped criminal from British Columbia (Sherwood 1965a, 319-20). Dr. Robert White (1880, 37) reported that the Indians learned the process from both Russian and American soldiers, although there seems to be no documented reference to the home-manufacture of liquor in southeastern Alaska prior to 1867. Whatever the origin, hootch was very much a fact of life by the time the Army pulled out its troops in 1877 (Morris 1879, 58).

Hootch took its name from the village of Hoochinoo, or Kootznahoo, not far from the present village of Angoon on Admiralty Island. As Dr. White (1880, 37) described the process, "An old coal-oil or other can of sufficient size furnishes a still, and a gun-barrel, or the long hollow arms of a species of kelp growing in great abundance on the coast, is used as a worm, while the sugar or molasses procured from the trader, or in the absence of this, fermented flour or potatoes, with berries, supplies the material." The worm was either packed in snow or placed in the cold water of a running stream. Initially molasses was the preferred ingredient, but when this item was restricted in trade, potatoes became the basis of the recipe. The potatoes were cooked, dumped into a tub, and allowed to ferment with the addition of sugar or a small amount of molasses. The mash was then distilled, following which the product was ready to drink (Niblack 1888, 346).

Contemporary observers, all of them presumably non-users, outdid themselves in describing the taste and effects of hootch, a word that has come into the American language to mean "bootleg liquor." Dr. Robert White (1880, 37) called it "very rank in taste and odor, and violently stimulant in their effects; their use is quickly followed by marked irritation of the urinary organs. After drinking, the natives may often be seen stupidly wallowing about on the ground and evidently suffering from strangury [slow, painful attempts to urinate]." Another wrote that the horrible product was drunk in its raw state and almost immediately robbed the drinker of his senses (Niblack 1888, 346). Special agents for the customs described it as "a vile, poisonous, life and soul destroying concoction, . . . which saps the very essence of the human system, producing crime, disease, insanity, and death" (Morris 1879, 58). In Wrangell the missionary S. Hall Young found whole villages drunk, where "murderous quarrels were frequent, and unspeakable scenes of debauchery and sin were enacted." And finally this vivid description from the naturalist John Muir (1915, 131-32), who visited the village of Kootznahoo itself in 1879:

> While we were yet half a mile or more away, we heard sounds I had never before heard—a storm of strange howls, yells, and screams rising from a base of gasping, bellowing grunts and groans. Had I been alone, I should have fled as from a pack of fiends, but our Indians quietly recognized this awful sound, simply as the 'whiskey howl' and quietly pushed on. . . . The whole village was afire with bad whiskey.

The Army, the Navy, the Customs Service, and the Revenue Cutter Service all tried to prevent the spread and abuse of alcohol among the Indians, but with notably little success. Many small trading vessels brought cheap whiskey to the Tlingit villages, where the large and cumbersome government vessels could not navigate (De Lorme 1975, 146). When it became too risky to sell alcohol as such, the traders switched to molasses and sugar as staple items. Molasses, the principal ingredient of hootch, became a major trade commodity. In a single five-month period of 1877, 4889 gallons were imported into Sitka and another 1635 gallons into Wrangell, nearly all of which was ultimately converted into hootch, gallon for gallon (Morris 1879, 58). As early as 1875 the Army tried to limit the sale of molasses, but this restriction drew criticism from many businessmen and government officials (U.S. Army Alaska 1962, 16); besides, when molasses could not be obtained, the stills were simply fed with potatoes and berries instead.

Drunkenness was by no means confined to the Indians. Stepan Ushin's diary (*in* University of Alaska 1936-1938, 12, 16-17, 34, 41) contains many entries describing the prevalence of drinking in Sitka. The 1880 census figures indicated that sixteen of the 215 Caucasians in the town were saloon-keepers (Brooks 1973, 267). Prior to 1877 the soldiers not only patronized these bars freely, but also manufactured their own hootch on occasion. It would appear that sometimes the soldiers and others even purchased hootch from the Indians (U.S. Army Alaska 1962, 16). The citizenry of Sitka, which came to include more and more "prospectors" with time on their hands, also freely patronized the saloons. The victims of these drunken men were not infrequently Indian women, who themselves often found easy access to alcohol. Ugly incidents occurred when rowdy gangs of drunken men roamed the streets late at night looking for excitement (Morris 1879, 2, 4-5).

Failing to control the importation of alcohol, government officials and missionaries concentrated on controlling the manufacture of hootch, whether in Sitka or in the many Tlingit villages in the Panhandle. When the Navy assumed the reins of Alaska government in 1877, it moved quickly to crack down on the homebrew problem. In July 1877 Captain Beardslee of the U.S.S. *Jamestown* ordered a raid that put some forty-one stills out of operation in Sitka, most of them in Indian homes. A couple of years later he enlisted the help of twenty-three Indians who broke up about forty stills with axes, clubs, and stones (Hanable 1978, 322-23). The missionaries employed similar tactics. Young (1927, 166) pursued his "Carrie [sic] Nation campaign" of destroying stills in the villages, even though he often received threats of violent retaliation. Young also deputized one village to destroy stills in another, a practice that nearly led to open warfare (Muir 1915, 202-3).

Civil government first came to Alaska with the passage of the Organic Act of 1884, section 16 of which prohibited the manufacture, importation, or sale of alcohol in Alaska, except for mechanical, scientific, or medical purposes. The first governor was able to state optimistically that although much bootleg alcohol was still finding its way into Alaska, little was getting into the Indian villages (Kinkead 1884, 8). His successor was less sanguine. Governor Swineford (1885; 1886, 46; 1889a, 49-50) could not see how the prohibition could be enforced with the endless Alaskan coastline. Violators made huge profits and few citizens were willing to make a complaint about them. Nor would grand juries indict obvious offenders. By 1888 prohibition was a dead letter and the governor was urging its repeal in favor of a strict licensing law that could bring needed revenue into the territory. One of his underlying concerns was that the White population of Alaska deeply resented not being able to obtain liquor legally. "Prohibition," he concluded prophetically in 1888, "does not prohibit" (1889b, 50).

The law, in fact, was not repealed until 1899 (Gruening 1954, 108), and until then the government continued efforts to suppress the alcohol trade. Meanwhile, lawlessness and violence went on in many communities of southeastern Alaska, for liquor, either imported or homemade, always found its way to those who wanted it badly enough. Large quantities of legal alcohol were imported by pharmacists "for medicinal purposes," and then resold to the public (De Lorme 1975, 150; Ushin *in* University of Alaska 1936-1938, 3:16). Considerable amounts of bootleg alcohol also continued to be successfully smuggled into the territory. Once past the customs officers it could be sold at retail, since the law prohibited only the importation, not the retail sale of liquor (Kinkead 1884, 8). Ushin (*in* University of Alaska 1936-1938, 3:63) expressed his frustration in 1885 that people were being unlawfully arrested for buying alcohol, while no action was ever taken against the many saloon-keepers, who were obviously obtaining their supplies illegally.

During the 1890s the governors continued to voice their concern about the liquor laws. In 1892 alone 102 permits were issued to land liquor legally for physicians, pharmacists, clergymen, the U.S. Navy, and others (Knapp 1892, 23). The following year the governor complained that large amounts of alcohol were being smuggled from British Columbia and that the existing law was a continuing source of "irritation and discontent" (Knapp 1893). Over the next few years Governor James Sheakley (1894, 5-6; 1895, 19; 1896, 203) repeatedly vented his frustration about the situation. Despite the best efforts of the Revenue Marine Service, customs officers and others, "intoxicating liquors are imported, landed, and sold without stint in every White settlement in Alaska." Despite many arrests, the courts could not obtain any convictions except, rather hypocritically, in cases where alcohol was being sold to an Indian. This disregard for the alcohol laws bred contempt for all laws and was thus a legitimate concern for the governor, whose resources for law enforcement were marginal at best. When Congress finally overturned the 1884 restrictions, southeastern Alaska was already in the throes of the Klondike stampede, and the law was truly a dead letter.

Alcohol overflowed the gold rush towns of Skagway and Dyea like the Yukon behind a spring ice jam. Bars sprang up everywhere, both to help the joyous gold-strikers to celebrate and to drown the sorrows of the many disappointed and lonely prospectors who had not found their El Dorado. A great deal of alcohol found its way beyond the settlements of Taiya Inlet, too, both as trail comfort in the outfits of the miners and as incentive for trade with the Chilkats and other Indians. Much the same situation developed around this period in the boom town of Valdez.

WESTERN ALASKA IN THE AMERICAN PERIOD

Shortly after the American purchase of Alaska, liquor was being freely traded in the Aleutians. When Capt. Alfred L. Hough visited the islands in

1869 he found the Aleuts getting drunk whenever they could obtain alcohol (Athearn 1949, 59). A report from Unalaska that same year indicated that ships of the American-Russian Ice Company were landing large amounts of whiskey and brandy at Belkofski (and presumably other villages) and making the Aleuts drunk (Colyer 1869, 1022). The lack of patrol vessels led to smuggling throughout the islands, except in the Pribilofs, where the use of alcohol, aside from medicinal purposes, was strictly forbidden by the terms of the lease with the Alaska Commercial Company (H. Elliott 1880, 108).

The Aleuts, however, did not need smuggled liquor, for since over a century they had adapted to their own use the art of making *kvass,* which they prepared by fermenting sugar, flour, hops, dried apples, and perhaps berries together with water in a large barrel. Before the mixture worked clear they drew off a thick, sour liquid that was an effective source of alcohol. Drunken orgies from the use of *kvass* were widespread throughout the early American years, causing much violence, destruction, and sometimes even leading to murder (H. Elliott 1886, 137; 1875, 25). Captain Healy of the *Rush* in the summer of 1881 became alarmed by the prevalence of drunkenness due to *kvass* throughout the Aleutians, and besides destroying many barrels of the brew, he also tried in vain to limit the sale of the brown sugar used in its manufacture. It must be said, however, that in the Aleutians and elsewhere, by no means everyone abused strong drink. Colyer (1869, 1042), for example, spoke of "many sober, steady men" at Unalaska during his stay there.

The alcohol situation was similar on Kodiak Island. Whiskey was freely available from trading ships, as elsewhere, but in addition alcohol became a common item of trade with the Chinese employed in the large salmon canneries that sprang up in Kodiak and elsewhere toward the end of the century (Jackson 1893a, 1248-49). An Orthodox priest who worked at Karluk in these years deplored the impact of this Chinese liquor, known as "shamsha," which could be legally imported from San Francisco for the use of the workers. The result of this pernicious trade not infrequently was violence and lechery, although toward the end of the century the priest was pleased to note that drunkenness and its attendant vices were declining (Shalamov *in* University of Alaska 1936-1938, 2:848). For most Koniag users, however, *kvass* remained the staple drink. It was prepared in much the same way as in the Aleutians, with seemingly more emphasis on the use of potatoes and berries (Howard 1900, 51; Huggins 1981, 8).

In Bristol Bay the whiskey traders moved in shortly after the purchase. When the Revenue Steamer *Lincoln* landed at Nushagak in July 1869, the special agent on board found two Russians and a Native priest drunk, having apparently just received a supply of liquor from a visiting schooner (Colyer 1869, 1021-22). The same vessel was implicated the following year in the establishment of a still on Cook Inlet (Hinckley 1972, 95). The Kenaitze Indians were soon distilling their own hootch, according to an Orthodox priest (Nikita *in* University of Alaska 1936-1938, 2:67), and by 1881 he considered drunkenness their "chief vice." A later priest (J. Bortnovsky *in* University of Alaska 1936-1938, 2:70) gave it as his opinion that no physician would find it necessary to use an anesthetic to perform surgery on them.

When canneries were established in Bristol Bay in the 1890s, alcohol abuse greatly increased. The Moravian mission at Carmel established a temperance society in 1894-1895, and urged all fishermen and other Whites to support its efforts to restrict the flow of alcohol to the Eskimos. By 1900, however, great quantities of alcohol were being brought in by the cannery workers. To make matters worse, the Chinese workers were teaching the local Natives how to distill a new type of liquor from graham flour, sugar, and water. Although efforts were made to restrict the sale of sugar, the Eskimos often saved it up until they had enough for a batch of hootch (VanStone 1967, 42-43, 76-77, 130).

The use of alcoholic beverages in the Yukon-Kuskokwim area apparently did not become widespread during the nineteenth century. In one of the earliest reports from the Moravian mission at Bethel (Jackson 1886, 69), the Kuskokwim Eskimos were said to know nothing of intoxicating liquors. Both the church and the Alaska Commercial Company had a stake in ensuring that this situation not change. Captain Hooper (1881, 5) of the *Corwin* records that a Nunivak Islander did not know the taste of brandy or whiskey, and when offered some spat it out in evident disgust. Along the lower Yukon Captain Raymond (1900, 33) in 1869 observed no evidence of intoxication among the Eskimos, and in fact was told that they sometimes sold alcohol to the Russians, among whom alcohol abuse was very prevalent.

At St. Michael the situation was different, since alcohol had long been known at the Russian post. It became even more readily available after the Americans arrived, as the town became an important dispatch point both for the Yukon River trade and for all of Norton Sound, including Nome. Just before the American takeover, Henry Bannister of the Telegraph Expedition (*in* James 1942, 233) wrote in his diary that "all the men had a big drunk and a regular Irish time of it, fighting, etc." on the occasion of the departure of a friend. A few years later Dall observed an umiak with two barrels of rum leaving an American schooner that was beginning regular trading runs to St. Michael (Dall 1870, 239). In 1873 an Indian agent, whose duty it was to abolish the liquor trade to the Natives, was stationed at St. Michael. During his short stay he heard of several traders who were distilling liquor or selling it to the Eskimos in the surrounding regions, but affirmed that the more serious problems were further north (D. Ray 1975, 189). Control efforts finally seem to have succeeded, at least among the Eskimos, for around the turn of the century Dr. Edmonds (1966, 66) was able to report that there was not much open drunkenness around the post, except among the mixed-blood Russians, some of whom were chronic drunkards.

THE INTRODUCTION OF ALCOHOL
TO NORTHERN ALASKA AND THE INTERIOR

According to Seemann (1853, 55) alcohol was unknown to the northern Eskimos by the middle of the nineteenth century, although he acknowledged that the people around Norton Sound had acquired a taste for it by "constant intercourse" with the Russian traders, presumably from St. Michael and perhaps Unalakleet. As early as 1851 several trading ships were operating in the Bering Strait region, at least one of them having wintered at St. Lawrence Bay on the Siberian side. That year vessels from Australia, Honolulu, and Hong Kong were trading for furs and ivory around the strait, and at least some of them had rum on board, in defiance of the prohibition of the Russian-American Company (Bockstoce 1986, 182). That same year a whaler that had grounded on the Chukchi Peninsula was boarded by a large group who made straight for the captain's rum supply and soon plundered the wreck (Bockstoce 1986, 183). Soon, unfortunately, liquor was found throughout the North, brought first by the trading ships and later by American whalers.

Even in 1850 Captain Collinson (1889, 74) of the British Royal Navy had reported that the Diomede Islanders were asking for rum, and when half a pint was offered in exchange for walrus tusks, the head man held it to his breast and stroked it with affection. A few years later, in 1854, Collinson found rum and brandy were the major items requested in trade at Wales. By 1867, liquor could be obtained by the barrel at Kotzebue Sound. Alcohol-spawned mischief was spreading, as evidenced by an attack by drunken King Islanders on an American boat (D. Ray 1975, 155, 166, 179).

The traders and whalers were eager to obtain ivory, baleen, fox pelts, and Eskimos crafts in exchange for brandy, whiskey, and rum. Alcohol became the most sought after of Western goods. A tragic incident occurred in 1871 when dozens of ships, mostly whalers, were caught in the ice of Point Belcher and abandoned. The Eskimos quickly boarded the ships looking for alcohol and took home everything they could find in bottles, including the contents of the medicine chests. The wild orgy that followed ended in death by poisoning for many of the villagers (Hadley 1915, 907).

In 1879 Special Treasury Agent H. A. Otis went north on the steamer *St. Paul* and found evidence that many ships were supplying rum and breech-loading rifles to the Eskimos. Such trading vessels usually fitted out in San Francisco, then proceeded to Honolulu to take on a cargo of rum and whiskey intended for the "Siberian trade," at least according to the ship's papers. On the voyage most of the tax-free liquor was adulterated with water and then sold or traded at a huge profit in Plover Bay or East Cape on the Siberian side, or in any number of Alaskan villages from Unalakleet to the arctic coast. Once on shore the liquor was retailed into the surrounding area, causing much drunkenness, violence, and misery. In Kotzebue Sound the previous year no fewer than six vessels had arrived in one day, one of them with fifty barrels of liquor, all of which was quickly sold. When the Eskimos saw the crew distilling a new supply on board the ship, they asked that stills be brought for them on the next voyage, so that they too could manufacture it (*in* Bailey 1880, 43-48).

Beginning also in 1879, ships of the Revenue Marine Service began making regular voyages into the Bering Sea. That first year Captain Bailey (1880, 17-18) reported that some thirty barrels of rum had been landed at Cape Rodney and from thence distributed widely. Bailey detained and searched a number of ships at sea and heard of others carrying as much as 1600 gallons of rum for the arctic trade. The following year the *Corwin* made the first of its many northern voyages. Captain Hooper (1881, 20) reported in some detail on two major tragedies that he attributed to the abuse of liquor (*see* Chapter 18). He told of boarding one schooner near Kotzebue Sound, the *Leo*, which was carrying cases of bottles marked as "Florida Water," "Bay-rum," "Painkiller," "Jamaica ginger," and other forms of alcohol, almost none of which was shown on the manifest. At Cape Espenberg he observed the Eskimos to be very poor, since "they can get all the whisky they can pay for" (Hooper 1881, 25). The next year Hooper (1884, 38) stopped a schooner that was selling whiskey by the drink to the Eskimos for one fox pelt each.

John Muir (1917, 25, 29, 206) traveled north on the *Corwin* in 1881 and feelingly described the devastation that alcohol was causing. On St.

Lawrence Island the Eskimos insisted on liquor as the only acceptable medium of exchange. Often they were deluded by the traders, who gave a sample of nearly pure alcohol to a "tester," but then sold a keg which was soon found to be well watered, "much to their disgust and surprise." When the officers of the *Corwin* once threw a keg of rum from a wrecked whaling ship over the side, with the intention of breaking it on the ice, an Eskimo seized it and sped away to his village, where it disappeared "as far beyond recovery as if it had been poured into a hot sand bank."

The revenue steamers continued to police the long arctic coast against whiskey traders through to the close of the nineteenth century. Capt. Michael. A. Healy, who took over the *Corwin* from Hooper and later became famous as skipper of the *Bear,* was almost fanatic in his effort to control the deadly traffic. In 1884 Healy (1889, 17) was able to report that the "whisky traffic in northern Alaska has almost entirely ceased," adding with obvious satisfaction that the *Corwin* had become known as "Oomiak-puck pe-chuck tonli-ka" or "no whisky ship." The following year he was equally upbeat, having found no evidence of drinking along the American coast, although it was still a big problem on the Siberian side (Healy 1887, 15). In later years Healy, as captain of the *Bear,* formed a unique relationship with the missionary Sheldon Jackson, who as commissioner of education for Alaska and later founder of the reindeer project went north nearly every summer on an inspection tour. Jackson (1893a, 1274) approved warmly of Healy's enthusiasm in chasing liquor violators, writing in 1889: "During the past ten years hundreds of barrels of vile liquors have been emptied into the sea as a result of the vigilance of Capt. Healy. . . . The country and all who are interested in saving the natives of this coast from the demoralization of rum owe a large debt of gratitude to Capt. Healy, who has practically broken up the traffic on this northwest coast." It is both sad and bitterly ironic that, according to his medical officer (but perhaps unbeknownst to Jackson), this same man that same year was so drunk he endangered his ship (J. White 1889). A few years later he was suspended from command for five years because of alcoholism, and in 1900 he suffered a suicidal depression brought on by alcohol and had to be relieved of command while at sea (Stein 1985).

Despite the best efforts of the Revenue Marine Service, alcohol continued to plague the northen Eskimos. Although by no means all whalers engaged in the whiskey trade, many did (Aldrich 1889, 114-15), to the continuing detriment of the people. When the whaling ships began overwintering in the mid-1880s, their crews distilled their own liquor on shore, an art soon learned by the Eskimos. Capt. John A. Cook (Cook and Pederson 1937, 176-

77) told the story of an Eskimo woman who bought flour and molasses from him, ostensibly for food, and then tried unsuccessfully to distill rum from them. Whatever she was doing wrong, word got around that Cook's molasses was no good and he had little further demand for it. Soon, however, the correct recipe diffused widely and molasses and sugar once more became leading articles of trade around Kotzebue Sound (VanStone 1958, 8-9; VanStone 1962a, 126-27) Making home brew became particularly popular because it could be carried out in the wintertime, when the revenue ships could not interfere.

By 1889 local manufacture of liquor was becoming an increasing problem. That past winter the northern coastal Eskimos had learned the secret of manufacture, and the following spring drunkenness seriously interfered with their subsistence whaling. A couple of years later three men were killed as a result of alcohol-induced violence (Gubser 1965, 8). A particularly nasty situation developed at Wales, where liquor was distilled at least as early as 1889 (Lopp 1892, 390), and difficulties were continually developing as a result of drunken rowdyism. The teachers' house was broken into on several occasions and the teachers subjected to much verbal abuse (Thornton 1931, 52). Hootch continued to be a serious problem at Wales in later years. In 1897 the winter was unparalleled in the memory of the villagers for drunkenness, disorder, and bloodshed (D. Ray 1975, 193).

The home manufacture of hootch came to St. Lawrence Island only in 1896, when a whaler brought a Point Hope woman to the island. According to her recipe, five quarts of molasses and three quarts of flour yielded about one quart of whiskey. That winter many of the islanders distilled their own alcohol and the teachers reported that drunken men were not uncommon in the village (Jackson 1898a, 1605).

As late as 1898 an officer of the *Bear* reported that he had searched all the villages from Cape Thompson to Point Hope and found six stills. At Point Hope itself he destroyed nine stills and later heard of five others broken up by a concerned Eskimo woman. He saw no answer to the problem but to restrict the sale of molasses and flour to the Eskimos (Bertholf *in* Jackson 1898b, 101).

Despite the serious problem it should not be assumed that all Eskimos—or even a majority—drank, or that many did not recognize the harm it was causing in their families and villages. Captain Hooper (1881, 62-63) related that at many places where the *Corwin* stopped the people told him that they would be glad if the whiskey trade could be stopped. At Barrow a few years before, the Eskimos had bought a large quantity of liquor from a trader, and while under its influence had neglected to hunt for the winter, with the result that many starved. Following this tragedy the people themselves asked the traders and whalers not to bring any more alcohol to the village.

The introduction of alcohol to the interior was relatively late and largely followed the arrival of American traders and prospectors during the 1870s and later. Both the Hudson's Bay Company and the Russian-American Company did not believe it was in the interest of the fur trade to allow the use of alcohol, nor did the larger American companies such as the Alaska Commercial Company. Reports of alcohol abuse are indeed scarce for the Athapaskans except for those who lived around the Cook Inlet posts (Brady 1900, 59), and by no means all of these were users (Learnard 1900, 666). As late as 1892 alcohol was virtually unknown around the Episcopalian mission field in the lower Yukon and in the upper Yukon near the Canadian border, but it was causing some trouble along other parts of the river (Brady 1900, 56-57), probably due to the increasing numbers of prospectors in the region. By the turn of the century the Indians along the Yukon were able to obtain all the whiskey they wanted, either through unscrupulous middlemen or in the saloons that had sprouted up to serve the ever-thirsty miners (U.S. Senate 1904, 131, 198). Even U.S. Army posts in the interior themselves could be sources of liquor for the Indians (Farnsworth 1977, 215).

Alcohol abuse flourished in the raucous mining towns along the Yukon such as Rampart and Circle City (Wickersham 1938, 41, 123). At Nome gambling halls, saloons, and houses of prostitution sprang up like mushrooms. Not a few of the barroom brawls involved none other than Wyatt Earp, who had opened a bar himself in 1899 (Cole 1984, 74-75). In 1900, thirsty residents could choose from some fifty saloons (Hunt 1974, 113). Somewhat belatedly, the local government got control of the situation, and drunken and disorderly conduct was promptly tried and punished, usually by a fine and imprisonment (Schrader and Brooks 1900, 45). The nineteenth century, however, had closed with alcohol abuse at an all-time high and still climbing.

HEALTH IMPLICATIONS OF ALCOHOL ABUSE

It is difficult to exaggerate the harm that alcohol caused in people in the early history of Alaska. The Russian settlers, particularly the soldiers and workers, were far from home, bored, lonely, and with few pleasures outside their allowance of grog. They were often abused, and their food, clothing, and shelter left much to be desired. Not surprisingly the men turned to alcohol whenever they could get it, not only because it immediately cheered their spirits, but because drunkenness offered oblivion.

For the Natives, except possibly the Koniag, alcohol was a totally new experience that they were unable to cope with right away. It offered a briefly altered perception of life, often pleasurable, and it heightened and fostered social relationships, although sometimes to the point of aggression and violence.

Most Russian workers, Creoles, or Natives probably did not reach the point of what we would call today chronic alcoholism, mainly because alcohol was not readily available most of the time. Opportunities to drink in the settlements were limited to holidays and feast days, or, in the villages, to when the traders were in the vicinity. In both of these situations all the available alcohol was quickly consumed in a binge. Russian officers and company officials, on the other hand, were much more at risk of a true alcohol addiction, because they had access to strong drink throughout the year. They too were subjected to boredom and depression, added to which some probably fiercely resented being posted to what they regarded as a God-forsaken place.

In the American period binge drinking was still the predominant pattern, not only among the Natives but among the settlers, especially the miners. Complicating the situation was that by this time the Tlingit and probably the northern Eskimos had learned how to distill "hootch," just as the Aleuts and Koniag had for years manufactured their *kvass*. Fortunately, the ingredients were not always at hand.

The point should be stressed that by no means all Alaskans drank. Probably the majority of Russian and American men did, but many parts of the vast territory remained totally free of alcohol, particularly the Native villages of the interior. It is easy to be misled about the extent of Native drinking, because it was reported primarily by Whites in notorious drinking towns such as Sitka, Skagway, St. Michael, and Nome, on the periphery of which many drunken Natives were indeed to be found.

If most who drank were binge drinkers, what were the principal health implications? Most important, of course, was violence and trauma, which might take the form of cuts, bruises, fractures, and head injuries. Drowning, falls, frostbite, accidental burns, and pneumonia were more indirect results of intoxication. The failure to hunt or fish during crucial animal and fish migrations could lead to hunger and even starvation in the winter that followed. Drinking also frequently led to social stresses in the home, such as spouse and child abuse, or family breakup. Finally, those who were repeatedly drunk, or who were suffering from chronic alcoholism, were also an easy prey for chronic infections, particularly tuberculosis.

18

Abuse, Hunger, and Violence

ABUSE OF THE ALASKA NATIVES

The Alaska Natives, especially the Aleuts but also the Koniag, Chugach, and Tanaina Indians, suffered much abuse at the hands of the Russians during the eighteenth and early nineteenth centuries. Such ill-treatment was never openly sanctioned by the imperial government; indeed, even Bering had specific instructions on his expedition of 1741 to treat all indigenous peoples with special kindness and not to burden them in any way (Fisher 1977, 125).

Once regular trading voyages were begun to the Aleutians in the 1750s, however, the people of the islands were subjected to many types of harassment and abuse, ultimately leading to a state of virtual enslavement. The Russians, although few in number, had great superiority in weaponry, by which they were rapidly able to cow even the warlike Aleuts into submission. The cruelty with which they treated the Natives doubtless resulted in part from insecurity and the fear of reprisal, which indeed occurred on several occasions. Hector Chevigny (1965, 37) has suggested that the cruelty and contempt shown by the early Russians toward the Aleuts also may have resulted from racial prejudice on the part of mixed-blood Russians from eastern Siberia. Be that as it may, the Russians must have seen as their only economic hope a diminution of the population so that a manageable number could be forced to work as hunters and skin processors (Okun 1979, 194).

After numerous bloody skirmishes in the early 1760s, the Russians systematically exterminated the Aleuts from many villages, especially on Unalaska and Umnak islands, and often took wives and children as hostages to ensure the cooperation and docility of the men (Shelikhov 1981, 128-29; Sauer 1802, 275). Most of the children, elderly, and infirm were left behind in the villages to be "employed in domestic drudgery, and digging edible roots," while the women were forced to make or mend clothing from inferior skins of animals or birds (Sauer 1802, appendix 56). Another early visitor said that sometimes the men of a village were forcibly sent hundreds of miles away for many months at a time, leaving the women to process fish and perform other duties without pay (Okun 1979, 195; Golovnin 1985/86, 65).

From the earliest contacts, the Russians were known to have appropriated for their own pleasure any Aleut or Koniag women who took their fancy. Captain Billings (*in* Burney 1819, 284) described the arrival of a gang of hunters: "They send the natives out on the chace, and then took by force the youngest and most handsome of the women for their companions." And from a document of the same period from the oppressed people of Unalaska: "Not a little do we suffer from the seizure of our girls, wives, daughters, and sisters, practised in general by all companies. . . Though seeing our women kept as mistresses and cruelly treated and knowing the beastly temperament of the hunters, we can not oppose, can not even raise our voices against it" (University of Alaska 1936-1938, 3:238).

In their relentless pursuit of profit the *promyshlenniki* sent the Aleut men out to hunt in all kinds of weather, including the worst winter storms, resulting in many drownings (University of Alaska 1936-38, 3:237). Many others, among both the hunters and those left at home, succumbed to sickness or starvation (Merck 1980, 80; Golovnin 1985/86, 63-64).

Physical abuse of the Aleuts was widespread, especially on the part of the men of certain trading companies, such as those of Ocheredin and Polutov (Shelikhov 1981, 128). Veniaminov (1984, 255) related cases where Aleuts were thrown from cliffs, beaten with axe handles, or slashed with knives for trivial offenses. One Russian was said to have ripped open the belly of an Aleut girl because she ate a piece of whale meat without his permission. One of the worst offenders was a man named Pshenichnoy, who mercilessly whipped the Aleuts with ropes and sticks, thereby causing the death of at least six. Another named Popov murdered with a spear all the girls and two men in the village of Bobrovoy (University of Alaska 1936-1938, 3:237). Golovnin (1985/86, 63-64) in 1818 recorded the complaints of an Aleut named Makar who was cruelly beaten on one occasion because a dog had chewed the sleeve of his birdskin parka, and at another time because he had laughed at a *promyshlennik*.

The true extent of these early abuses will never be known, but it is clear that the Aleut and Koniag populations greatly diminished in the latter half of the eighteenth century, due to murder, drownings, disease, and starvation. Besides those who died, families were broken up and permanently dispersed, women were raped, and children and elderly forced to work far beyond their capacity. Of one group of a hundred Aleut men and women taken to the Alaska Peninsula, only a few remained alive after four years of oppression. What happened to the women, children, and elderly left behind to fend for themselves on the islands is not recorded (University of Alaska 1936-1938, 3:237).

In the 1780s the government in St. Petersburg had instructed Captain Billings to investigate and report on the rumors of cruel behavior by the hunters and merchants in the far-off islands. Billings and his officers not only collected testimony from the Natives but were themselves eyewitnesses to the abuses. His and other such reports reached the higher levels of government and from time to time new instructions were handed down to forbid further cruelties and excesses (Tikhmenev 1978, 143-44). In 1796 the monk Makarii, who had arrived in Kodiak only two years before, returned to St. Petersburg with six Aleuts to plead the cause of the Natives who were being abused. They were able to get an audience with Tsar Paul I himself, but nothing specific came of it, except that Makarii was severely reprimanded by the Holy Synod for having left his post without permission (Barbara Smith 1980, 4; Black 1980, 99). Of the original delegation of six Aleuts none returned to Alaska, the last two survivors dying under suspicious circumstances at Irkutsk (Okun 1979, 195-97). Someone had apparently taken notice, however, for within a few years a church official, Father Gedeon, was sent to look into the matter (Barbara Smith 1980, 4).

The first charter of the Russian-American Company in 1799 had made no specific reference to the treatment of Natives (Bancroft 1886, 379-80). Within only a couple of years, however, Krusenstern on his round-the-world voyage was accusing the company of improper conduct toward the Aleuts and Koniag. Upon hearing of these charges the directors of the company immediately ordered Baranov to respond to them. They then set forth detailed rules designed to prevent further abuses and laid on the chief manager the "sacred duty" of properly carrying them out (Tikhmenev 1978, 143-44).

Following his arrival in 1801, Father Gedeon (*in* Pierce 1978, 54) described in vivid detail how the Russians forced reluctant Koniag to go out to hunt sea otters by threatening them with neck and leg shackles, birch rods, whips, and loaded guns. When one protested, "they seized him, put him in irons, and flogged him until he was hoarse from screaming." Even the sick and elderly were given jobs. A few years later Gedeon reported that Koniag mothers were killing their babies in the womb or deliberately starving them to death to spare them a life of slavery (*in* Pierce 1978, 58).

In 1805 Count Rezanov was appalled by the mistreatment of the Natives by company employees both at Kodiak and in the Aleutians, and took severe measures in response. Despite his own efforts and his authority from the tsar himself, abuses went on throughout Baranov's administration. Among the most frequent later complaints from the Natives was the Russian practice of forcibly taking concubines, although higher officials sometimes required their employees to marry their unwilling mistresses. On his inspection voyage of 1818 Golovnin visited several villages and collected further evidence of mistreatment and abuse (Sarafian 1971, 181-87; Golovnin 1985/86, 63-64).

The company charters of 1821 and again of 1844 made specific reference to relations between the company and the Natives and charged the chief manager with the responsibility for preventing abuse. Although physical mistreatment probably decreased during these years, the Natives had few privileges and continued to be exploited as a work force. For example, men between eighteen and fifty were under obligation to serve the company as hunters, yet they were not permitted to sell or even give away furs except to the company. When selling their furs, they could accept only company merchandise or scrip. One provision of the statutes read "The Company has the right or obligation to prevent the growth of luxury among the Aleuts, such as the use of bread, tea, and similar items" (Okun 1979, 197-98). The company also issued clothing and footgear of poor quality to the Native hunters, an economy which probably contributed to a high prevalence of sickness among the Koniag hunters (Pierce 1984, 167).

Although the Natives bore the brunt of Russian cruelty, the rank and file employees of the company also had a difficult lot, particularly in the earlier years. For the most part they were ill-fed, ill-clothed, ill-housed, and frequently beaten. According to Dr. Langsdorff (1814, 2:92-94), who saw conditions not only in Sitka but also in Kodiak and even Kamchatka, "many of these needy and diseased beings, who were kept daily to very hard work, were unfortunately in debt to the Company, and it not infrequently happened, that when totally exhausted, and lying on a sick-bed, they were driven to their work with blows." Another report around the same period told of an official threatening the Russian workers with a whip (Tikhmenev 1979, 133).

The foregoing description of mistreatment of the Natives under the Russian administration applies primarily to the Aleuts and Koniag, and to some extent also to the people of Cook Inlet and Prince William Sound (*see* Sherwood 1974, 54). In southeastern Alaska the Russians transplanted and used these same peoples for most of their unpleasant work. The Tlingit escaped much of this abuse, largely because the Russians never had the numerical strength to subdue them completely by force of arms. Relatively few Indians were employed by the company until the later years, their contacts with the Russians being primarily as independent hunters and traders. By the time of the company's second charter, many of the Native employees were in fact Creoles, who on the whole were better treated and even sometimes attained positions of respect and authority. When the company expanded its operations to the Yukon-Kuskokwim Delta and Norton Sound in the 1820s and 1830s, there was probably little systematic abuse of the Natives, although individual episodes doubtless occurred.

Nor was there regular harassment or mistreatment of the Natives during the early American period. Alaska Natives were left largely undisturbed in their own homes and villages, although often treated with condescension or contempt. Most of those who came in regular contact with White Americans were hunters, fishermen, or craftsmen interested in trade, although a few were employed in rather menial positions in the larger towns, or later in the century in the canneries and mines. Working conditions were poor and the hours were long, but the employment was at least voluntary and sometimes at a good rate of pay.

The missionaries had a special relationship with the Natives. As teachers, doctors, nurses, and of course ministers, missionary families lived in Native villages for years on end, often learning the local language and customs quite thoroughly. By and large the missionaries had a sincere commitment and respect toward Natives, although sometimes in their zeal for order, discipline, and rapid cultural change, they became seriously at odds with the people they served. Violence might result, as it did at Wales in 1893 (*see* below), but more likely negative outcomes were a sullen passive resistance on the part of the Natives and sometimes overexuberant school discipline by the missionaries (University of Alaska 1936-1938, 3:41).

SCURVY, HUNGER, AND FAMINE

The early history of Alaska is replete with stories of malnutrition and starvation affecting not only individuals and small groups, but also on occasion whole populations. As in aboriginal times, food was a precious and often precarious commodity.

Scurvy was probably the most important single disease affecting the Whites who visited or lived in Alaska during this period. Scurvy, although now known to be caused solely by a deficiency of vitamin C, or ascorbic acid, in the diet, was believed as late as the end of the nineteenth century to be related also to such factors as a lack of potassium, diminished alkalinity of the blood, a specific microorganism, overcrowding, a damp environment, fatigue, depression, and even nostalgia (Osler 1895, 337-38). The disease was a debilitating one, characterized by weakness, bleeding gums, loosened teeth, swollen painful joints, and hemorrhagic bruising of the skin.

As early as the seventeenth century scurvy had been recognized as being somehow related to a lack of fresh fruits and vegetables in the diet, and more enlightened sea captains, notably Cook, took special precautions to prevent it (Watt 1979, 130-32). Most, however, considered the disease to be an inevitable hazard of a long voyage, as the trip to Alaska almost always was. Chapter 5 has recounted some of the disastrous consequences of a steady diet of salt meat and hardtack on the voyages of Bering, Chirikov, Glotov, Krenitsyn, Arteaga, Meares, Billings, and Zaikov (Fortuine 1988a).

Nor was scurvy by any means confined to ships' crews. Shelikhov's infant colony at Three Saints' Bay nearly failed because of a severe outbreak of scurvy in the winter of 1784-1785 (Shelikhov 1981, 46). Likewise, the early Russian settlement at Yakutat suffered overwhelming losses from the disease during the winter of 1795-1796. In the following years similar gloomy reports came from the company post at Unalaska (Bancroft 1886, 357, 417).

Perhaps the most significant outbreak of scurvy during the Russian period was that occurring at New Archangel in the winter and spring of 1805-1806 (*see* Chapter 6). By the begining of February eight had died and 60 out of the 150 who remained were laid up in their barracks totally unfit for work. "The scurvy," according to Dr. Langsdorff (1814, 2:94), "commonly showed itself first by debility, listlessness and melancholy; inflammatory spots, sometimes larger, sometimes smaller, then appeared on the legs from the knees to the toes, which in a short time turned to sores." Those who were thus affected were made to stand guard duty and even forced to exercise, in the mistaken belief that it was helpful. When the doctor applied to the overseers to find better food and lodging for those who were suffering, "They laughed at me, and said 'That must be a pretty doctor who could cure his patients with good eating and drinking, instead of medicine'" (Langsdorff 1814, 2:97). Count Rezanov (*in* Tikhmenev 1979, 175) wrote in February of that year that despite the use of spruce beer as a preventative, "Some are walking, but look bad; men who looked better have sometimes been put in a coffin." With the colony faced with starvation, Rezanov (1926, 5-8, 69) took a ship in March to buy provisions from the Spanish settlement in San Francisco. By the time of his return the situation was somewhat improved because of the availability of green plants and fresh fish once more. But that winter seventeen Russians had died at Sitka and sixty more were incapacitated. In his report Rezanov also noted that many of "our Americans" (presumably Aleut and Koniag employees) had died of the disease. Scurvy also decimated the settlement at St. Paul's Harbor in Kodiak that year (Tikhmenev 1979, 222; Fortuine 1988a).

In the later years of the company scurvy was rare, largely because provisioning ships arrived with much greater regularity, including those from the Fort Ross colony in California. In 1853, however, sixty-four cases occurred at Sitka, resulting in nine deaths. Typhoid fever was also unusually prevalent that year (Andrews 1916, 293). In the outlying posts scurvy was a much greater hazard because of the uncertainty of travel; for example, in 1856 eighteen of forty laborers at the coal mine on the Kenai Peninsula developed scurvy and one died (Pierce 1975, 106). In 1863 Father Netsvetov (1984, 459-62) himself contracted scurvy at St. Michael.

Scurvy again became a scourge in the last decade of the nineteenth century among the many ill-provisioned miners and prospectors who trekked through the interior of Alaska seeking instant wealth. Although scattered cases occurred in the Yukon and Tanana river valleys and along the Chilkoot Trail, the worst disaster was that which overtook the many hopefuls who tried to reach the Klondike by crossing the Valdez Glacier in the spring of 1899 (*see* Chapter 9). Many succumbed to scurvy, frostbite, and accidents either on the glacier or in the Copper River basin. Dr. Leroy Townsend (*in* Abercrombie 1900a, 44-47) attended numerous scurvy victims and wrote in arresting clinical detail about the natural history of the disease. His prescriptions for cure make excellent sense still: "Supply fresh fruit and vegetables, lemons, oranges, apples, potatoes, cabbage, etc., together with fresh meat if available. . . . Divert the mind of the patient and inspire hope and cheerfulness." A chronicle of the sufferings of the miners on the Copper River route in 1898-1899 is that of Horace Conger, whose diary has recently been published (1983).

The Alaska Natives rarely suffered from scurvy on their traditional diet, since they normally ingested adequate vitamin C in greens, berries, fresh meat, and fish. Despite many episodes of hunger and even starvation, scurvy was encountered principally when the Natives were depending on the diet of the Russians or Americans. For example, scurvy was mentioned among the hunters at Sitka in 1806 (Tikhmenev 1979, 175), among the Eskimos near St. Michael in 1898 (Edmonds 1966, 29), and notably among nearly all of the boarding school children at the Holy Cross Mission in 1890 (Calasanctius 1947, 142).

Scurvy develops when caloric intake is adequate but ascorbic acid is insufficient. During the early historical period in Alaska food shortages led to several episodes of frank starvation and widespread hunger, but without the development of scurvy, among both Natives and Caucasians.

Although the Aleuts had suffered periodic hunger throughout their life on the islands, famine and starvation became a constant specter with the arrival of the *promyshlenniki*. Families were broken up, with the men being forcibly sent out to hunt sea otter for furs instead of for food for their wives and children, who were left in the villages without support for months or years at a time. The worst recorded famine in the eighteenth century was in and around Unalaska in 1762, and this greatly diminished the Aleut population (Coxe 1787, 215; Masterson and Brower 1948, 58). Times of hunger affecting smaller groups, however, occurred throughout the latter part of the eighteenth century (Merck 1980, 80). The situation was no better in the villages of Kodiak Island, as Father Gedeon wrote (*in* Pierce 1978, 55): "Because of the onerous company duties the Aleuts in all the villages are in the winter subjected to great hunger: they eat the seal bladders in which they store fat and salmon roe, laftoks, cord and other articles made from gut, because they have no shellfish and seaweed when the beaches are covered with ice. . . . They look more like corpses than living people." Conditions improved after the establishment of the Russian-American Company in 1799, but even well into the nineteenth century occasional reports of starvation were known in the Aleutians (Kashevaroff 1927, 55).

The Russians probably did not take enough game on the mainland coast and in the interior to upset seriously the food cycles of the Natives, and the occasional reports of famine that occurred in the early nineteenth century (e.g., Wrangell 1970, 7; Oswalt 1960, 102, 106; University of Alaska 1936-1938, 2:90) were probably due to the periodic fluctuations in the abundance of animals and fish that had been known for centuries. Likewise, in the American period some episodes of famine among the Natives were doubtless caused by natural cycles of traditional food supplies (Spurr 1899, 73; Schwalbe 1951, 47; Nelson 1978, 39).

New factors, however, were entering the equation. The introduction of firearms on the north coast and in the interior profoundly changed Native hunting methods and increased the kill of sea mammals as well as of large land mammals, such as caribou and moose. Competition in shooting game also came from whalers, miners, and traders. Shooting sea mammals from a boat or from the shore ice was deadly efficient but frequently resulted in non-recovery of the carcass. It is clear, however, that the major decline in bowhead whales and walrus, at least, must be attributed to the unrestricted killing by the commercial whalers, not by the Natives.

Another significant cause of hunger was the consequence of the introduction of epidemic or debilitating diseases among the Natives. Hunger occurred after all major epidemics because the hunters and fishermen were left without the strength to provide for their families (e.g., Petroff 1882, 114; Brower 1960, 37; Brady 1900, 32, 51). Another external factor was probably alcohol abuse (Petroff 1882, 45), especially in a few coastal villages where the food supply was precarious even in the best of times. It was certainly possible that extended drunkenness could prevent the hunters and fishermen from profiting from the best salmon runs or the critical migrations of the walrus or caribou.

By all odds the best documented and most tragic episode of starvation in historical times was that which occurred on St. Lawrence Island in the winter and spring of 1878-1879. The first rumors of wholesale starvation reached Captain Bailey (1880, 26) during the 1879 voyage of the *Rush,* when a trading schooner called at the island in September and found all the people dead at three settlements. According to survivors at other villages, the people had starved from their inability to hunt seals, walrus, and whales because of an unusually early ice breakup. The following summer Capt. C. L. Hooper (1881, 10-11) of the *Corwin* had orders to investigate this incident more fully. He visited some four villages on the north side of the island, finding no one living except at the fourth one, which was probably the present village of Gambell. In each of the first three he found mostly bodies of adult males, the women and children probably having died first and been buried, a view confirmed by a whaleman who had visited the previous year (Bockstoce 1986, 138). Estimating from the number of bodies found, and from the stories of survivors, Hooper guessed that over four hundred persons had died that winter. At the large village some three hundred people remained, most of whom had barely survived by eating their dogs and the walrus hides covering their boats. The people attributed the tragedy to persistent cold, stormy weather that prevented hunting walrus and seal. Although the Eskimos did not implicate alcohol in the tragedy, Hooper noted that the islanders would trade only for whiskey, breech-loading rifles, and cartridges.

The *Corwin* stopped at St. Lawrence Island again the following year, and this time Hooper (1884, 100-101) was able to investigate the situation more thoroughly. He visited five out of six villages on the island. At three all inhabitants were dead, at the fourth sixteen people of two families survived, and at the fifth (which was not visited) nearly all had died. At the large village two hundred out of six hundred perished. In one house they counted some thirty bodies, and in one of the settlements found eight or nine bodies in a summer house, suggesting that the people had survived the winter. Nowhere did they find evidence of cannibalism. (*See* Figure 24.)

John Muir (1917, 107-8) traveled on the *Corwin* in 1881 and left his own account of the events of that terrible year of famine. He estimated that about 1000 out of an original population of 1500 had perished, including every inhabitant of seven villages. His moving description is unsurpassed:

> We found twelve desolate huts close to the beach with about 200 skeletons in them or strewn about on the rocks and rubbish heaps within a few yards of the doors. The scene was indescribably ghastly and desolate, though laid in a country purified by frost as by fire. Gulls, plovers, and ducks were swimming and flying about in happy life, the pure salt sea was dashing white against the shore, the blooming tundra swept back to the snow-clad volcanoes, and the wide azure sky bent kindly over all—nature intensely fresh and sweet, the village lying in the foulest and most glaring death.

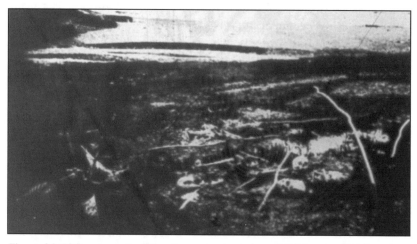

Figure 24. Human remains from the mass starvation of Eskimos on St. Lawrence Island in the winter of 1878-79. (Healy 1889.)

Muir went ashore with the naturalist E. W. Nelson, who was collecting for the ethnological museum of the Smithsonian Institution. Nelson obviously had a different perspective of the grisly scene for he, according to Muir (1917, 110), "went into this Golgotha with hearty enthusiasm, gathering the fine white harvest of skulls spread before him, and throwing them in heaps like a boy gathering pumpkins. He brought nearly a hundred on board."

Controversy still exists on the cause of this grim tragedy. Hooper had no specific evidence for any part played by alcohol, although he suspected the whiskey trade as the ultimate cause. Muir (1917, 109) stated that starvation could not have been the whole story, since some families seem to have died despite some edible objects, such as skins, lying around the dwellings. Dr. Rosse (1883, 21), who also visited the scene, pointed out that alcohol could hardly have been the whole answer, since the hunger affected every village on the island, and the Eskimos could not have obtained enough alcohol to last for more than a few days' drunk. He himself suspected that an epidemic may have been the problem, especially since a whaler who visited in 1878 had spoken of "measles or black tongue," which he was supposed to have seen among the dying. Such signs, however, also could have resulted from the hemorrhages of scurvy. The Eskimos themselves steadfastly maintained that the weather and resulting ice conditions were the ultimate cause of the disaster.

NEW FORMS OF VIOLENCE AND INJURY

With the arrival of Europeans in Alaska in the mid-eighteenth century, violence and personal injury took on added dimensions. As detailed in Chapter 5, the early Russian traders were an unscrupulous lot who did not hesitate to use firearms and other "modern" weapons to force their will first on the Aleuts and later on the Koniag. As early as 1745 gunfire rang out at Agattu and a musket ball tore open the hand of a hapless Aleut (Berkh 1974, 4-5), only the first volley in many uneven encounters that occurred in the islands over the next half-century.

After numerous bloody incidents and minor skirmishes, the Aleuts by 1762 had had their fill and rose up in armed resistance at several places, perhaps with the vain hope of driving off the Russians once and for all. Several prominent Russians were killed during a coordinated uprising in 1763-1764, in which the Aleuts attacked hunting parties and overwintering ships on Unalaska and the surrounding islands. Terrible reprisals followed, led by Soloviev and Glotov, who systematically murdered hundreds of islanders and destroyed their means of subsistence (Black 1980, 94-95).

Bloody hostilities also occurred between the Koniag and Russians, beginning with the first visit by Glotov in 1763. When Shelikhov arrived in 1784 to establish a permanent settlement, the Koniag resolutely defended their island with spears and arrows, but were quickly overwhelmed by the force of superior weaponry, including ship's cannon.

In southeastern Alaska the warlike Tlingit annihilated the first Russian settlement near Sitka in 1802, for which the Russians took fearful vengeance two years later, aided by the guns of the warship *Neva*. In 1805 the Tlingit destroyed the Russian colony at Yakutat, leaving few to tell the tale (Khlebnikov 1973, 56). For most of the next few decades an uneasy peace reigned in southeastern Alaska. The Russians were always prepared for trouble, while the Tlingit for their part kept a weather eye for any military weakness on the part of the outsiders. In 1852 the Stikine Tlingit destroyed the buildings around the hot springs near Sitka and three years later the Sitka Tlingit even attacked the capital itself, where they were repulsed with heavy losses by musketry and cannon (Bancroft 1886, 574-75; Tikhmenev 1978, 353).

The Russians were able to maintain their hegemony with harsh measures in Sitka, Kodiak, and the Aleutians, while rather peaceably extending their rule to the Eskimo areas of Bristol Bay, the Yukon-Kuskokwim Delta and Norton Sound. A notable exception to this peaceful expansion was the Russian attempt to penetrate the Copper River basin in the first half of the nineteenth century. The hostile Ahtna more than once showed armed resistance to the outside intrusion and in 1848 wiped out the entire exploring party of Serebrennikov (*See* Chapter 6).

A further bloody encounter took place in 1851 at the isolated Russian settlement at Nulato, on the middle Yukon River, where twelve years earlier another episode of violence had occurred (Zagoskin 1967, 275). Lieutenant John Barnard, a junior officer on Collinson's ship *Enterprise*, had accompanied a Russian party inland to the post about a hundred miles away. From there he sent a Russian employee to a Koyukon village about twenty miles further upriver to make some inquiries, but the man was set upon and killed by the Indians. Almost immediately a war party descended on an Indian village about one mile from the Russian post, burning the houses and killing all the inhabitants. Early next morning, February 15, 1851, the Koyukon party attacked the trading post at Nulato. They killed the trader Deriabin as he came outside, then rushed into the quarters, where Barnard was shot in the abdomen during the ensuing struggle. He lingered for a day or two, long enough to write a brief message to Mr. Adams, the ship's surgeon, who was waiting at St. Michael. Adams hurried to the scene but Bernard was already dead (Collinson 1889, 126-28; Whymper 1868, 183-85; Netsvetov 1984, 259). The cause of the attack remains obscure, but it may be that Lieutenant Barnard just happened to be in the wrong place and was caught in the cross-fire of an internecine struggle, or perhaps of a war party directed at the Russians.

Although the American soldiers who enforced the peace after 1867 were fresh from the battlefields of the Civil War and the western Indian frontier, they encountered little more than sullen hostility from the Tlingit and other Alaska Natives, who by this time had reluctantly resigned themselves to sharing their ancestral lands with the Whites. Although no pitched battles are recorded in southeastern Alaska between American military forces and the Indians, the Americans were always edgy and probably expected a general uprising. As recounted in Chapter 8, an incident occurred in 1869 in which two White traders were killed by the Kake Indians in reprisal for an Indian shot by a sentry at Sitka. When the Kakes refused to give up the "murderers," the military commander ordered the destruction of several of their villages by naval gunfire (Bancroft 1886, 611-12). Another ugly incident of the same nature occurred in 1882 when compensation was refused to the Indians for some of their men killed accidentally on the job. When the traditional indemnity payment was refused, the Indians captured several White men, which in turn led to the naval bombardment of the village of Angoon, an event that even today is deeply ingrained in the consciousness of these people (De Laguna 1960, 158-61).

On a smaller scale were the many isolated incidents of violence that occurred throughout the nineteenth century, some of them secondary to the effects of alcohol. Three such notable events during the American period were the murder of a trader's wife, Mrs. Bean, by the Indians on the Tanana River in 1878 (C. Hooper 1881, 17; Mercier 1986, 20-21), the murder by one of his assistants of the Bishop of Vancouver, Charles-Jean Seghers, near Nulato in 1886 (Mercier 1986, 51), and the murder of the schoolteacher-missionary Thornton at Wales in 1893.

This last incident deserves special mention because Thornton was one of the first missionary-teachers in northern Alaska. The whole episode demonstrated the tragic outcome of a clash of cultures, with neither side willing to compromise. Arriving at Wales in July 1890, he and his colleague William T. Lopp had a difficult time in a village that by its location had felt many of the bad effects of frequent contacts with the illicit liquor traders. Thornton had suffered from depression in the past and was known as a strict disciplinarian, even carrying a gun at all times. After limited success the first year, Thornton left for a year, returning in 1892 with a new wife. His mental condition was unchanged, however, and soon he was in trouble with the Eskimos again. Thornton and his wife remained as the only missionaries in 1893-1894. Since he constantly felt that his life was in danger from drunken Eskimos, he asked Captain Healy of the *Bear* to make a show of force at the village. Healy demurred and later in the summer Thornton was killed with a whaling gun at his home. Three young men were implicated by the villagers and all three were ultimately executed by the village elders in accordance with their own canons of justice (D. Ray 1975, 217-22; Strickland 1986).

The bloodiest alcohol-related incident has come to be known as the "Gilley affair," which occurred offshore near Wales in 1877. Several conflicting accounts exist of this encounter between the Eskimos and the crew of a Hawaiian trading brig *Wm. H. Allen,* which was trading foxskins for liquor one evening some distance from shore. According to Captain Gilley (or Gilly, or Gillie) himself (*in* Brower 1960, 78), who is not necessarily the most reliable witness of the event, the Eskimos who paddled out to the ship in umiaks the following day were intoxicated. They demanded ammunition and more alcohol, but having nothing further to trade, they were refused. Tempers flared, and the mate hit one of the unruly Eskimos, whereupon another stabbed the mate to death with a knife. The crew, who were mostly Hawaiians, then grabbed axes, boat-hooks, and other weapons and attacked the Eskimos, driving them into the fo'c's'le. One by one the sailors yanked them out, clubbed them to death and threw the bodies over the side. The only survivor was a woman who had hid under some canvas in one of the umiaks. Another account from a whaling captain (*in* Jenness 1957, 158-9) said the the row started when an Eskimo was struck down by a sailor as he was about to stab the captain from behind. In addition to killing those who had come on board, Gilley was said to have fired on and sunk the umiaks around the ship. Captain Bailey (1880, 20) of the Revenue Marine Service reported that fifteen persons, including one woman, died in the melee, whereas Captain Hooper (1881, 20) the following year mentioned well over thirty victims. In still another version Gilley himself (*in* Aldrich 1889, 143-6) reported twenty killed.

Epilogue

In brief summary, the early history of Alaska properly begins before Bering's voyages and thus before written records are available. The traditions relating to health and hygiene in daily life go back many centuries and to some degree are carried on today in the lives of many Alaska Natives, although probably in modified form.

The health of the Native peoples of Alaska was not always good in aboriginal times, although it was probably better then than following contact. In earlier times the Natives were subject to many hazards associated with their pattern of living. In the home and village burns, falls, cuts, and bruises took their toll and many suffered from chronically sore eyes from smoke irritation in the home. Subsistence activities were especially dangerous and not infrequently led to drowning, cold injury, or mutilation by wild animals. Food was scarce in the winter and spring months, sometimes leading to frank starvation. Other foods were toxic, either due to contamination or methods of preparing them. Snowblindness was a common problem in the spring and the summer brought unbelievable hordes of biting insects.

Poor personal hygiene and the unwholesome home and village environment contributed to the spread of infectious diseases among the people. Boils and open skin sores were prevalent at all ages and nearly every person suffered from head and body lice. Gastrointestinal upsets often resulted from contaminated food, and internal parasites were frequently the consequence of inadequately cooked food or of close contact with animals and their products. Infections of the respiratory tract were fostered by crowded, poorly ventilated homes, and included colds, ear infections, bronchitis, pneumonia, and pleurisy.

Nor were the Natives spared degenerative diseases. Chronic arthritis was aggravated by the cold, damp climate. Cancer occurred sporadically, as did arteriosclerotic disease and probably stroke. Congenital disorders were relatively frequent because of the inbreeding resulting from small isolated populations. Blindness, deafness, and various crippling disorders were also common.

The arrival of Europeans in Alaska changed none of these morbidity and mortality patterns, but only added new health problems to an already burdened people. The newcomers brought first of all violence and cruelty, which led to deaths in their own right. They also brought alcohol and, indirectly, tobacco, both of which were to cause slow but certain death to many who abused them.

Most deadly of all, of course, were the infectious diseases to which the Alaska Natives had had no prior exposure and hence no immunity. The first great plague was probably smallpox, brought into southeastern Alaska from the southward in the 1770s. Syphilis likewise reached epidemic proportions in the eighteenth century in the Aleutians, Kodiak, and other regions under Russian influence. Throughout the nineteenth century influenza and measles swept repeatedly through the Native villages of Alaska, culminating in the dreadful epidemic of 1900, in which both diseases simultaneously ravaged the whole of western Alaska from the Aleutians to the Arctic Circle. Even more destructive was the great smallpox epidemic of 1835 to 1840, which laid waste the entire southern half of Alaska, causing the deaths of an estimated one-third of the Native population. There were other introduced infectious diseases, including diphtheria, whooping cough, gonorrhea, and typhoid, but none so ruinous as tuberculosis, which moved more slowly but no less surely through the susceptible population, causing death, disability, and misery.

Adding new and terrible diseases to peoples already in precarious health led to a rapid decline of what had been a stable population, to the extent that by 1900 there were some fears of the extinction of the original inhabitants of the land.

But the failing health of the Alaska Natives was not the only dimension of Alaskan medical history, albeit the most significant. Many of those who came to Alaska from far-off lands, sometimes half a world away, themselves found injury, sickness, and not infrequently death. Some brought sickness with them and passed it on to the Natives, unknowingly and of course unintentionally. Others developed sickness from the cold, damp climate, lack of fresh food, poorly ventilated quarters, and hard labor. Of all the diseases affecting the Europeans, scurvy was perhaps the most important, decimating many ships' crews, fur-trading posts, and later the mining camps. Alcoholism was another major cause of disability and death among the lonely Alaskan settlers.

The history of medical care in Alaska is also an integral part of the story. The Native people for centuries had depended on their shamans for treatment of the more severe and mysterious illnesses. For the care of the minor injuries and illnesses of everyday life, however, they turned to family members, village elders, skilled midwives, herbalists, and surgeons, all of whom over time had developed useful methods of treatment, some of which still seem reasonable today.

The early ships' surgeons provided little care to the Native people, but by their writings they did contribute much to our understanding of Native culture, including health practices and disease patterns.

The Russian-American Company first assigned a physician to Alaska in 1820 and over the next few decades evolved a very sophisticated health care system for the benefit of their employees. The system included hospitals in Sitka and Kodiak, and several smaller health facilities under the supervision of *feldshers* in the more remote posts. The physicians at Sitka not only supervised the whole program, but also were responsible for training surgeons' apprentices and midwives for service in outlying areas. Treatment as well as prevention was stressed, as evidenced by a vigorous smallpox vaccination program and measures taken to prevent the spread of syphilis. Although the program was designed for the employees of the company, some Natives benefited directly or indirectly.

Medical care took a step backward during the early years of American administration, as the Russian health care system was dismantled and nothing took its place. Although the Army and Navy offered limited services in the earlier years, the first consistent but episodic medical care for the Natives was provided by the doctors of the Revenue Marine Service ships that regularly patrolled the Alaskan waters, especially after 1879. In the last decade of the nineteenth century several medical missionaries arrived in Alaska and devoted their full energies to the Natives. For the rest of the population, care was available sporadically from private physicians who set up shop in Sitka and later in the gold-mining towns such as Juneau, Circle City, and Nome.

And what of Alaska's health and history after 1900? By the turn of the century, Alaska's future course was already irrevocably determined. Economic development—first of furs and minerals, later of fish and timber, and in our own day of petroleum—has been and still is the dominant theme of the twentieth century. More and more outsiders have streamed in, first to make their fortune and later to make their home. The two world wars, especially the second, brought a great influx of new Alaskans, as did the oil boom of the 1970s.

By 1900, nearly all the important diseases of the twentieth century had already been introduced. Infectious diseases continued to plague the territory, particularly the more remote areas, which were suffering "virgin soil" epidemics of polio, measles, rubella, and mumps as late as the 1960s. The Spanish influenza pandemic of 1918-1919 also struck Alaska hard, this time not only devastating the Natives but the Caucasian population as well.

The greatest epidemic of the twentieth century, however, was one of the legacies of earlier times, tuberculosis, which probably reached its peak around the end of World War II. The disease killed, maimed, or disabled thousands of Natives and not a few Whites, until it was gradually brought under control in the 1960s by a combination of intensive case-finding and the development of new antituberculosis drugs, notably isoniazid, which could be used not only as a treatment but also as a preventative. (Fortuine 1975a, 21-22; Fortuine 1986, 5-6, 21-24). In the 1980s some "new" infections, such as hepatitis A and B, *Haemophilus influenzae* type b infection ("Hib"), herpes simplex type II, and *Chlamydia* have taken center stage in the area of communicable disease. Perhaps one day acquired immune deficiency syndrome (AIDS) will become the greatest plague of them all.

Over the last few decades the health of all Alaskans has greatly improved, due to higher incomes, better housing, improved water supplies, more effective treatment methods, and the greater availability of medical care. These changes have been particularly evident in the Native population. Infectious diseases, including tuberculosis, are no longer the terrible threat they once were. Accident rates remain high, and now cancer, hypertension, emphysema, heart disease, and diabetes are gaining ground, just as they are in the general population. Among the major health indicators, infant mortality and general mortality rates have fallen almost to the level of the rest of the Alaskan population. Of the prominent diseases of an earlier era, only alcoholism remains a deadly threat to the health of all Alaskans.

Shortly after the turn of the century the federal government finally recognized a responsibility for the health care of the Natives and began to provide doctors, nurses, and later hospitals through the U.S. Bureau of Education. In 1931 federal health services for the Natives were transferred to the Bureau of Indian Affairs, which built several new hospitals in remote areas over the next two decades. On July 1, 1955 all Native health facilities and programs were taken over by the U.S. Public Health Service, which continues to operate or fund them today. A particularly encouraging development has been the passage by Congress in 1975 of the Indian Self-Determination and Education Assistance Act (P.L. 93-638). This law has allowed Native regional non-profit corporations or health corporations to contract with the federal goverment for the management of many of the health programs that serve the Native people.

What then may we conclude from studying the history of health and disease in Alaska? Is it any more than an arcane nook of scholarly endeavor? In reply, may I suggest the following:

1. For the Alaska Natives themselves, the original occupants of the land, the study of health conditions resulting from contact with the outside is important for a better understanding of their own heritage. Some Natives lean to the view that their ancestors lived in a state of pristine good health, unencumbered by infection or degenerative disease. According to this view, infants were born healthy, survived the manifold dangers of infancy and childhood, and lived long, productive lives, the minor indispositions along the way being successfully treated by family members, traditional practitioners, or shamans. In this admittedly exaggerated perspective, serious disease and disability arrived only with the Russians and other Europeans from beyond the horizon. Such a perception is obviously distorted, as this book has tried to prove.

2. For the eighty percent or more of the Alaskan population who were born elsewhere or who are the descendants of earlier settlers, the study of health and disease in former times may provide greater insight into their own history. The history of Alaska contains some painful truths about the impact that Europeans, and later Americans, had on Native societies, which had over centuries achieved a remarkable balance with the realities of life in the Subarctic and Arctic. Alaska, like the West, was not simply "won;" it was settled at a terrible cost to its original inhabitants, by means of the force of numbers and of superior technology. Hunger and disease among the Native peoples, brought on as the indirect result of this settlement, greatly hastened the outcome.

3. Finally, for historians generally, the study of the impact of health and disease on peoples and events can add an important dimension to the social, political, and economic history of a region. Nearly everyone will concede that health and disease often have been crucial factors leading to the subjection, decline, and even threatenened cultural extinction of populations. That more attention has not been paid to these forces—by historians both in Alaska and elsewhere—is unfortunate, but may reflect the view that the determinants of health and disease, at least until recently, lay almost completely beyond human control.

References Cited

Abercrombie, W. R.
  1900a   *Alaska, 1899. Copper River exploring expedition.*
                  Washington, D.C.: Government Printing Office.
  1900b   A supplementary expedition into the Copper River Valley,
                  Alaska. In *Compilation of narratives of explorations in
                  Alaska. See* U.S. Senate, 1900:383-408.

A'Court, H. Holmes
  1976   H.M.S. *Osprey* at Sitka 1879. *Alaska Journal* 6(2):124-27.

Adams, George R.
  1982   *Life on the Yukon 1865-1867.* Edited by Richard A. Pierce.
                  Kingston, Ontario: Limestone Press.

Ager, Thomas A. and Lynn Price Ager
  1980   Ethnobotany of the Eskimos of Nelson Island, Alaska.
                  Arctic Anthropology 17(1):27-47.

Alberts, Laurie
  1977   Petticoats and pickaxes. *Alaska Journal* 7(3):146-59.

Aldrich, Herbert L.
  1889   *Arctic Alaska and Siberia, or, eight months with the arctic
                  whalemen.* Chicago and New York: Rand, McNally and
                  Co.

Allen, Henry T.
  1887   *Report of an expedition to the Copper, Tanana, and
                  Koyukuk rivers in the Territory of Alaska, in the year 1885.*
                  Washington, D.C.: Government Printing Office.

Almquist, L. Arden
  1962   *Covenant missions in Alaska.* Chicago: Covenant Press.

Anderson, Eva Greenslit
  1942   *Dog-team doctor: The story of Dr. Romig.* Caldwell, Idaho:
                  Caxton Printers.

Anderson, J. P.
  1939   Plants used by the Eskimos of the northern Bering Sea and
                  arctic regions of Alaska. *American Journal of Botany*
                  26:714-16.

Andrews, Clarence L.
  1916   Alaska under the Russians—industry, trade and social life.
                  Washington Historical Quarterly 7(4):278-95.
  1945   Settlement of Sitka. Reprinted in *Alaska and its history.*
                  See Sherwood 1967:46-55.

Andreyev, A. I., ed.
1952   *Russian discoveries on the Pacific and in North America in the eighteenth and nineteenth centuries*. Trans. by Carl Ginsburg. Ann Arbor, Mich.: American Council of Learned Societies.

Archer, Christon I.
1980   Russians, Indians, and passages: Spanish voyages to Alaska in the eighteenth century. In: *Exploration in Alaska. Captain Cook commemorative lectures, June-November 1978,* edited by Antoinette Shalkop and Robert L. Shalkop. Anchorage, Alaska: Cook Inlet Historical Society, 1980: 128-143.

Arctander, John W.
1909   *The apostle of Alaska: The story of William Duncan of Metlakahtla*. Toronto: Fleming H. Revell Co.

Arndt, Katherine L.
1985   The Russian-American Company and the smallpox epidemic of 1835 to 1840. Paper presented at the 12th Annual Meeting, Alaska Anthropological Association. Anchorage, Alaska, March 2, 1985.

Aronson, Joseph D.
1940   The history of disease among the natives of Alaska. *Transactions and Studies of the College of Physicians of Philadelphia*. 8(series 4):27-34.

Arteaga, Ygnacio
n.d.   Spain claims Alaska 1779. Diary of the commander, Don Ygnacio Arteaga. Trans. by Katrina Moore. Typescript. M3-E3, box 2, binder 8, Spanish exploration of Alaska. Fairbanks, Alaska: Archives, Alaska and Polar Region Dept., University of Alaska Fairbanks.

Athearn, Robert G., ed.
1949   An army officer's trip to Alaska in 1869. *Pacific Northwest Quarterly* 40(1):44-64.

Austin, Basil
1968   *The diary of a ninety-eighter*. Mt. Pleasant, Mich.: John Cumming.

Bailey, George W.
1880   *Report on Alaska and its people*. Washington, D.C.: Government Printing Office.

Balcom, Mary G.
1970   *The Catholic Church in Alaska*. Chicago: Adams Press.

Bancroft, Hubert Howe
1886   *History of Alaska 1730-1885*. Reprint 1959. New York: Antiquarian Press.

Bank, Theodore P. II
1953   Botanical and ethnobotanical studies in the Aleutian
                         Islands II. Health and medical lore of the Aleuts. *Papers of
                         the Michigan Academy of Science* 38:415-31.
Beardslee, L. A.
1882   *Reports relative to affairs in Alaska and the operations of
                         the U.S.S.* Jamestown. Washington, D.C.: Government
                         Printing Office.
Beechey, Frederick W.
1831   *Narrative of a voyage to the Pacific and Beering's Strait,
                         to cooperate with the polar expeditions: Performed in His
                         Majesty's Ship* Blossom, *under the command of Captain F.
                         W. Beechey, R.N., F.R.S. etc., in the years 1825, 26, 27, 28.*
                         Two volumes. Reprint 1967. Amsterdam: N. Israel; New
                         York: Da Capo Press.
Belcher, Edward, and Francis Guillemard Simpkinson
1979   *H.M.S.* Sulphur *on the northwest and California coasts,
                         1837 and 1839.* Edited by Richard A. Pierce and John H.
                         Winslow. Kingston, Ontario: Limestone Press.
Bender, Thomas R., T. S. Jones, W. E. De Witt, G. J. Kaplan, A. R. Saslow,
       S. Edward Nevius, Paul S. Clark, and E. J. Gangarosa
1972   Salmonella associated with whale meat in an Eskimo
                         community: Serologic and bacteriologic methods as
                         adjuncts to an epidemiological investigation. *American
                         Journal of Epidemiology* 96(2):153-60.
Benjamin, Anna Northend
1898   The Innuit of Alaska. *Outlook* 58:857-64.
Bensin, Basil M.
n.d.   *Russian Orthodox Church in Alaska 1794-1967.* Sitka:
                         Russian Orthodox Greek Catholic Church of North
                         America, Diocese of Alaska.
Berkh, Vasilii Nikolaevich
1974   *A chronological history of the discovery of the Aleutian
                         Islands or the exploits of Russian merchants.* Translated by
                         Dmitri Krenov. Edited by Richard A. Pierce. Kingston,
                         Ontario: Limestone Press.
1979   *The wreck of the* Neva. Translated by Antoinette Shalkop.
                         Anchorage, Alaska: Alaska Historical Society and Sitka
                         Historical Society.
Birket-Smith, Kaj
1953   *The Chugach Eskimos.* Nationalmuseet Skrifter.
                         Etnografisk Raekke VI. Copenhagen: Nationalmuseets
                         Publikationsfond.

Birket-Smith, Kaj, and Frederica De Laguna
1938   *The Eyak Indians of the Copper River Delta, Alaska.*
                             Copenhagen: Levin and Munksgaard.
Black, Lydia T., trans. and ed.
1977   The Konyag (the inhabitants of the Island of Kodiak) by
                             Iosaf [Bolotov] (1794-1799) and by Gideon (1804-1807).
                             Arctic Anthropology 14(2):79-108.
1980   Early history. *Alaska Geographic* 7(3):82-105.
1984   *Atka. An ethnohistory of the western Aleutians.* Kingston,
                             Ontario: Limestone Press.
Blaschke, Eduard Leontjevich
1842   *Topographia medica portus Novi-Archangelscensis, sedis
                             principalis coloniarum rossicarum in Septentrionali
                             America.* St. Petersburg, Russia: K. Wienhöber and Son.
Blee, Catherine Holder
[1986]   *Wine, yaman and stone: The archeology of a Russian
                             hospital pit.* Sitka National Historical Park, Sitka, Alaska.
                             Denver: U.S. Department of the Interior, National Park
                             Service.
Bockstoce, J. R.
1977   *Eskimos of northwest Alaska in the early nineteenth
                             century.* Oxford: University of Oxford, Pitt River's
                             Museum.
1986   *Whales, ice, and men. The history of whaling in the
                             western Arctic.* Seattle and London: University of
                             Washington Press, in association with the New Bedford
                             Whaling Museum.
Bodega y Quadra, Juan Francisco de la
n.d.   The first Spanish landing in Alaska. Bodega's narrative of
                             the voyage of the *Sonora,* 1775. Trans. by Katrina Moore.
                             Typescript. M3-E3, box 2, binder 7, Spanish explorations
                             of Alaska. Fairbanks, Alaska: Archives, Alaska and Polar
                             Regions Dept., University of Alaska Fairbanks.
Book, Patricia A., Mim Dixon, and Scott Kirchner
1983   Native healing in Alaska. Report from Serpentine Hot
                             Springs. *Western Journal of Medicine* 139(6):923-27.
Boyd, William L.
1972   Jarvis and the Alaskan reindeer caper. *Arctic* 25(2):74-82.
Brady, John G.
1900   *Report of the Governor of the District of Alaska to the
                             Secretary of the Interior: 1900.* Washington, D.C.:
                             Government Printing Office.

1901   *Report of the Governor of Alaska, 1901*. U.S. Department of the Interior. Washington, D.C.: Government Printing Office.

1904   Witchcraft in Alaska. *The Independent* 57:1498-99. (December 29)

Brevig, Tollef L.

1901   Epidemic among natives. Letters to Sheldon Jackson. In *Tenth annual report on introduction of domestic reindeer into Alaska. 1900. See* Jackson 1901b:141-42.

Brickey, James, and Catherine Brickey

1975   Reindeer, cattle of the Arctic. *Alaska Journal* 5(1):16-24.

Brooke, John

1875   Report of Assistant Surgeon John Brooke, United States Army. In *A report on the hygiene of the United States Army, with descriptions of military posts*. War Department. Surgeon-General's Office. Circular No. 8, May 1, 1875. Washington, D.C.: Government Printing Office. Pp. 478-83.

Brooks, Alfred Hulse

1899   A reconnaissance in the White and Tanana river basins, Alaska, in 1898. In: *Twentieth annual report of the U.S. Geological Survey to the Secretary of the Interior 1898-99. Part VII. Explorations in Alaska in 1898. See* U.S. Geological Survey, 1899:425-94.

1973   *Blazing Alaska's Trails*. Second edition. Fairbanks: University of Alaska Press.

Brower, Charles D.

1960   *Fifty years below zero: A lifetime of adventure in the Far North*. In collaboration with Philip J. Farrelly and Lyman Anson. New York: Dodd, Mead.

Bruce, Miner W.

1894   Some of the habits and customs of the Eskimos (June 30, 1893). In *Report on introduction of domesticated reindeer into Alaska. 1894. See* Jackson 1894c:96-116.

Burch, Ernest S., Jr.

1974   Eskimo warfare in northwest Alaska. *Anthopological Papers of the University of Alaska.* 16(2):1-14.

1981   *The traditional Eskimo hunters of Point Hope, Alaska: 1800-1875*. Barrow, Alaska: North Slope Borough.

1984   Kotzebue Sound Eskimo. In *Handbook of North American Indians. See* Sturtevant 1984, 5:303-19.

Burlingame, Virginia S.
1978   John J. Healy's Alaskan adventure. *Alaska Journal* 8(4):310-19.

Burney, James
1819   *A chronological history of north-eastern discovery; and of the early eastern navigations of the Russians.* Reprint 1969. Amsterdam: N. Israel; New York: Da Capo Press.

Calasanctius, Mary Joseph
1947   *The voice of Alaska. Memoirs of a missioner.* La Chine, Quebec: Saint Ann's Press.

Caldwell, Francis E.
1986   Dr. Goddard's medicinal hot springs. Building a sanitarium at Goddard Hot Springs. In *Alaska Journal. A 1986 collection. See* Cole 1986:188-93.

Campbell, Archibald
1819   *A voyage round the world from 1806 to 1812; in which Japan, Kamschatka, the Aleutian Islands, and the Sandwich Islands were visited. . . .* Second American edition. New York: Broderick and Kitter.

Cantwell, J. C.
1887   A narrative account of the exploration of the Kowak River, Alaska. In *Report of the cruise of the Revenue Marine Steamer* Corwin *in the Arctic Ocean in the year 1885. See* Healy 1887:21-52.
1889   A narrative account of the exploration of the Kowak River, Alaska. In *Report of the cruise of the Revenue Marine Steamer* Corwin *in the Arctic Ocean in the year 1884. See* Healy 1889:47-98.
1902   *Report of the operations of the U.S. Revenue Steamer* Nunivak *on the Yukon River Station, Alaska, 1899-1901.* Washington, D.C.: Government Printing Office.

Carlson, L. H.
1946   The discovery of gold at Nome, Alaska. In *Alaska and its history. See* Sherwood, 1967:352-80.

Carroll, Ginger A.
1972   Traditional medical cures along the Yukon. *Alaska Medicine* 14(2):50-53.

Castner, J. C.
1900   A story of hardship and suffering in Alaska. In *Compilation of narratives of explorations in Alaska. See* U.S. Senate, 1900:686-709.

Chamisso, Adelbert von
1986   *The Alaska Diary of Adelbert von Chamisso, naturalist on
                        the Kotzebue voyage 1815-18.* Translated with introduction
                        and notes by Robert Fortuine, with editorial assistance
                        from Eva R. Trautmann. Anchorage, Alaska: Cook Inlet
                        Historical Society.
Chapman, John W., and Bertha W. Sabine
1895   The Alaska mission in 1894-95. *Spirit of Missions* 60:378-
                        80.
1899   Alaska annual report of the Christ Church Mission. *Spirit
                        of Missions* 64:572-73.
Chevigny, Hector
1965   *Russian America: The great Alaskan venture 1741-1867.*
                        New York: Viking Press.
Chirikov, Alexei
1922   The journal of Chirikov's vessel, the "St. Paul." In
                        *Bering's voyages. An account of the efforts of the Russians
                        to determine the relation of Asia and America. See* Golder
                        1922, 1:283-311.
Choris, Louis
1822   *Voyage pittoresque autour du monde, avec des portraits de
                        sauvages d'Amérique, d'Asie, d'Afrique, et des Iles du
                        grand Océan; des paysages, des vues martimes, et
                        plusieurs objets d'Histoire naturelle.* . . . Paris.
Clark, Annette McFayden
1981   Koyukon. In *Handbook of North American Indians. See*
                        Sturtevant 1981, 6:582-601.
Clark, Donald W.
1984   Pacific Eskimo: Historical ethnography. In *Handbook of
                        North American Indians. See* Sturtevant 1984, 5:185-97.
Cocke, Albert J.
1974   Dr. Samuel J. Call. *Alaska Journal* 4(3):181-88.
Cole, Terence, ed.
1984   City of the golden beaches. *Alaska Geographic* 11(1):1-
                        183.
1986   *The Alaska Journal. A 1986 collection.* Anchorage: Alaska
                        Northwest Publishing Co.
Collinson, Richard
1889   *Journal of H.M.S.* Enterprise, *on the expedition in search
                        of Sir John Franklin's ships by Behring Strait 1850-55.*
                        London: Sampson Low, Marston, Searle, and Rivington.

Collis, Septima M.
1890   *A woman's trip to Alaska: Being an account of a voyage through the inland seas of the Sitkan archipelago in 1890.* New York: Cassell Publishing Co.

Colyer, Vincent
1869   Report of the Hon. Vincent Colyer, United States Special Indian Commissioner, on the Indian tribes and their surroundings in Alaska Territory, from personal observation and inspection in 1869. In *Report of the Secretary of the Interior 1869.* Washington, D.C.: Government Printing Office. Pp. 975-1058.

Conger, Horace S.
1983   *In search of gold. The Alaska journals of Horace S. Conger 1898-1899.* Edited by Carolyn Jean Holeski and Marlene Conger Holeski. Anchorage: Alaska Geographic Society.

Cook, James
1967   *The journals of Captain James Cook on his voyages of discovery.* Three volumes. Edited by J. C. Beaglehole. Vol. 3. *The voyage of the* Resolution *and* Discovery *1776-1780* (two parts). Cambridge, U.K.: Hakluyt Society.

Cook, John A. and Samson S. Pederson
1937   *"Thar she blows." Experiences of many voyages chasing whales in the Arctic.* Boston: Chapman and Grimes.

Corney, Peter
1965   *Early voyages in the north Pacific 1813-1818.* Fairfield, Wash.: Ye Galleon Press.

Coxe, William
1787   *Account of the Russian discoveries between Asia and America.* Third edition. London: J. Nichols.

Cracroft, Sophia
1981   *Lady Franklin visits Sitka, Alaska, 1870: The journal of Sophia Cracroft, Sir John Franklin's niece.* Edited by R. N. De Armond. Anchorage: Alaska Historical Society.

Cutter, Donald C.
1972   Malaspina at Yakutat Bay. *Alaska Journal* 2(4):42-49.

Dall, William Healy
1870   *Alaska and its resources.* Boston: Lee and Shepherd.

Davydov, G.I.
1977   *Two voyages to Russian America, 1802-1807.* Translated by Colin Bearne. Edited by Richard A. Pierce. Kingston, Ontario: Limestone Press.

De Armond, R. N., ed.
1973   Letter to Jack McQuesten: "Gold on the Fortymile." *Alaska Journal* 3(2):114.

De Laguna, Frederica
1956   *Chugach prehistory. The archeology of Prince William Sound, Alaska.* Seattle and London: University of Washington Press.
1960   *The story of a Tlingit community: A problem in the relationship between archeological, ethnological and historical methods.* Smithsonian Institution. Bureau of American Ethnology Bulletin No. 172. Washington, D.C.: Government Printing Office.
1972   *Under Mount Saint Elias: The history and culture of the Yakutat Tlingit.* Smithsonian Contributions to Anthropology. Vol. 7. Three parts. Part I. Washington, D.C.: Smithsonian Institution Press.

De Laguna, Frederica and Catherine McClellan
1981   Ahtna. In *Handbook of North American Indians. See* Sturtevant 1981, 6:641-63.

DeLapp, Tina, and Elizabeth Ward
1981   *Traditional Inupiat health practices.* Barrow, Alaska: North Slope Borough Health and Social Services Area.

Del'Isle de la Croyère, Louis
1914   A report in Russian, with the translation, on the inhabitants found on September 20, 1741, in a port near Kamchatka by Captain Alexis Chirikof and my brother in the voyage which they made to America. In *Russian Expansion on the Pacific 1641-1850. See* Golder 1914:314-23.

De Lorme, Roland L.
1975   Liquor smuggling in Alaska, 1867-1899. *Pacific Northwest Quarterly* 66(4):145-52.

Dixon, George
1789   *A voyage round the world, but more particularly to the north-west coast of America: Performed in 1785, 1786, 1787, and 1788. . . .* London: George Goulding.

Dixon, Mim, and Scott Kirchner
1982   "Poking", an Eskimo medical practice in northwest Alaska. *Etudes/Inuit/Studies* 6(2):109-25.

Dmytryshyn, Basil, E. A. P. Crownhart-Vaughan, and Thomas Vaughan, eds.
1986   *Russian penetration of the north Pacific Ocean, 1700-1799.* Portland: Oregon Historical Society.

Doty, William Furman
1900   The Eskimo on St. Lawrence Island, Alaska. In *Ninth annual report on the introduction of domestic reindeer into Alaska. 1899. See* Jackson 1900b:186-223.

Down, Mary Margaret
1966   *1858-1958. A century of service.* Victoria, B.C.: The Sisters of Saint Ann.

Driggs, John B.
1894   The work at Point Hope, Alaska, in 1893-4. *Spirit of Missions* 59(12):562-64.

1897   Dr. Driggs's report from Point Hope, Alaska. *Spirit of Missions* 62(11):607-8.

Drucker, Philip
1955   *Indians of the northwest coast.* Reprint 1963. Garden City, NY: Natural History Press.

Dubos, René, and Jean Dubos
1952   *The white plague. Tuberculosis, man and society.* Boston: Little, Brown and Co.

Dumond, Don E.
1986   Demographic effects of European expansion. A nineteenth-century native population on the Alaska Peninsula. *University of Oregon Anthropological Papers.* No. 35. [Eugene, Ore.].

D'Wolf, John
1861   *A voyage to the north Pacific.* Reprint 1968. Fairfield, Wash.: Ye Galleon Press.

Dyerberg, J., and H. O. Bang
1979   Haemostatic function and platelet polyunsaturated fatty acids in Eskimos. *Lancet* 2:433-35.

Edmonds, H. M. W.
1966   The Eskimos of St. Michael and vicinity, as related by H. M. W. Edmonds. Edited by Dorothy Jean Ray. *Anthropological Papers of the University of Alaska* 13(2).

Edwards, Stan
1959   *Brucella suis* in the Arctic. *Alaska Medicine* 1(1):41-44.

Eisenberg, Mickey S., and Thomas R. Bender
1976   Plastic bags and botulism: A new twist to an old hazard of the North. *Alaska Medicine* 18(4):47-49.

Elliott, Charles P.
1900   Salmon fishing grounds and canneries. In *Compilation of narratives of explorations in Alaska. See* U.S. Senate 1900:738-41.

Elliott, Henry W.

1875   *A report on the condition of affairs in the Territory of Alaska.* Washington, D.C.: Government Printing Office.

1880   *Report on the Seal Islands of Alaska.* Washington, D.C.: Government Printing Office.

1886   *Our arctic province: Alaska and the Seal Islands.* New York: Charles Scribner.

Ellis, William

1782   *An authentic narrative of a voyage performed by Captain Cook and Captain Clerke in His Majesty's Ships* Resolution *and* Discovery *during the years 1776, 1777, 1778, 1779 and 1780; in search of a north-west passage between the continents of Asia and America.* Two volumes. Reprint 1969. Amsterdam: N. Israel; New York: Da Capo Press.

El-Najjar, Mahmoud Y.

1979   Human treponematosis and tuberculosis: Evidence from the New World. *American Journal of Physical Anthropology* 51(4):599-618.

Emmons, George T.

1905   *Conditions and needs of the natives of Alaska.* 58th Congress, 2nd session. Senate Document No. 106. Washington, D.C.: Government Printing Office.

Eschscholtz, Frederick

1821   On the diseases of the crew during the three years of the voyage. In *A voyage of discovery into the South Sea and Beering's Straits. . . . See* Kotzebue 1821, 2:315-47.

Farnsworth, Robert J.

1977   An army brat goes to Alaska. Conclusion. Building Fort Gibbon. *Alaska Journal* 7(4):211-19.

Fedorova, Svetlana G.

1973   *The Russian population in Alaska and California: Late 18th century-1867.* Translated and edited by Richard A. Pierce and Alton S. Donnelly. Kingston, Ontario: Limestone Press.

Feltz, Elmer T., B. List-Young, Donald G. Ritter, P. Holden, Gary R. Noble, and Paul S. Clark

1972   California encephalitis virus: Serological evidence of human infections in Alaska. *Canadian Journal of Microbiology* 18(6):757-62.

Fienup-Riordan, Ann

n.d.   The real people and the children of thunder. Typescript of unpublished book, used by permission of author.

1988   *The Yup'ik Eskimos, as described in the travel journals
                             and ethnographic accounts of John and Edith Kilbuck who
                             served the Alaska mission of the Moravian Church 1886-
                             1900.* Kingston, Ontario: Limestone Press.

Fisher, Raymond H.
1977   *Bering's voyages: Whither and why.* Seattle and London:
                             University of Washington Press.

Fleurieu, C. P. Claret
1801   *A voyage round the world performed during the years
                             1790, 1791, and 1792, by Etienne Marchand.* Two
                             volumes. Reprint 1969. Amsterdam: N. Israel; New York:
                             Da Capo Press.

Foote, Don C.
1964   American whalemen in northern arctic Alaska. *Arctic
                             Anthropology* 2(2):16-20.

Fortuine, Robert
1971   The health of the Eskimos, as portrayed in the earliest
                             written accounts. *Bulletin of the History of Medicine*
                             45(2):97-114.

1975a   Health care and the Alaska Native: Some historical
                             perspectives. *Polar Notes* 14:1-42.

1975b   Paralytic shellfish poisoning in the North Pacific: Two
                             historical accounts and implications for today. *Alaska
                             Medicine* 17(5):71-76.

1984a   Ships' surgeons and naturalists in the early history of
                             Alaska. Part 1. Voyages of discovery, 1741-1786. *Alaska
                             Medicine* 26(2):57-61.

1984b   Ships' surgeons and naturalists in the early history of
                             Alaska. Part 3. Voyages for Empire and the Northwest
                             Passage, 1814-1850. *Alaska Medicine* 26(4):117-21.

1985   Lancets of stone: Traditional methods of surgery among
                             the Alaska Natives. *Arctic Anthropology* 22(1):23-45.

1986   *Alaska Native Medical Center. A history 1953-1983.*
                             Anchorage: Alaska Native Medical Center, Indian Health
                             Service.

1986/87   Early evidence of infections among Alaska Natives.
                             Alaska History 2(1):39-56.

1988a   Scurvy in the early history of Alaska: The haves and the
                             have-nots. *Alaska History* 3(2):21-44.

1988b   The use of medicinal plants by the Alaska Natives. *Alaska
                             Medicine* 30(6): 185-226.

Foulks, Edward F.
1972   *The arctic hysterias of the North Alaskan Eskimo.*
                      Washington, D.C.: American Anthropological Association.
Fournelle, Harold J., V. Rader, and C. Allen
1966   A survey of enteric infections among Alaskan Indians.
                      Public Health Reports 81(9):797-803.
Fournelle, Harold J., I. L. Wallace, and V. Rader
1958   A bacteriological and parasitological survey of enteric
                      infections in an Alaskan Eskimo area. *American Journal
                      of Public Health* 48(11):1489-97.

Fox, Carroll
1902   Tuberculosis among the Indians of southeast Alaska.
                      Public Health Reports 16:1615-16.

Fraser, J. D.
1923   *The gold fever, or two years in Alaska.* Privately printed.
French, L .H.
1901   *Nome nuggets. Some of the experiences of a party of gold
                      seekers in northwestern Alaska in 1900.* New York:
                      Montross, Clarke and Emmons.
Fritz, Milo H., and Philip Thygeson
1951   Phlyctenular keratoconjunctivitis among Alaskan Indians
                      and Eskimos. *Public Health Reports* 66(29):934-39.

Gambell, F. H.
1900   Reports, Eaton reindeer station. In *Ninth annual report on
                      introduction of domestic reindeer into Alaska. 1899.* See
                      Jackson, 1900b:69-73.

Gambell, V. C.
1898   Notes with regard to the St. Lawrence Island Eskimo. In
                      *Report on introduction of domestic reindeer into Alaska,
                      1898. See* Jackson 1898c:141-45.
Geist, Otto William, and Froelich G. Rainey
1936   *Archeological excavations at Kukulik, St. Lawrence Island,
                      Alaska.* Misc. Publications of the University of Alaska.
                      Washington, D.C.: Government Printing Office.

Gibson, James R.
1976   *Imperial Russia in frontier America. The changing
                      geography of supply of Russian America, 1784-1867.* New
                      York: Oxford University Press.
1982-83   Smallpox on the northwest coast 1835-1838. *British
                      Columbia Studies* 36:61-81.

Giddings, J. Louis
1961   *Kobuk River people.* College: University of Alaska Press.

| 1964 | *The archeology of Cape Denbigh*. Providence, R.I.: Brown University Press. |

1967   *Ancient men of the Arctic*. New York: Alfred A. Knopf.

Glushankov, I. V.

1973   The Aleutian expedition of Krenitsyn and Levashov. Translated by Mary Sadouski and Richard A. Pierce. *Alaska Journal* 3(3):204-10.

Golder, Frank A.

1914   *Russian expansion on the Pacific 1641-1850*. Reprint 1960. Gloucester, Mass.: Peter Smith.

1916   Mining in Alaska before 1867. Reprinted in: *Alaska and its history. See* Sherwood 1967:148-56.

1922   *Bering's voyages. An account of the efforts of the Russians to determine the relation of Asia and America*. Two volumes. New York: American Geographical Society.

Golovin, P. N.

1979   *The end of Russian America. Captain P. N. Golovin's last report 1862*. Translated by Basil Dmytryshyn and E. A. P. Crownhart-Vaughan. Portland: Oregon Historical Society.

1983   *Civil and savage encounters. The worldly travel letters of an Imperial Russian Navy officer 1860-1861*. Translated and annotated by Basil Dmytryshyn and E. A. P. Crownhart-Vaughan. Portland: Oregon Historical Society.

Golovnin, V. M.

1979   *Around the world on the* Kamchatka, *1817-1819*. Translated with introduction and notes by Ella Lury Wiswell. Honolulu: The Hawaiian Historical Society and the University Press of Hawaii.

1985/86   Memorandum of Captain 2nd Rank Golovnin on the condition of the Aleuts in the settlements of the Russian-American Company and on its *promyshlenniki*. Translated by Katherine L. Arndt. *Alaska History* 1(2):59-71.

Govorlivyi, Z.

n.d.   Diseases prevalent among the Kolosh Indian inhabitants of the island of Sitka. Translated by Tanya DeMarsh. Kingston, Ontario: Limestone Press, forthcoming.

Green, J. S.

1984   Extracts from the report of an exploring tour on the northwest coast of North America in 1829. In *Warriors of the north Pacific. Missionary accounts of the northwest coast, the Skeena and Stikine rivers and the Klondike, 1829-1900*, edited by Charles Lillard. Victoria, B.C.: Sono Nis Press. Pp. 29-62.

Griffiths, C. E.
1900   Explorations in and about Cook Inlet, 1899. Subreport of
                     topographer C. E. Griffiths. In *Compilation of narratives
                     of explorations in Alaska. See* U.S. Senate 1900:724-33.

Grinnell, Joseph
1901   *Gold hunting in Alaska.* Edited by Elizabeth Grinnell.
                     Chicago: David C. Cook Publishing Co.

Gruening, Ernest
1954   *The state of Alaska.* New York: Random House.

Gubser, Nicholas J.
1965   *The Nunamiut Eskimos: Hunters of caribou.* New Haven
                     and London: Yale University Press.

Hadley, Jack R.
1915   Whaling off the Alaskan coast. *Bulletin of the American
                     Geographical Society* 47(11):905-21.

Hall, Edwin S.
1975   Kutchin Athapaskan/Nunamiut Eskimo conflict. An
                     ethnohistorical study. *Alaska Journal* 5(4):248-52.
1984   Interior north Alaska Eskimo. In *Handbook of North
                     American Indians. See* Sturtevant 1984, 5:338-46.

Hanable, William S.
1973   New Russia. *Alaska Journal* 3(2):77-80.
1978   When quarterdeck was capitol. *Alaska Journal* 8(4):320-
                     25.
1982   *Alaska's Copper River. The 18th and 19th centuries.*
                     Anchorage: Alaska Historical Commission.

Healy, Michael L.
1887   *Report of the cruise of the Revenue Marine Steamer*
                     Corwin *in the Arctic Ocean in the year 1885.* Washington,
                     D.C.: Government Printing Office.
1889   *Report of the cruise of the Revenue Marine Steamer*
                     Corwin *in the Arctic Ocean in the year 1884.* Washington,
                     D.C.: Government Printing Office.

Heller, Christine A.
1963   Poisonous plants in Alaska. *Alaska Medicine* 5(4):94-99.
1981   *Wild edible and poisonous plants of Alaska.* Publication
                     No. 28. Revised. Fairbanks: University of Alaska
                     Extension Service.

Henkelman, James W., and Kurt H. Vitt
1985   *Harmonious to dwell. The history of the Alaska Moravian
                     Church 1885-1985.* Bethel, Alaska: Moravian Seminary
                     and Archives.

Herron, Joseph S.
1901   *Explorations in Alaska, 1899, for an all-American overland route from Cook Inlet, Pacific Ocean, to the Yukon.* U.S. Adjutant-General's Office. Washington, D.C.: Government Printing Office.

Hill, Beth
1977   The Sisters of St. Ann. *Alaska Journal* 7(1):40-45.

Hinckley, Ted C.
1972   *The Americanization of Alaska, 1867-1897.* Palo Alto, Cal.: Pacific Books.

1979   Some biased observations on the Christian missionary. In *The church in Alaska's past: Conference proceedings.* Office of History and Archaeology. Anchorage: Alaska Division of Parks.

1984   Alaska pioneer and west coast town builder, William Sumner Dodge. *Alaska History* 1(1):1-26.

Hitchcock, Dorothy
1950   Parasitological study on the Eskimos in the Bethel area of Alaska. *Journal of Parasitology* 36(3):232-34.

1951   Parasitological study on the Eskimos in the Kotzebue area of Alaska. *Journal of Parasitology* 37(3):309-11.

Holcomb, Richmond C.
1940   Syphilis of the skull among Aleuts, and the Asian and North American Eskimo about Bering and Arctic Seas. *U.S. Naval Medical Bulletin* 38(4):177-92.

Holmberg, Heinrich Johan
1985   *Holmberg's ethnographic sketches.* Edited by Marvin W. Falk. Translated by Fritz Jaensch. The Rasmuson Library Historical Translation Series. Vol. I. Fairbanks: University of Alaska Press.

Hooper, Calvin L.
1881   *Report of the cruise of the U.S. Revenue-Steamer* Corwin *in the Arctic Ocean.* 1880. Washington, D.C.: Government Printing Office.

1884   *Report of the cruise of the U.S. Revenue Steamer* Thomas Corwin *in the Arctic Ocean, 1881.* Washington, D.C.: Government Printing Office.

Hooper, William H.
1853   *Ten months among the tents of the Tuski, with incidents of an arctic boat expedition in search of Sir John Franklin, as far as the Mackenzie River, and Cape Bathurst.* London: John Murray.

Hopkins, Donald R.
1983   *Princes and peasants. Smallpox in history.* Chicago and London: University of Chicago Press.

Hosley, Edward H.
1981   Environment and culture in the Alaska Plateau. In *Handbook of North American Indians. See* Sturtevant 1981, 6:533-45.

Howard, O. O.
1900   A visit to Alaska in June, 1875. In *Compilation of narratives of explorations in Alaska. See* U.S. Senate 1900:45-52.

Hrdlička, Aleš
1930   *Anthroplogical survey in Alaska.* Smithsonian Institution, Bureau of American Ethnology. 46th Annual Report. Washington, D.C.: Government Printing Office.

1931   *Anthropological work on the Kuskokwim River, Alaska.* Smithsonian Institution Publication No. 3111. Washington, D.C.: Government Printing Office.

1940   Diseases and artifacts on skulls and bones from Kodiak Island. *Smithsonian Miscellaneous Collections* 101(4):1-25.

Huggins, Eli Lundy
1981   *Kodiak and Afognak life, 1868-1870.* Edited by Richard A. Pierce. Kingston, Ontario: Limestone Press.

Hulley, Clarence C.
1958   *Alaska: Past and present.* Portland, Ore.: Binfords and Mort.

Hunt, William R.
1974   *North of 53°. The wild days of the Alaska-Yukon mining frontier 1870-1914.* New York: Macmillan.

Ivashintsov, N. A.
1980   *Russian round-the-world voyages, 1803-1849, with a summary of later voyages to 1867.* Translated by Glynn R. Barratt. Edited by Richard A. Pierce. Kingston, Ontario: Limestone Press.

Jackson, Sheldon
1880   *Alaska, and missions on the north Pacific coast.* New York: Dodd, Mead & Co.

1881   Education in Alaska. 47th Congress, 1st Session. Senate Exec. Doc. No. 30. Washington, D.C.: Government Printing Office.

1884   Education in Alaska. In *Report of the commissioner of education for the year 1882-'83.* Washington, D.C.: Government Printing Office.

1886   *Report on education in Alaska, 1886.* 49th Congress, 1st Session. Senate Exec. Doc. No. 85. Washington, D.C.: Government Printing Office.

1893a   Education in Alaska. In *Report of the commissioner of education for 1889-90.* Washington, D.C.: Government Printing Office. Pp. 1245-1300.

1893b   Education in Alaska. In *Report of the commissioner of education for 1890-91.* Washington, D.C.: Government Printing Office. Pp. 923-60.

1894a   Education in Alaska. 1891-92. In *Report of the commissioner of education for 1891-92.* Washington, D.C.: Government Printing Office. Pp. 873-92.

1894b   *Facts about Alaska: Its people, villages, missions, schools.* New York: Woman's Executive Committee of Home Missions of the Presbyterian Church.

1894c   *Report on introduction of domesticated reindeer into Alaska. 1894.* Washington, D.C.: Government Printing Office.

1895   Education in Alaska. 1892-93. In *Report of the commissioner of education for 1892-93.* Washington, D.C.: Government Printing Office. Pp. 1705-48.

1896a   Report on education in Alaska. In *Report of the commissioner of education for 1893-94.* Washington, D.C.: Government Printing Office. Pp. 1451-92.

1896b   *Report on introduction of domestic reindeer into Alaska. 1895.* 54th Congress, 1st session. Senate Doc. No. 111. Washington, D.C.: Government Printing Office.

1897a   Education in Alaska. 1895-96. In *Report of the commissioner of education for 1895-96.* Washington, D.C.: Government Printing Office. Pp. 1435-68.

1897b   *Report on introduction of domestic reindeer into Alaska. 1896.* Washington, D.C.: Government Printing Office.

1898a   Education in Alaska. 1896-97. In *Report of the commissioner of education for 1896-97.* Washington, D.C.: Government Printing Office. Pp. 1601-46.

1898b   *Report on introduction of domestic reindeer into Alaska. 1897.* 55th Congress, 2nd Session. Senate Doc. No. 30. Washington, D.C.: Government Printing Office.

1898c   *Report on introduction of domestic reindeer into Alaska. 1898.* 55th Congress, 3rd Session. Senate Document No.

34. Washington, D.C.: Government Printing Office.

1899   Education in Alaska. 1897-98. In *Report of the commissioner of education for 1897-98.* Washington, D.C.: Government Printing Office. Pp. 1753-71.

1900a   Education in Alaska. 1898-99. In *Report of the commissioner of education for 1898-99.* Washington, D.C.: Government Printing Office. Pp. 1373-1402.

1900b   *Ninth annual report on introduction of domestic reindeer into Alaska. 1899.* Washington, D.C.: Government Printing Office.

1901a   Education and reindeer in Alaska. 1899-1900. In *Report of the commissioner of education for 1899-1900.* Washington, D.C.: Government Printing Office. Pp. 1733-62.

1901b   *Tenth annual report on introduction of domestic reindeer into Alaska. 1900.* Washington, D.C.: Government Printing Office.

1903a   Education and reindeer in Alaska. 1901. In *Report of the commissioner of education for 1900-1901.* Washington, D.C.: Government Printing Office. Pp. 1459-80.

1903b   *Facts about Alaska: Its people, villages, missions, schools.* New York: Women's Board of Home Missions of the Presbyterian Church.

Jacobsen, Johan Adrian
1977   *Alaskan voyage 1881-1883. An expedition to the northwest coast of America.* Translated by Erna Gunther from the German text of Adrian Woldt. Chicago and London: University of Chicago Press.

James, James Alton
1942   *The first scientific exploration of Russian America and the purchase of Alaska.* Evanston and Chicago: Northwestern University Press.

[Jarvis, D. H.]
1899   *Report of the cruise of the U.S. Revenue Cutter* Bear *and the overland expedition for the relief of the whalers in the Arctic Ocean from November 27, 1897 to September 13, 1898.* U.S. Treasury Department Doc. No. 2101. Washington, D.C.: Government Printing Office.

Jenkins, Thomas
1943   *The man of Alaska: Peter Trimble Rowe.* New York: Morehouse-Gorham Co.

Jenness, Diamond
1957   *Dawn in arctic Alaska.* Minneapolis: University of Minnesota Press.

1962   *Eskimo administration: I. Alaska.* Arctic Institute of North
                             America. Technical Paper No. 10. Montreal.

Jetté, Julius
1907   On the medicine-men of the Ten'a. *Journal of the Royal
                             Anthropological Institute of Great Britain and Ireland*
                             37:157-88.

1911   On the superstitions of the Ten'a Indians (middle part of
                             the Yukon Valley, Alaska). *Anthropos* 6(1):95-108,
                             (2):241-59, (3,4):602-15, (5):699-703.

Jones, Livingston F.
1914   *A study of the Thlingets of Alaska.* London and Edinburgh:
                             Fleming H. Revell Co.

Justice, James W.
1966   Use of devil's club in southeast Alaska. *Alaska Medicine*
                             8(2):36-39.

Kari, Priscilla Russell
1987   *Tanaina plantlore. Dena'ina K'et'una.* Second edition,
                             revised. [Anchorage}: National Park Service, Alaska
                             Region.

Kashevaroff, A. P.
1927   Ivan Veniaminov, Innocent, metropolitan of Moscow and
                             Kolomna. *Alaska Magazine* 1:45-46, 145-50, 217-24.

Kashevarov, A. F.
1977   A. F. Kashevarov's coastal explorations in northwest
                             Alaska, 1838. Edited by James W. VanStone. Translated by
                             David H. Kraus. *Fieldiana: Anthropology* 69. (Sept. 28,
                             1977).

Kempton, Phyllis E., and Virginia L. Wells
1968   Mushroom poisoning in Alaska: *Helvella. Alaska
                             Medicine* 10(1):32-34.

Khlebnikov, Kyrill T.
1973   *Baranov: Chief manager of the Russian colonies in
                             America.* Translated by Colin Bearne. Edited by Richard
                             A. Pierce. Kingston, Ontario: Limestone Press.

1976   *Colonial Russian America. Kyrill T. Khlebnikov's reports
                             1817-1832.* Translated by Basil Dmytryshyn and E. A. P.
                             Crownhart-Vaughan. Portland: Oregon Historical Society.

Khromchenko, V. S.
1973   V. S. Khromchenko's coastal explorations in southwestern
                             Alaska, 1822. Edited by James W. VanStone. Translated by
                             David J. Kraus. *Fieldiana: Anthropology* 64. (Nov. 23,
                             1973).

Kinkead, John H.
1884   *Report of the Governor of Alaska, for the year 1884.* Washington, D.C.: Government Printing Office.

Knapp, Lyman E.
1889   *Report of the Governor of Alaska for the fiscal year 1889.* U.S. Department of the Interior. Washington, D.C.: Government Printing Office.

1890   *Report of the Governor of Alaska for the fiscal year 1890.* U.S. Department of the Interior. Washington, D.C.: Government Printing Office.

1892   *Report of the Governor of Alaska for the fiscal year 1892.* U.S. Department of the Interior. Washington, D.C.: Government Printing Office.

1893   *Report of the Governor of Alaska for the fiscal year 1893.* (Typescript available in the Elmer E. Rasmuson Library, University of Alaska Fairbanks).

Kotzebue, Otto von
1821   *A voyage of discovery into the South Sea and Beering's Straits, for the purpose of exploring a north-east passage, undertaken in the years 1815-1818. . . .* Three volumes. Reprint 1967. Amsterdam: N. Israel; New York: Da Capo Press.

1830   *A new voyage round the world in the years 1823, 24, 25, and 26.* Two volumes. Reprint 1967. Amsterdam: N. Israel; New York: Da Capo Press.

Koutsky, Kathryn
1981   *Early days on Norton Sound and Bering Strait.* Six volumes. Anthropological and Historic Preservation Cooperative Park Unit. Occasional Paper No. 29. Vol. 2. Fairbanks: University of Alaska.

Krasheninnikov, S. P.
1764   *The history of Kamchatka, and the Kurilski Islands, with the countries adjacent.* Translated by James Grieve. Reprint 1962. Chicago: Quadrangle Books.

Krause, Aurel
1956   *The Tlingit Indians: Results of a trip to the northwest coast of America and the Bering Straits.* Translated by Erna Gunther. Seattle and London: University of Washington Press.

Krauss, Michael E.
1982   *Native peoples and languages of Alaska.* Map. Fairbanks: Alaska Native Language Center, University of Alaska.

Krusenstern, Adam J. von
1813   *Voyage round the world in the years 1803, 1804, 1805, and 1806, by order of His Imperial Majesty Alexander the First, on board the ships* Nadeshda *and* Neva. Two volumes. Reprint 1968. Ridgewood, NJ: Gregg Press.

L., C. ("C. L.")
1789   *A voyage round the world in the years 1785, 1786, 1787, and 1788: Performed in the* King George, *commanded by Captain Portlock, and the* Queen Charlotte, *commanded by Captain Dixon.* Reprint 1984. Fairfield, Wash.: Ye Galleon Press.

Lada-Mocarski, Valerian
1969   *Bibliography of books on Alaska published before 1868.* New Haven and London: Yale University Press.

Lagier, R., C. A. Baud, G. Arnaud, S. Arnaud, and R. Menk
1982   Lesions characteristic of infection or malignant tumor in paleo-Eskimo skulls. An anatomical and radiological study of two specimens. *Virchows Archiv* 395(3):237-43.

Lain, B. D.
1977   The Fort Yukon affair. *Alaska Journal* 7(1):12-17.

Langdon, Steve J.
1987   *The Native people of Alaska.* Anchorage, Alaska: Greatland Graphics.

Langsdorff, Georg H. von
1814   *Voyages and travels in various parts of the world during the years 1803, 1804, 1805, 1806, and 1807.* Two volumes. Reprint 1968. Amsterdam: N. Israel; New York: Da Capo Press.

Lantis, Margaret
1946   The social culture of the Nunivak Eskimo. *Transactions of the American Philosophical Society* n.s. 35(3):153-323.

1959   Folk medicine and hygiene: Lower Kuskokwim and Nunivak-Nelson Island areas. *Anthropological Papers of the University of Alaska* 8(1):1-76.

1980   Changes in the Alaskan Eskimo relation of man to dog and their effect on two human diseases. *Arctic Anthropology* 17(1):2-25.

1984a   Aleut. In *Handbook of North American Indians. See* Sturtevant 1984, 5:161-84.

1984b   Nunivak Eskimo. In *Handbook of North American Indians. See* Sturtevant 1984, 5:209-23.

La Pérouse, J. F. G. de
1799   *A voyage round the world performed in the years 1785, 1786, 1787, 1788, by the* Boussole *and* Astrolabe. Two volumes. Reprint 1968. Amsterdam: N. Israel; New York: Da Capo Press.

Larkin, Jack
1988   The secret life of a developing country (ours). *American Heritage* 39(6):44-67.

Laughlin, William S.
1963   Eskimos and Aleuts: Their origins and evolution. *Science* 142(3593):633-45.

1980   *Aleuts: Survivors of the Bering land bridge.* New York: Holt, Rinehart and Winston.

Laughlin, William S., and Jean S. Aigner
1974   Burial of an aged Chaluka adult male. *Arctic Anthropology* 11(1):47-60.

Lazell, J. Arthur
1960   *Alaskan apostle. The life story of Sheldon Jackson.* New York: Harper and Brothers.

Learnard, H. G.
1900   A trip from Portage Bay to Turnagain Arm and up the Sushitna. In *Compilation of narratives of explorations in Alaska. See* U.S. Senate 1900:648-71.

Ledyard, John
1963   *John Ledyard's journal of Captain Cook's last voyage.* Edited by James Kenneth Mumford. Corvallis: Oregon State University Press.

Leonhardt, Saul C.
1901   End of smallpox at Juneau and Douglas City, Alaska. *Public Health Reports* 16:1616.

Lerrigo, P. H. J.
1901   Report from St. Lawrence Island. In *Tenth annual report on introduction of domestic reindeer into Alaska. 1900. See* Jackson 1901b:98-114.

Lichtenfels, J. R., and F. P. Brancato
1976   Anisakid larvae from the throat of an Alaskan Eskimo. *American Journal of Tropical Medicine and Hygiene* 25(5):691-93.

Lisiansky, Urey
1814   *A voyage round the world in the years 1803, 4, 5, and 6; Performed by order of His Imperial Majesty Alexander the First, Emperor of Russia, in the ship* Neva. London: John Booth, Longman, Hurst, Rees, Orme, and Brown.

Litke, F. P.
1987   *A voyage around the world 1826-1829.* Translated by
                       Renee Marshall. Edited by Richard A. Pierce. Kingston,
                       Ontario: Limestone Press.
Llorente, Segundo
1969   *Jesuits in Alaska.* Portland, Ore.: Service Office Supply.
Lobdell, John E.
1980   Prehistoric human population resource utilization in
                       Kachemak Bay, Gulf of Alaska. Ph.D. dissertation,
                       University of Tennessee, Knoxville.
Lopp, William Thomas
1892   A year alone in Alaska. The *American Missionary* 46:386-
                       91.
Loree, David R.
1935   Notes on Alaskan medical history. *Northwest Medicine*
                       34(7):262-68.
Lucier, Charles V., James W. VanStone, and Della Keats
1971   Medical practices and human anatomical knowledge
                       among the Noatak Eskimos. *Ethnology* 10(3):251-64.
Maguire, Rochfort
1857   Narrative of Commander Maguire, wintering at Point
                       Barrow. In *The discovery of the north-west passage. See*
                       M'Clure 1857:351-405.
Mallory, Charles E.
1986   Nome fever. My trip to Alaska in 1900. In *Alaska Journal.
                       A 1986 collection. See* Cole 1986:216-19.
Margolis, H. S., John P. Middaugh, and Robert D. Burgess
1979   Arctic trichinosis: Two Alaskan outbreaks from walrus
                       meat. *Journal of Infectious Diseases* 139(1):102-5.
Marsh, Gordon H., and William S. Laughlin
1956   Human anatomical knowledge among the Aleutian
                       islanders. *Southwestern Journal of Anthropology* 12(1):38-
                       78.
Masterson, James R. and Helen Brower
1948   *Bering's successors 1745-1780. Contributions of Peter
                       Simon Pallas to the history of Russian exploration toward
                       Alaska.* Seattle: University of Washington Press.
Matson, B., E. B. Larsson, and W. D. Thornbloom
1941   *Covenant frontiers. Fifty years in China, fifty-three years
                       in Alaska, three years in Africa.* Chicago: Evangelical
                       Mission Covenant Church of America.

Maynard, James E., and Frank P. Pauls

1962   Trichinosis in Alaska: A review and report of two outbreaks due to bear meat with observations of serodiagnosis and skin testing. *American Journal of Hygiene* 76(3):252-61.

M'Clure, Robert Le M.

1857   *The discovery of the north-west passage, by H.M.S. Investigator, Capt. R. M'Clure 1850, 1851, 1852, 1853, 1854.* Edited by Sherard Osborn. Reprint 1969. Edmonton, Alberta: M. G. Hurtig.

McGregor, Marianna

1981   Native medicine in southeast Alaska: Tsimshian, Tlingit, Haida. *Alaska Medicine* 23(6):65-69.

McKee, Lanier

1902   *The land of Nome.* New York: Grafton Press.

McKennan, Robert A.

1959   *The upper Tanana Indians.* Yale University Publications in Anthropology No. 55. New Haven, Conn.

1965   *The Chandalar Kutchin.* Arctic Institute of North America Technical Paper No. 17. Montreal.

Meares, John

1790   *Voyages made in the years 1788 and 1789 from China to the north-west coast of America.* Reprint 1967. Amsterdam: N. Israel; New York: Da Capo Press.

Mendenhall, W. C.

1899   A reconnaissance from Resurrection Bay to the Tanana River, Alaska, in 1898. In *Twentieth annual report of the U.S. Geological Survey to the Secretary of the Interior 1898-99. Part VII. Explorations in Alaska in 1898. See* U.S. Geological Survey 1899: 265-340.

Mercier, Francois Xavier

1986   *Recollections of the Youkon. Mémoires from the years 1868-1885.* Translated and edited by Linda Finn Yarborough. Anchorage: Alaska Historical Society.

Merck, Carl Heinrich

1980   *Siberia and northwestern America 1788-1792. The journal of Carl Heinrich Merck, naturalist with the Russian scientific expedition led by Captains Joseph Billings and Gavril Sarychev.* Edited by Richard A. Pierce. Translated by Fritz Jaensch. Kingston, Ontario: Limestone Press.

Middleton, W. Vernon

1958   *Methodism in Alaska and Hawaii: New patterns for living together.* New York: Board of Missions of the Methodist Church.

Miertsching, Johann
1967   *Frozen ships: The arctic diary of Johann Miertsching 1850-1854*. Trans. by L. H. Neatby. New York: St. Martin's Press.

Milan, Frederick A.
1962   Racial variations in human response to low temperatures. In *Proceedings. Symposium on Arctic Biology and Medicine*. College: University of Alaska. Pp. 335-88.

Milan, Leda Chase
1974   Ethnohistory of disease and medical care among the Aleut. *Anthropological Papers of the University of Alaska* 16(2):15-40.

Miller, L. G.
1974   Further studies on tularemia in Alaska: Human tularemia. *Canadian Journal of Microbiology* 20(1):1539-44.

Miller, L. G., Paul S. Clark, and G. A. Kunkle
1972   Possible origin of *Clostridium botulinum* contamination of Eskimo foods in northwestern Alaska. *Applied Microbiology* 23(2):417-18.

Moore, Katrina
1986   The captain who claimed Alaska for Spain. Bodega's narrative of the voyage of the Sonora in 1775. In *Alaska Journal. A 1986 collection. See* Cole 1986:162-69.

Morris, William Gouverneur
1879   *Report upon the Customs District, public service and resources of Alaska Territory*. Washington, D.C.: Government Printing Office.

Mortimer, George
1791   *Observations and remarks made during a voyage to the islands of Teneriffe, Amsterdam . . . the Fox Islands on the north west coast of America, Tinian, and from thence to Canton, in the brig* Mercury, *commanded by John Henry Cox, Esq.* Reprint 1975. Amsterdam: N. Israel; New York: Da Capo Press.

Mourelle, Francisco Antonio
1920   *Voyage of the* Sonora *in the second Bucareli expedition. To explore the northwest coast, survey the port of San Francisco, and found Franciscan missions and a presidio and pueblo at that port. The journal kept in 1775 on the* Sonora. Reprint 1975. Millwood, N.Y.: Kraus Reprint Co.

Muir, John
1915   *Travels in Alaska*. Boston and New York: Houghton Mifflin Co.

1917   *The cruise of the* Corwin. *Journal of the arctic expedition of 1881 in search of De Long and the* Jeannette. Boston and New York: Houghton Mifflin Co.

Murdoch, John
1892   Ethnological results of the Point Barrow expedition. International Polar Expedition to Point Barrow, Alaska 1881-83. In *Smithsonian Institution, Bureau of Ethnology, 9th annual report 1887-1888.* Washington, D.C.: Government Printing Office. Pp. 3-441.

Nelson, Edward W.
1899   *The Eskimo about Bering Strait.* Reprint 1983. Washington, D.C. Smithsonian Institution Press.
1978   E. W. Nelson's notes on the Indians of the Yukon and Innoko rivers, Alaska. Edited by James W. VanStone. *Fieldiana: Anthropology* 70. April 28, 1978.

Netsvetov, Iakov
1980   *The journals of Iakov Netsvetov: The Atkha years, 1828-1844.* Translated by Lydia Black. Kingston, Ontario: Limestone Press.
1984   *The journals of Iakov Netsvetov: The Yukon years, 1845-1863.* Translated by Lydia T. Black. Edited by Richard A. Pierce. Kingston, Ontario: Limestone Press.

Niblack, Albert P.
1888   *The coast Indians of southern Alaska and northern British Columbia.* Reprint 1970. New York: Johnson Reprint Corp.

Noble, Dennis L., and Truman R. Strobridge
1979   The *Thetis* in Alaskan waters. *Alaska Journal* 9(1):50-57.

Nome News
1899   Oct. 9, Nome, Alaska.
1900   Jan. 20, Nome, Alaska.

North Star
1887-92   *The North Star. A monthly publication in the interests of schools and missions in Alaska.* Reprint 1973. Seattle: Shorey Bookstore.

Oberg, Kalervo
1966   Crime and punishment in Tlingit society. In *Indians of the north Pacific coast,* edited by Tom McFeat. Seattle and London: University of Washington Press. Pp. 209-22.

Okun, S. B.
1979   *The Russian-American Company.* Edited by B. D. Grekov. Translated by Carl Ginsburg. New York: Octagon Books.

Oleksa, Michael, ed.
1987   *Alaskan missionary spirituality.* New York and Mahwah,
                        N.J.: Paulist Press.
Osgood, Cornelius
1936   *Contributions to the ethnography of the Kutchin.* Reprint
                       1970. New Haven, Conn.: Human Relations Area Files
                       Press.
1937   *The ethnography of the Tanaina.* Yale University
                       Publications in Anthropology No. 16. New Haven, Conn.
1958   *Ingalik social culture.* Yale University Publications in
                       Anthropology No. 53. New Haven, Conn.
1971   *The Han Indians. A compilation of ethnographic and
                       historical data on the Alaska-Yukon boundary area.* Yale
                       University Publications in Anthropology No. 74. New
                       Haven, Conn.
Osler, William
1895   *The principles and practice of medicine.* Second edition.
                       New York: D. Appleton and Co.
Oswalt, Wendell H.
1957   A western Eskimo ethnobotany. *Anthropological Papers
                       of the University of Alaska* 6(1):16-36.
1960   Eskimos and Indians of western Alaska 1861-1868:
                       Extracts from the diary of Father Illarion. *Anthropological
                       Papers of the University of Alaska* 8(2):100-118.
1963   *Mission of change in Alaska. Eskimos and Moravians on
                       the Kuskokwim.* San Marino, Cal.: Huntington Library.
1967   *Alaskan Eskimos.* San Francisco: Chandler Publishing Co.
1979   *Eskimos and explorers.* Novato, Cal.: Chandler and Sharp,
                       Publishers.
1980   *Kolmakovskiy Redoubt. The ethnoarchaeology of a
                       Russian fort in Alaska.* Los Angeles: Institute of
                       Archaeology, University of California.
Pauls, Frank P.
1957   A possible case of rabies. *Science in Alaska, 1954.
                       Proceedings of the 5th Alaskan Science Conference.*
                       Alaska Division, American Association for the
                       Advancement of Science. College, Alaska. Pp. 89-90.
Petajan, J. H., Glen L. Momberger, Jon Aase, and D. Gilbert Wright
1969   Arthrogryposis syndrome (Kuskokwim disease) in the
                       Eskimo. *Journal of the American Medical Association*
                       209(10):1481-86.

Petroff, Ivan
1882   *Report on the population, industries, and resources of Alaska.* U.S. Bureau of the Census, 10th Census, 1880. Washington, D.C.: Government Printing Office.
Philip, R. N., B. Huntley, D. B. Lackman, and George W. Comstock
1962   Serologic and skin-test evidence of tularemia infection among Alaskan Eskimos, Indians and Aleuts. *Journal of Infectious Diseases* 110(3):220-30.
Pierce, Richard A.
1963   Georg Anton Schäffer, Russia's man in Hawaii, 1815-1817. Reprinted In *Alaska and its history.* See Sherwood 1967:71-81.
1975   The Russian coal mine on the Kenai. *Alaska Journal* 5(2):104-8.
1986   *Builders of Alaska. The Russian governors 1818-1867.* Kingston, Ontario: Limestone Press.
Pierce, Richard A., ed.
1974   Five years of medical observations in the colonies of the Russian-American Company (1843-1848), by (Doctors) Romanovskii and Frankenhaeuser. Translated by Richard A. Pierce. [Juneau]: Alaska Division of State Libraries (Microfiche).
1976   *Documents on the history of the Russian-American Company.* Translated by Marina Ramsay. Kingston, Ontario: Limestone Press.
1978   *The Russian Orthodox religious mission in America 1794-1837, with material concerning the life and works of the Monk German, and ethnographic notes by the Hieromonk Gedeon.* Translated by Colin Bearne. Kingston, Ontario: Limestone Press.
1984   *The Russian-American Company. Correspondence of the governors. Communications sent: 1818.* Translated by Richard A. Pierce. Kingston, Ontario: Limestone Press.
Portlock, Nathaniel
1789   *A voyage round the world; but more particularly to the north-west coast of America: Performed in 1785, 1786, 1787, and 1788, in the* King George *and* Queen Charlotte, *Captains Portlock and Dixon.* London: Stockdale and Goulding.
Rausch, Robert L.
1972   Observations on some natural-focal zoonoses in Alaska. *Archives of Environmental Health* 25(10):246-52.

Rausch, Robert L., B. B. Babero, R. V. Rausch, and E. L. Schiller
1956   Studies on the helminth fauna of Alaska XXVII. The occurrence of larvae of *Trichinella spiralis* in Alaskan mammals. *Journal of Parasitology* 42(3):259-71.

Rausch, Robert L., and D. K. Hilliard
1970   Studies on the helminth fauna of Alaska XLIX. The occurrence of *Diphyllobothrium latum* (Linnaeus, 1758) (Cestoda: Diphyllobothriidae) in Alaska, with notes on other species. *Canadian Journal of Zoology* 48(6):1201-19.

Ray, Dorothy Jean
1964   Nineteenth century settlement and subsistence patterns in Bering Strait. *Arctic Anthropology* 2(2):61-95.

1975   *The Eskimos of Bering Strait, 1650-1898.* Seattle and London: University of Washington Press.

1983   *Ethnohistory in the Arctic: The Bering Strait Eskimo.* Kingston, Ontario: Limestone Press.

1984   Bering Strait Eskimo. In *Handbook of North American Indians. See* Sturtevant 1984, 5:285-302.

Ray, P. Henry.
1885   *Report of the International Polar Expedition to Point Barrow, Alaska, in response to the resolution of the U.S. House of Representatives of December 11, 1884.* Washington, D.C.: Government Printing Office.

Raymond, Charles W.
1870-71   The Yukon River region, Alaska. In *Annual Report, American Geographical Society of New York.* Pp. 158-92.

1900   *Reconnoissance of the Yukon River.* 1869. In *Compilation of narratives of explorations in Alaska. See* U.S. Senate 1900:19-41.

Reinicker, Juliette C. ed.
1984   *Klondike letters: The correspondence of a gold seeker in 1898.* Anchorage: Alaska Northwest Publishing Co.

Renner, Louis J.
1979   Farming at Holy Cross Mission on the Yukon. *Alaska Journal* 9(1):32-37.

Rezanov, Nikolai
1926   *The Rezanov voyage to Nueva California in 1806. The report of Count Nikolai Petrovich Rezanov of his voyage to that provincia of Nueva España from New Archangel.* Translated by Thomas C. Russell. San Francisco: Privately printed.

Richardson, W. P.
1900   Alaska—1899. Yukon River exploring expedition. Winter conditions along the Yukon, 1899. In *Compilation of narratives of explorations in Alaska. See* U.S. Senate 1900:743-751.

Rickman, John
1781   *Journal of Captain Cook's last voyage to the Pacific Ocean.* Reprint 1967. Amsterdam: N. Israel; New York: Da Capo Press.

Rininger, E. M.
1985   The scourge of the mining camps: Typhoid fever in Alaska. *Alaska Journal* 15(1):29-32.

Romig, Joseph H.
1962   Medical practice in western Alaska around 1900. *Alaska Medicine* 4(4):85-87.

Roppel, Patricia
1975   Loring. *Alaska Journal* 5(3):168-78.

Roquefeuil, Camille de
1981   *A voyage around the world 1816-1819, and trading for sea otter fur on the northwest coast of America.* Fairfield, Wash.: Ye Galleon Press.

Rosse, Irving C.
1883   Medical and anthropological notes on Alaska. In *Cruise of the Revenue-Steamer* Corwin *in Alaska and the N.W. Arctic Ocean in 1881. Notes and memoranda: Medical and anthropological; botanical; ornithological.* Washington, D.C.: Government Printing Office. Pp. 9-43.

Rowe, Peter T.
1897a   First annual report of the bishop of the Missionary District of Alaska. *Spirit of Missions* 62:19-25.

1897b   A letter from Bishop Rowe. *Spirit of Missions* 62:364-66.
1898   Second annual report of the missionary bishop of Alaska. *Spirit of Missions* 63:14-23

Sarafian, Winston Lee
1971   Russian-American Company employee policies and practices 1799-1867. Ph.D. dissertation, University of California, Los Angeles.

1977a   Alaska's first Russian settlers. *Alaska Journal* 7(3):174-77.
1977b   Smallpox strikes the Aleuts. *Alaska Journal* 7(1):46-49.
Sarychev, Gavriil
1802   *Puteshestvie flota kapitana Sarycheva po sieverovostochnoi chasti Sibiri Ledovitomu moriu i*

Vostochnomu okeanu v prodolzhenie vośmi liet pri geograficheskoi i astronomicheskoi morskoĭ ekspeditsii. . . . . St. Petersburg.

1807   *Account of a voyage of discovery to the north-east of Siberia, the Frozen Ocean and the North-east Sea.* Two volumes in one. Reprint 1969. Amsterdam: N. Israel; New York: Da Capo Press.

Satterfield, Archie
1973   *Chilkoot Pass: Then and now.* Anchorage: Alaska Northwest Publishing Co.

Sauer, Martin
1802   *An account of a geographical and astronomical expedition to the northern parts of Russia,* . . . *by Commodore Joseph Billings in the years 1785, &c. to 1794.* Reprint 1972. Surrey, U.K.: Richmond Publishing Co., Ltd.

Savage, A. H.
1942   *Dogsled apostles.* New York: Sheed and Ward.

Schrader, Frank C.
1899   A reconnaissance of a part of Prince William Sound and the Copper River District, Alaska, in 1898. In *Twentieth annual report of the U.S. Geological Survey to the Secretray of the Interior 1898-99. Part VII. Explorations in Alaska in 1898.* See U.S. Geological Survey 1899:341-424.

Schrader, Frank C., and Alfred H. Brooks
1900   *Preliminary report on the Cape Nome gold region, Alaska.* 56th Congress, 1st Session. Senate Doc. No. 236. Washington, D.C.: Government Printing Office.

Schuhmacher, W. Wilfred
1979   Aftermath of the Sitka massacre of 1802. *Alaska Journal* 9(1):58-61.

Schwalbe, Anna Buxbaum
1951   *Dayspring on the Kuskokwim. The story of Moravian missions in Alaska.* Bethlehem, Pa.: Moravian Press.

Schwatka, Frederick
1885   *Report of a military reconnaissance in Alaska made in 1883.* Washington, D.C.: Government Printing Office.
1891   *A summer in Alaska.* Philadelphia: John Y. Huber Co.

Scidmore, Eliza Ruhamah
1885   *Alaska, its southern coast and the Sitkan Archipelago.* Boston: D. Lothrop and Co.

Scott, Edward M.
1972   Genetic disorders in isolated populations. *Archives of Environmental Health* 26(1):32-55.

Seemann, Berthold Carl
1853   *Narrative of the voyage of H.M.S.* Herald *during the years 1845-51, under the command of Captain Henry Kellett . . . Being a circumnavigation of the globe, and three cruises to the arctic regions in search of John Franklin.* Two volumes. London: Reeve.

Shalkop, Antoinette
1977   Stepan Ushin, citizen by purchase. *Alaska Journal* 7(2):103-8.

Sheakley, James
1894   *Report of the Governor of District of Alaska to the Secretary of the Interior. 1894.* Washington, D.C.: Government Printing Office.
1895   *Report of the Governor of Alaska to the Secretary of the Interior. 1895.* Washington, D.C.: Government Printing Office.
1896   *Report of the Governor of Alaska to the Secretary of the Interior. 1896.* Washington, D.C.: Government Printing Office.

Shelikhov, Grigorii I.
1981   *A voyage to America 1783-1786.* Translated by Marina Ramsay. Edited by Richard A. Pierce. Kingston, Ontario: Limestone Press.

Shepard, Isabel S.
1889   *The cruise of the U.S. Steamer* Rush *in Behring Sea. Summer of 1889.* San Francisco: Bancroft Co.

Sherwood, Morgan B.
1965a   Ardent spirits: Hooch and the *Osprey* affair at Sitka. *Journal of the West* 4(3):301-44.
1965b   *Exploration of Alaska 1865-1900.* New Haven and London: Yale University Press.

Sherwood, Morgan B. ed.
1967   *Alaska and its history.* Seattle and London: University of Washington Press.
1974   *The Cook Inlet collection. Two hundred years of selected Alaskan history.* Anchorage: Alaska Northwest Publishing Co.

Sigerist, Henry E.
1951   *A history of medicine.* Two volumes. Vol. 1. *Primitive and archaic medicine.* New York: Oxford University Press.

Simpson, George
1847   *Narrative of a journey round the world during the years*
                             1841 and 1842. Two volumes in one. Philadelphia: Lea
                             and Blanchard.

Simpson, John
1855   *Further papers relative to the recent arctic expeditions in*
                             search of Sir John Franklin in the cruise of the H.M.S.
                             Erebus *and* Terror. Admiralty, Great Britain. London: H.M.
                             Stationery Office.

Simpson, Thomas
1843   *Narrative of the discoveries on the north coast of America,*
                             effected by the officers of the Hudson's Bay Company
                             during the years 1836-39. London: Richard Bentley.

Slobodin, Richard
1981   Kutchin. In *Handbook of North American Indians. See*
                             Sturtevant 1981, 6:514-32.

Smith, Barbara
1980   *Russian Orthodoxy in Alaska. A history, inventory, and*
                             analysis of the church archives in Alaska with an
                             annotated bibliography. Anchorage: Alaska Historical
                             Commission.

Smith, Becky
1973   Prohibition in Alaska—when Alaskans voted "dry."
                             Alaska Journal 3(3):170-79.

Snow, W. P.
1867   Russian America. *Hours at Home* 5:254-64.

Spencer, Robert F.
1959   *The north Alaskan Eskimo. A study in ecology and society.*
                             Smithsonian Institution. Bureau of Ethnology Bulletin No.
                             171. Washington, D.C.: Government Printing Office.
1984   North Alaska coast Eskimo. In *Handbook of North*
                             American Indians. See Sturtevant 1984, 5:320-37.

Spurr, J. E.
1899   A reconnaissance in southwestern Alaska in 1898. In
                             Twentieth annual report of the U.S. Geological Survey to
                             the Secretary of the Interior 1898-99. Part VII.
                             Explorations in Alaska in 1898. See U.S. Geological
                             Survey 1899:31-264.

State of Alaska
1988   Tularemia. *State of Alaska Epidemiology Bulletin.* Bulletin
                             No. 25, December 16, 1988.

Stein, Gary C.
1985   A desperate and dangerous man: Captain Michael A.
                        Healy's arctic cruise of 1900. *Alaska Journal* 15(22):39-
                        45.

Steller, Georg Wilhelm
1988   *Journal of a voyage with Bering 1741-1742.* Edited by O.
                        W. Frost. Trans. by Margritt A. Engel and O. W. Frost.
                        Stanford, Cal.: Stanford University Press.

Stewart, T. Dale
1979   Patterning of skeletal pathologies and epidemiology. In
                        The first Americans: Origins, affinities, and adaptations,
                        edited by William S. Laughlin and A. B. Harper. New York
                        and Stuttgart: Gustav Fischer. Pp. 257-74.

Stoney, George M.
1900   *Naval explorations in Alaska. An account of two naval
                        expeditions to northern Alaska, with official maps of the
                        country explored.* Annapolis, Md.: U.S. Naval Institute.

Strickland, Dan
1986   Murder at the mission. The death of H. R. Thornton at
                        Cape Prince of Wales in 1893. In *The Alaska Journal. A
                        1986 collection. See* Cole 1986:208-15.

Stuck, Hudson
1920   *The Alaskan missions of the Episcopal Church. A brief
                        sketch, historical and descriptive.* New York: Domestic
                        and Foreign Missionary Society.

Sturtevant, William C., ed.
1981   *Handbook of North American Indians.* Vol. 6. *Subarctic.*
                        Edited by June Helm. Washington, D.C.: Smithsonian
                        Institution.
1984   *Handbook of North American Indians.* Vol. 5. *Arctic.*
                        Edited by David Damas. Washington, D.C.: Smithsonian
                        Institution.

Suría, Tomás de
1936   *Journal of Tomás de Suría of his voyage with Malaspina to
                        the northwest coast of America in 1791.* Translated and
                        edited by Henry R. Wagner. Glendale, Cal.: Arthur H.
                        Clark Co.

Swanton, John R.
[1908]   *Social condition, beliefs, and linguistic relationship of the
                        Tlingit Indians.* Reprint 1970. New York: Johnson Reprint
                        Corp.

Swineford, Alfred P.

1885   *Report of the Governor of Alaska to the Secretary of the Interior. 1885.* Washington, D.C.: Government Printing Office.

1886   *Report of the Governor of Alaska for the fiscal year 1886.* U.S. Department of the Interior. Washington, D.C.: Government Printing Office.

1887   *Report of the Governor of Alaska for the fiscal year 1887.* U.S. Department of the Interior. Washington, D.C.: Government Printing Office.

1889a   *Report of the Governor of Alaska for the fiscal year 1888.* U.S. Department of the Interior. Washington, D.C.: Government Printing Office.

1889b   *Report of the Governor of Alaska for the fiscal year 1889.* U.S. Department of the Interior. Washington, D.C.: Government Printing Office.

Teichmann, Emil

1963   *A journey to Alaska in the year 1868: Being a diary of the late Emil Teichmann.* Edited by Oskar Teichmann. New York: Argosy-Antiquarian Ltd.

Tero, Richard D.

1973   Alaska: 1779. Father Riobo's narrative. *Alaska Journal* 3(2):81-88.

Thomas, George B.

1900   From Middle Fork of Sushitna River to Indian Creek. In *Compilation of narratives of explorations in Alaska. See* U.S. Senate 1900:733-35.

Thorborg, N. B., S. Tulinius, and H. Roth

1948   Trichinosis in Greenland. *Acta Pathologica et Microbiologica Scandinavica* 25:778-94.

Thornton, Harrison Robertson

1931   *Among the Eskimos of Wales, Alaska 1890-93.* Baltimore: Johns Hopkins Press.

Tikhmenev, Petr Aleksandrovich

1978   *A history of the Russian-American Company.* Translated and edited by Richard A. Pierce and Alton S. Donnelly. Seattle and London: University of Washington Press.

1979   *A history of the Russian-American Company. Vol. 2. Documents. Period 1783-1807.* Translated by Dmitri Krenov. Edited by Richard A. Pierce and Alton S. Donnelly. Kingston, Ontario: Limestone Press.

Torrey, Barbara Boyle
1978   *Slaves of the harvest.* [St. Paul, AK]: TDX Corporation.

Townsend, Joan Brown
1965   Ethnohistory and culture change of the Iliamna Tanaina. Ph.D. dissertation, University of California, Los Angeles.

U.S. Army Alaska.
1962   *Building Alaska with the U.S. Army: 1867-1962.* Pamphlet No. 355-5. Anchorage, Alaska: U.S. Army.

U.S. Department of the Interior
1893   *Report of population and resources of Alaska at the eleventh census: 1890.* Census Office. Washington, D.C.: Government Printing Office.

U.S. Geological Survey
1899   *Twentieth annual report of the U.S. Geological Survey to the Secretary of the Interior 1898-99. Part VII. Explorations in Alaska in 1898.* Washington, D.C.: Government Printing Office.

U.S. House of Representatives
1882   *Report of United States naval officers cruising in Alaska waters.* 47th Congress, 1st Session. House Doc. 81. Washington, D.C.: Government Printing Office.

U.S. Senate
1880   *Letter from the Secretary of the Treasury.* 46th Congress, 2nd Session. Senate Executive Document No. 179. Washington, D.C.: Government Printing Office.

1900   *Compilation of narratives of explorations in Alaska.* 56th Congress, 1st Session. Senate Report No. 1023. Washington, D.C.: Government Printing Office.

1904   *Conditions in Alaska.* 58th Congress, 2nd Session. Senate Report No. 282. Parts I and II. Washington, D.C.: Government Printing Office.

University of Alaska
1936-1938 *Documents relative to the history of Alaska.* Typescript. Fifteen volumes. Fairbanks: Alaska History Research Project, University of Alaska.

Vancouver, George
1798   *Voyage of discovery to the north Pacific Ocean and round the world.* Four volumes. Reprint 1967. Amsterdam: N. Israel; New York: Da Capo Press.

VanStone, James W.
1958   Commercial whaling in the Arctic Ocean. *Pacific Northwest Quarterly* 49(1):1-10.

1959 Russian exploration in interior Alaska. An extract from the journal of Andrei Glazunov. *Pacific Northwest Quarterly* 50(2):37-47.

1960 An early nineteenth-century artist in Alaska. Louis Choris and the first Kotzebue expedition. *Pacific Northwest Quarterly* 51(4):145-58.

1962a Notes on nineteenth century trade in the Kotzebue Sound area, Alaska, *Arctic Anthropology* 1(1):126-28.

1962b *Point Hope. An Eskimo village in transition.* Seattle and London: University of Washington Press.

1967 *Eskimos of the Nushagak River: An ethnographic history.* Seattle and London: University of Washington Press.

1971 Historic settlement patterns in the Nushagak River region, Alaska. *Fieldiana: Anthropology* 61. Feb. 25, 1971.

1972 Nushagak. *Alaska Journal* 2(3):49-53.

1974 *Athapaskan adaptations: Hunters and fishermen of the subarctic forests.* Chicago: Aldine Publishing Co.

1979 Ingalik contact ecology: An ethnohistory of the lower-middle Yukon, 1790-1935. *Fieldiana: Anthropology* 71. March 29, 1979.

1984 Mainland southwest Alaska Eskimo. In *Handbook of North American Indians. See* Sturtevant 1984, 5:224-42.

1988 *Russian exploration in southwest Alaska: The travel journals of Petr Korsakovskiy (1818) and Ivan Ya. Vasilev (1829).* Trans. by David H. Kraus. Fairbanks: University of Alaska Press.

Van Wagoner, Richard S., and Tong H. Chun
1974 Facial paralysis carved in Alaskan native masks. *Alaska Medicine* 16(6):123-25.

Veniaminov, Ivan [Innokentii]
1972 The condition of the Orthodox Church in Russian America. Translated and edited by Robert Nichols and Robert Croskey. *Pacific Northwest Quarterly* 63(2):41-54.

1984 *Notes on the islands of the Unalashka District.* Translated by Lydia T. Black and R. H. Geoghegan. Edited by Richard A. Pierce. Kingston, Ontario: Limestone Press.

Watt, James
1979 Medical aspects and consequences of Cook's voyages. In *Captain James Cook and his times,* edited by Robin Fisher and Hugh Johnston. Seattle and London: University of Washington Press. Pp. 129-57.

Waxell, Sven
1962   *The Russian expedition to America.* New York: Collier
                        Books.
Wells, E. H.
1975   From St. Michael to Katmai. Edited by Ro Sherman.
                        Alaska Journal 5(2):109-16.
Wells, Virginia L., and Phyllis E. Kempton
1961   The genus *Amanita* in Alaska. *Alaska Medicine* 3(1):1-20.
Wennekens, Alix Jane
1985   Traditional plant usage by Chugach natives around Prince
                        William Sound and on the lower Kenai Peninsula, Alaska.
                        M.A. thesis. University of Alaska Anchorage.
West, Ellsworth Luce (with Eleanor R. Mayhew)
1965   *Captain's papers. A log of whaling and other sea
                        experiences.* Barre, Mass.: Barre Publishers.
Weyer, Edward Moffat
1932   *The Eskimos: Their environment and folkways.* New
                        Haven, Conn.: Yale University Press
White, James T.
1889   Diary of cruise of Revenue Steamer *Bear* in 1889.
                        Typescript. Copy in John Wesley White-James Taylor
                        White Collection. Box VII, folder 40. University of Alaska
                        Archives, Fairbanks, Alaska.
1890   Diary of cruise of U.S. Marine Steamer *Rush,* 1890.
                        Typescript, from manuscript in the University of
                        Washington Archives, Seattle. Copy in John Wesley
                        White-James Taylor White Collection. Box VII, folder 41.
                        University of Alaska Archives, Fairbanks, Alaska.
1894   James Taylor White diary of cruise of U.S. Revenue
                        Steamer *Bear,* 1894. Typescript. Copy in John Wesley
                        White-James Taylor White Collection. Box VII, folder 42.
                        University of Alaska Archives, Fairbanks, Alaska.
1902   Report of the medical officer of the U.S. Steamer *Nunivak,*
                        Yukon River, Alaska, made under the direction of First
                        Lieutenant J. C. Cantwell, R.C.S., commanding. In *Report
                        of the operations of the U.S. Revenue Steamer* Nunivak *on
                        the Yukon River Station. See* Cantwell 1902:257-74.
White, Robert
1880   Notes on the physical condition of the inhabitants of
                        Alaska. In *Report on Alaska. See* Bailey 1880:41-49.
Whymper, Frederick
1868   *Travel and adventure in the territory of Alaska.* London:
                        John Murray.

Wickersham, James
1938   *Old Yukon: Tales—trails—and trials.* Washington, D.C.:
                            Washington Law Book Co.
Willard, Mrs. Eugene S.
1884   *Life in Alaska. Letters of Mrs. Eugene S. Willard.* Edited
                            by Eva McClintock. Philadelphia: Presbyterian Board of
                            Publication.
Williams, Ralph B.
1945   Tularemia. First case to be reported in Alaska. *Public
                            Health Reports* 61:875 (June).
Williams, Ralph B., and M. W. Dodson
1960   *Salmonella* in Alaska. *Public Health Reports* 75(10):913-
                            15.
Wilson, Joseph F., and Robert L. Rausch
1980   Alveolar hydatid disease: A review of clinical features of
                            33 indigenous cases of *Echinococcus multilocularis*
                            infection in Alaskan Eskimos. *American Journal of
                            Tropical Medicine and Hygiene* 29(6):1340-55.
Wirt, Loyal Lincoln
1937   *Alaskan adventures.* New York: Fleming H. Revell Co.
Wolfe, Robert J.
1982   Alaska's Great Sickness, 1900: An epidemic of measles
                            and influenza in a virgin soil population. *Proceedings of
                            the American Philosophical Society* 126(2):91-121.
Wrangell, Ferdinand Petrovich von
1970   The inhabitants of the northwest coast of America. *Arctic
                            Anthropology* 6(2):5-20.
1980   *Russian America. Statistical and ethnographic
                            information.* Trans. by Mary Sadouski. Edited by Richard
                            A. Pierce. Kingston, Ontario: Limestone Press.
Wright, Julia McNair
1883   *Among the Alaskans.* Philadelphia: Presbyterian Board of
                            Publication.
Wythe, W. T.
1871   Medical notes on Alaska. *Pacific Medical and Surgical
                            Journal* 4:337-42.
Young, S. Hall
1927   *Hall Young of Alaska. "The mushing parson."* New York
                            and Chicago: Fleming H. Revell Co.
Zagoskin, Lavrentii A.
1967   *Lieutenant Zagoskin's travels in Russian America, 1842-
                            1844; The first ethnographic and geographic*

investigations in the Yukon and Kuskokwim valleys of Alaska. Edited by Henry N. Michael. Arctic Institute of North America, Anthropology of the North. Translations from Russian Sources No. 7. Toronto: University of Toronto Press.

Zimmerman, Michael R., and Arthur C. Aufderheide
1984   The frozen family of Utqiagvik: The autopsy findings. *Arctic Anthropology* 21(1):53-64.

Zimmerman, Michael R., and George S. Smith
1975   A probable case of accidental inhumation of 1600 years ago. Bulletin of the New York Academy of Medicine 51(2nd series):828-37.

Zimmerman, Michael R., Erik Trinkaus, Marjorie Le May, Arthur C. Aufderheide, Theodore A. Reyman, Guy R. Marrocco, Wade Ortel, Jaime T. Benitez, William S. Laughlin, Patrick D. Horne, Richard E. Schultes and Elizabeth A. Coughlin.
1981   The paleopathology of an Aleutian mummy. *Archives of Pathology and Laboratory Medicine* 105(12):638-41.

Zimmerman, Michael R., Gentry W. Yeatman, Helmuth Sprinz, and Wesley P. Titterington.
1971   Examination of an Aleutian mummy. *Bulletin of the New York Academy of Medicine* 47(1):80-103.

Author Index

363

Subject Index

Abercrombie, William R., 14, 145, 176
Abortion, 40-41
Abscesses, 66, 67, 68, 137, 259
Abuse: general, 301-5; of Aleuts, 91, 92, 93, 94, 110, 113, 115, 301-2; appeal to tsar against, 303; break-up of families, 308; efforts to control, 110, 115,301, 303, 304; forced labor as, 94, 110, 116, 198, 302, 303, 304, 308; of Koniag, 9, 110, 115, 302; murder as, 92, 93, 302, 303;   physical methods of, 115, 303; sexual, 94, 110, 302, 303, 304; of workers, 298, 303, 304
Adak I., 90, 265
Adams, Dr., 313
Admiralty I., 287
Adrenogenital syndrome, congenital salt-losing, 83
Afognak I., 95, 207
Agattu I., 91, 311
Agriculture, 115
Ahtna, (Athapaskan) Indians, 21, 22, 78, 117, 207, 272, 312; contact, 116
AIDS, 318
Akutan Pass, 93, 256
Alaska Commercial Company, 150, 155, 168, 169, 171, 203, 204, 243, 249, 291, 292, 297
Alaska Natives. *See* individual groups
Alaska Peninsula, 6, 9, 11, 93, 101, 112, 113, 117, 161, 202, 203, 206, 233, 238, 262, 267, 303
Alaska, exploration of: American, 99, 122-23, 144-45, 148, 248; British, 93, 96, 99, 100, 101, 102, 120, 248, 267; French, 99, 102, 228, 282; Russian, 89-96, 98, 100-1, 102, 116-18, 120-22, 249, 267; Spanish, 95, 98, 99, 102, 228, 267
Alcohol abuse: among Americans, 146, 164, 177, 247, 285, 288, 289, 292, 295, 316; among Chinese cannery

workers, 170, 291, 292; among Creoles, 285, 293, 298; among Natives generally, 146, 157, 189, 282, 283, 285, 286, 288, 291, 292, 294, 295, 298, 309, 318; among Russians, 103, 109, 110, 112, 113, 127, 279, 280, 281, 282, 284, 285, 298, 309; concern of Natives about, 282, 286; health effects of, 1981, 259, 297-99; violence caused by, 144, 187, 198, 282, 283, 287, 288, 289, 291, 292, 294, 296, 297, 298
Alcohol: general, 243, 279-299, 316; as gift, 282; attempts to limit by missionaries, 192, imperial monopoly on trade of, 279; introduction of, Aleutians, 89, 265, 279; introduction of, interior, 297; introduction of, Kodiak, 279; introduction of, northern Alaska, 155, 293; introduction of, southeastern Alaska, 282; introduction of, western Alaska, 290-93; precontact use of, 279; prohibition of, in American period, 110, 144, 146, 167, 285, 289, 290, 297; prohibition of, in Russian period, 111, 112, 282, 283, 284, 285, 293; ration to hunters and workers, 281, 284; for sexual favors, 260, 285; smuggling of, 284, 289, 290; use as trade item, by Americans, 106, 108, 250, 283, 288, 292, 293, 295, 311; as trade item by British, 106, 283, 291; as trade item by Russians, 282. *See also* Hootch and Kvass
Alcoholism. *See* Alcohol abuse
Alegnagik Lake, 118
Aleutian Islands, 1, 6, 27, 79, 80, 89, 90, 94, 106, 113, 115, 150, 154, 155, 161, 166, 167, 189, 190, 204, 205, 238, 241, 252, 254, 256, 257, 259,

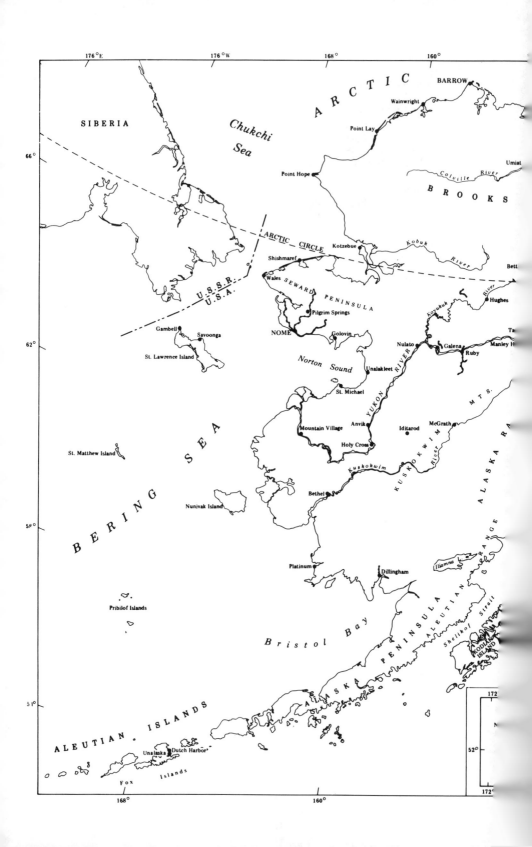

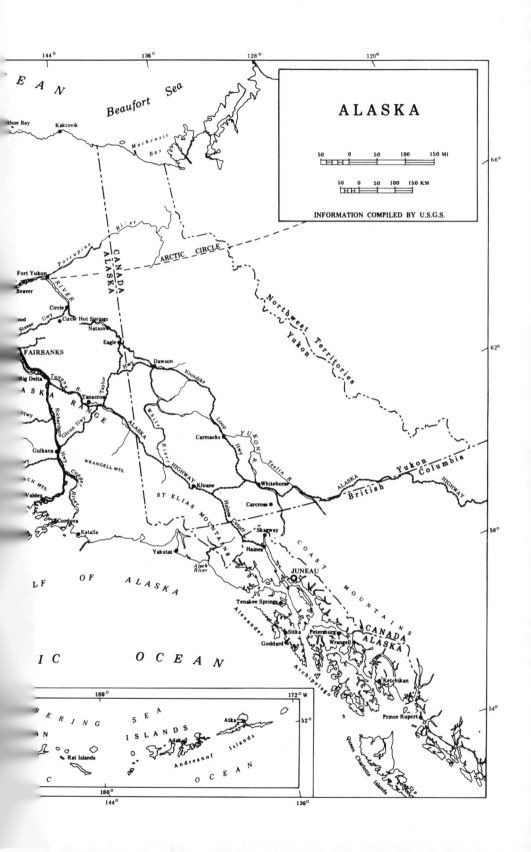

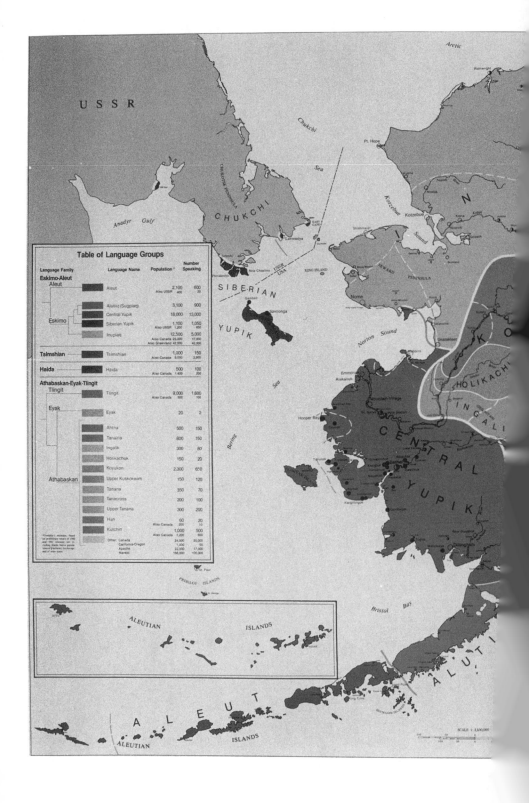

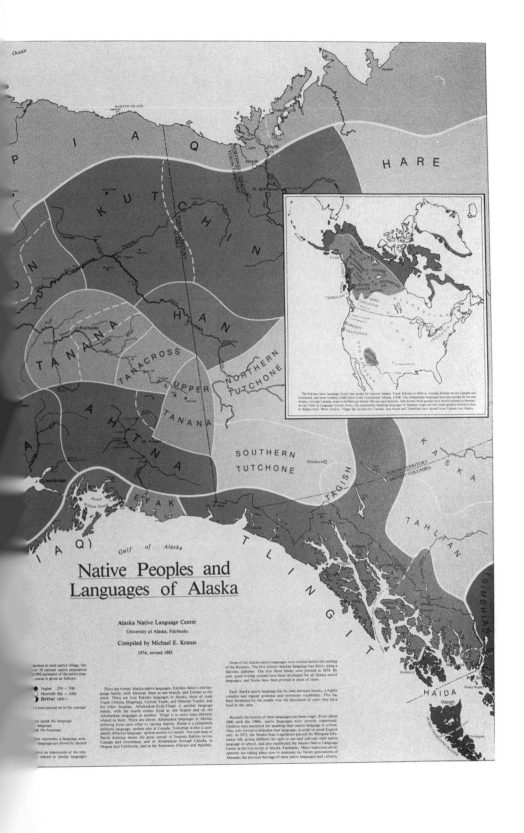

Native Peoples and Languages of Alaska

Alaska Native Language Center
University of Alaska, Fairbanks

Compiled by Michael E. Krauss

1974, revised 1982